NURSING LEADERSHIP AND MANAGEMENT

NURSING LEADERSHIP AND MANAGEMENT
CONTEMPORARY STRATEGIES

Gertrude K. McFarland, R.N., D.N.Sc.
Nurse Consultant
Nursing Education Branch
Division of Nursing
Health Resources and Services Administration
U.S. Department of Health and Human Services
Rockville, Maryland
Formerly, Chief, Nursing Education Section
Psychiatric Clinical Nurse Specialist
Saint Elizabeth's Hospital
National Institute of Mental Health
Department of Health, Education, and Welfare
Washington, D.C.

H. Skipton Leonard, Ph.D.
Organizational Consultant
President, Persona, Inc.
Reston, Virginia
Formerly, Adjunct Assistant Professor
State University of New York at Plattsburgh
Plattsburgh, New York

Martha M. Morris, R.N., Ed.D.
Chairman, Department of Nursing
Ball State University
Muncie, Indiana
Formerly, Assistant Professor
Louisiana State University Medical Center School of Nursing
New Orleans, Louisiana

A WILEY MEDICAL PUBLICATION
JOHN WILEY & SONS
New York • **Chichester** • **Brisbane** • **Toronto** • **Singapore**

The opinions expressed herein by Dr. Gertrude K. McFarland, R.N., are her own and do not necessarily reflect those of the Division of Nursing, Health Resources and Services Administration, U.S. Public Health Service, U.S. Department of Health and Human Services.

Library of Congress Cataloging in Publication Data:
McFarland, Gertrude K., 1941–
  Nursing leadership and management.

  (A Wiley medical publication)
  Includes index.
  1. Nursing service administration. 2. Leadership.
I. Leonard, H. Skipton. II. Morris, Martha M.
III. Title. IV. Series.

RT89.M43   1984   362.1'73'068   83-16724
ISBN 0-471-09097-2

Printed in the United States of America
10 9 8 7 6 5 4 3 2 1

CONSULTANTS

Barbara A. Hill, R.N., Ed. D.
Associate Professor
Indiana University-Purdue University
Fort Wayne, Indiana

Duane D. Walker, R.N., M.S., F.A.A.N.
Associate Administrator/
Director Nursing Service
Stanford University Hospital and Clinics
Stanford, California

Evelyn L. Wasli, R.N., D.N.Sc.
Psychiatric Nursing Coordinator
Saint Elizabeths Hospital
National Institute of Mental Health
U.S. Department of Health and Human Services
Washington, D.C.

FOREWORD

Increasingly, recognition is being given to the importance of nurses and nursing management in health care institutions. The turbulent environment in which the health care system is operating and the forces that are interacting to cause changes in the system have been instrumental in bringing about this increased recognition. Nursing is perceived as an element critical in keeping the fabric of health care institutions intact. This change in perception of the role and value of nursing places great demands upon the nursing leadership group.

Nursing Leadership and Management: Contemporary Strategies provides valuable assistance to nursing leaders. Its content reflects an understanding of the health care institution as a set of systems and subsystems, as an organization with its own culture and norms—often in need of change—and as a place where critical interactions and processes take place. Strategies for use by nursing leaders are proposed, and the institution is depicted as an entity whose characteristics are derived from the strengths and weaknesses of human beings. As nurses study the content of the text—which the authors have carefully synthesized from theories of many disciplines and from content found in many sources—they are encouraged to view it from their own clinical perspective and translate its meaning and value to the discipline of nursing.

The knowledge held by nursing leaders comes from at least two sources: the primary source is our own practice discipline, that is, nursing; the secondary source is management, which cuts across knowledge drawn from the social sciences. Knowledge and skill derived from management should be translated and integrated into nursing. Thus, in order to be effective, nursing leaders need advanced knowledge and skills in both disciplines.

Nursing is a clinical practice discipline and, as such, must develop ways to manage its own practitioners, practice, and resources. Such management requires nursing leaders who understand the environment in which nursing is practiced and how that environment should be changed to bring about more effective nursing practice. There is a need for nursing leaders who can establish nursing practice departments and subunits that are clinical and professional in nature and who perceive nurses as salaried professionals capable of growth and contribution. Likewise, nursing leaders must be astute, wise, and statesmanlike in behavior and be able to achieve the humanistic system that nurses desire for themselves, their clients, and all who are employed.

Nursing leaders need a broad perspective of health services and a long-range view of what is the desirable health care system of the future. Nurses serving as policymakers, power brokers, politicians, and communicators are essential in setting forth and implementing the ideas of the clinicians and clients they represent. An understanding of the various psychological, sociological, and managerial constructs upon which strategies rest will assist nursing leaders in the development and use of appropriate strategies.

The roles of nursing leaders are not easy ones. The remodeling of social institutions, which includes the professions, is indeed challenging. There is a great opportunity for nurses, regardless of their place in the nursing management structure, to be a part of that remodeling. Nursing as a profession can mature fully if we but learn what we need in order to be more effective in our practice, in the management of our resources, and in meeting our obligations as a citizen of the institution. Change is required. The authors of this text offer us a great source of power—the knowledge of management and strategies for our use, which we must invest the energy to learn and then to apply. Without this knowledge, nurses cannot move into their rightful leadership position.

This text emphasizes the use of management knowledge, skills, and strategies, complementary to nursing practice, to carve out a better system of care for patients and clients. The system will improve the quality of working life for all. The authors make a great contribution by assimilating a vast amount of rich and useful information, making this book a valuable resource for aspiring nursing leaders and those currently in leadership roles.

Myrtle K. Aydelotte, R.N., Ph.D., F.A.A.N.
Adjunct Professor of Nursing
University of Iowa
Executive Director (retired)
American Nurses' Association

PREFACE

Effective nursing leadership, management, and supervision require strategies to accomplish the goals and objectives of the organizational structure for which the nurse is responsible. At the same time, it requires maintaining job-satisfaction and motivation among nursing faculty or staff.

Nursing Leadership and Management: Contemporary Strategies explores the means of achieving effective nursing leadership, management, and supervision based on a synthesis of concepts, principles, and theories from organizational development, social psychology, organizational and industrial psychology, social systems theory, nursing management and leadership, psychology of groups, and sociology. Systems theory provides an overall framework for the text.

Designed as a guide for beginning to midlevel practicing nurse leaders, managers, or supervisors, this volume is directed to nurses in both educational and practice settings, including staff development educators. Part Three can be used as a handbook, utilizing the strategies needed, after Parts One and Two have been read. The book is also designed for upper-level undergraduate students in leadership courses and can be adapted for use by graduate nursing students in nursing management and supervision.

Our goal is to broaden the perspectives of both the practitioner and the student with concepts, principles, and theory for achieving effective nursing leadership, management, and supervision. Likewise, we wish to present the reader with a description of techniques and practical strategies for achieving organizational goals while maintaining job satisfaction and motivation, and to stimulate the reader to test these strategies in practice.

Theory, more heavily emphasized in Part One, is interwoven with descriptions of nursing management and leadership strategies and their application, including actual case examples. Chapter 1 provides a prospectus. A central theme of the book is introduced: Attempts at increasing productivity and goal achievement must consider human factors in order to achieve humanistic and effective nursing leadership and management. In addition, Chapter 1 traces the historical development of organizations and social systems theory—the organizing framework for the book. Chapter 2, focusing on the nature of social systems, describes an open system and its primary characteristics. The organization of social systems, task accomplishment, system maintenance, roles, norms, values, and hierarchies are explored in Chapter 3. The book proceeds in Chapter 4 with a treatment of organizational life cycles—growth, maturation, and decline—as well as subsystem development (product or technical, supportive, maintenance, adaptive, and managerial). Part One concludes with two chapters on processes within subsystems and team and group dynamics in nursing. Such topics as modes of communication, trust, reward structures, and covert processes including hidden agendas, basic assumption behavior, splitting, and scapegoating are presented in Chapter 5.

Group task dimensions, team development, along with implications for nursing teams and groups, are covered in Chapter 6.

Part Two, "The Processes of Nurse Leadership, Management, and Supervision," reviews the more traditional management and leadership processes. Situational leadership theory provides a framework for a comprehensive examination of leadership.

In Part Three strategies are examined for effective nursing leadership, management, and supervision. General systems theory, along with organization development and action research processes, provides the framework for the presentation of major strategies. Chapter 9 begins with an overview of the organization development process. The concept and process of planned change is covered in Chapter 10. System intervention strategies, described in Chapters 11 to 21, include communication techniques, the problem-solving process and idea generation, decision making, motivation and job satisfaction, methods of socialization, the acquisition and use of power, team building, conducting formal nursing meetings, time management, stress management, and conflict management. Application of these strategies to both service and educational settings is included throughout these chapters. Part Three concludes with Chapter 22 which presents an analysis of major social forces that may influence the future of the nursing profession and the role of nurse leaders, managers, and supervisors.

We believe that a humanistic management atmosphere, blended with an emphasis on methods to improve productivity, is essential for effective organizational goal achievement. A clear definition of organizational problems that impede goal attainment, an assessment of the consequences of proposed alternative intervention strategies, the selection and implementation of intervention strategies, along with an evaluation of their results, will continue to foster the development of a sound scientific base for nursing leadership and management.

We wish to acknowledge our families—Al McFarland and parents John and Emma Ramseier; Faith Leonard and daughters Allison and Christy; and daughter Lynn Chance—for their support and patience during the preparation of this project. Thanks also to our competent and supportive secretaries, Mrs. Dorothy Kustanborter and Mrs. Mary Lou Huber at Ball State University, and Mrs. Nancy Freil formerly at Catholic University of America. Finally, our appreciation is extended to Suzanne S. Resner, R.N., D.N.Sc., Program Analyst, U.S. Department of Health and Human Services, Rockville, Maryland, and to Janice F. Gosser, B.A., M.A., Muncie, Indiana, for their editorial assistance.

Gertrude K. McFarland
H. Skipton Leonard
Martha M. Morris

CONTENTS

NURSING LEADERSHIP AND MANAGEMENT

PART ONE
FOUNDATIONS FOR NURSING LEADERSHIP, MANAGEMENT, AND SUPERVISION

CHAPTER 1
PROSPECTUS AND
HISTORICAL FOUNDATIONS

PROSPECTUS

The Changing Environment

A changing, somewhat turbulent environment will confront nurse leaders and managers during the next several decades. Forces and trends (more fully explored in the concluding chapter of this text)—such as changing organizational structures, increasing knowledge/technology, increasing specialization/interdisciplinary collaboration, cost-containment, consumerism, shifting health problems, health care policy, women in the work force, and trends in higher education and in nursing education—are beginning and will continue to affect the nursing profession and the roles, functions, and skill requirements of nurse leaders, managers, and supervisors. In addition, nurse employees in both health care and educational systems are requesting more conducive work environments along with opportunities for continued professional growth/self-actualization and for delivery of quality patient care or provision of quality educational programs. At the same time, economic, political, and professional changes are serving as driving forces for cost containment and productivity, as well as accountability and quality control.

Changing Systems

Increasing organizational complexity; changing organizational structure; increasing availability of information; increased use of technology, interdisciplinary team work, or collaboration; competition for scarce resources; internal conflict and power struggles; and problems needing creative solutions are increasingly predicted to characterize organizational systems in which nurse leaders or managers find themselves. Effectively managing a system's input, throughput, and output processes in such a milieu demands competence in a number of processes and strategies, as well as a theoretical foundation. These traditional management processes include goal setting together with values clarification, planning, organizing, staffing, cost-effective budgeting, motivating, delegating, directing, and evaluating. These special strategies include planned change, communication skills, problem solving, idea generation, decision making, strategies to increase job satisfaction, strategies for socialization, use of power, team building, conducting groups and meetings, time management, stress management, and conflict management. Competence in the leadership process is an overall requirement.

Orientation of the Text

With general systems theory as the framework, concepts and theories from a number of sciences provide, in Part One, the theoretical foundation for understanding increasingly complex organizations and their environments. Part One introduces a central theme: Attempts at increasing productivity and goal achievement must reflect human factors *and* system maintenance. This dual emphasis on productivity and human factors contributes to achieving humanistic and effective nurse leadership and management. The more traditional processes of management and supervision, along with leadership, are presented in Part Two. Strategies for effective nurse leadership, management, and supervision—as identified earlier in this chapter—are examined in Part Three of this text. General systems theory continues to serve as an organizing framework in Part Three, along with the organization development and action research processes. Throughout the book, content, processes, and strategies are applied to both service and educational settings.

A humanistic management atmosphere, blended with an emphasis on methods to improve productivity, is essential for effective organizational goal achievement. A clear definition of organizational problems that impede goal attainment, an assessment of the consequences of proposed alternative intervention strategies, and the selection and implementation of intervention strategies, together with an evaluation of their results, will continue to foster the development of a sound scientific base for nurse leadership, management, and supervision.

Nursing Leadership, Management, and Supervision Defined

Nursing leadership is defined as interpersonal influence by which the efforts of nursing faculty or staff are directed, through the communication process, toward the achievement of organizational or subsystem goals. While nurses in management and supervisory roles are in positions to provide leadership, not all nursing managers or supervisors are leaders. It is equally true, that not all nursing leaders are in management or supervisory roles.

Nursing management and supervision, on the other hand, are administrative processes involved with the execution of policies and regulations in a specific social system. *Management* is defined as the mechanism that regulates and adjusts the system to produce optimal goal achievement through the use of technical, interpersonal, and conceptual skills. *Nursing supervision* involves the dynamic process in which the employee is encouraged to participate in activities designed to meet organizational goals and to develop professionally. The scope of impact of the supervisor is generally narrower than that of the manager. The supervisor is also more directly involved with employees performing the work of the organization.

Middle-level managers usually direct the activities of several units or subsystems and are responsible for the implementation of policy and procedures within those units. First-level managers, or supervisors, are concerned with the direct control of the work environment and the supervision of the actual performance of work in one or a few units. The content in this text is relevant for beginning to midlevel leaders, managers, and supervisors in both educational and clinical practice settings.

THE EVOLUTION OF SOCIAL SYSTEMS THEORY

The Industrial Revolution of the eighteenth and nineteenth centuries and the resultant rise in the importance of organizations demanded the creation of theories that explained not only how small groups of people worked together but also how many small work groups could be organized to perform increasingly more complicated and sophisticated tasks. Before this, only religious institutions and the military had required such concepts.

Early Systems Approaches

The Church

The church was concerned with adding to its membership, controlling doctrine, and increasing its influence over secular institutions. Some of its goals, such as the number of members or the laws establishing the power of the church, were easily quantifiable. Other goals—How well had the membership of the church assimilated church teachings? Had appropriate attitudes, values, and norms been developed? How committed was the membership to church-sponsored values?—were difficult to measure. The church believed that its goals would best be met by an organization that stressed control over ideas, norms, and values. The efficiency of these activities was of less concern than the degree of commitment to the teachings and values of the church.

The Military

The military, by comparison, was intensely concerned with control over and coordination of the activities of its members, the quality of their training, and their commitment to the cause for which they risked their lives. Military outcomes were easily measured and of crucial significance to soldiers, leaders, and states. In some areas, the efficiency of obtaining a goal—for example, teaching the use of weapons—was of little concern, as long as a high level of skill was obtained. The critical time frames for the exercise of military skills and tactics were small in comparison to the time available for training.

The Industrial Revolution

With the advent of the Industrial Revolution, emerging organizations were required to cope with an additional factor—economic efficiency. The church had traditionally been given special economic status and, in addition, disclaimed any interest in material gain. The military had to live grudgingly within the economic capability of its state. Industry, however, quickly learned that survival depended upon its capability of producing a needed product more efficiently and for less money. This was a relatively new concept for organizations developing from religious and military traditions.

The legacy from the church and the military to the emerging industrial organizations, nevertheless, was great. The importance of norms and values for developing commitment, discipline, and morale was demonstrated by both religious and military organizations. The concepts of unity of command and centralization of decision making were of great utility to both institutions. The military's experience with problems of quality control and span of control was of value to the emerging industrial organizations.

The legacy of both these institutions to emerging health care organizations is also considerable. Like the military, the ultimate success rate of a method is more critical for the survival of medicine than the relative cost. Rigorous and lengthy training is necessary to ensure quality control. Values and norms are carefully nurtured to protect against practices that violate prevailing cultural values or standards. Likewise, the authority of the team leader is reinforced so that lifesaving procedures may be conducted within limited time frames. For the same reasons, proven methods are valued over promising, innovative, but untested, procedures.

Leaders of these early organizations developed systems principles that helped them accomplish their specific organizational goals. They did not develop, however, comprehensive systems theories. It can be argued that the church proposed a system that organized all matters, religious and secular, scientific, military, and economic, within a single religious–philosophical perspective. The church had little success, however, in linking its systems principles to observable data and the scientific method. Much of its system had to be taken on faith alone. Later, systems theorists began to use the rapidly developing scientific method to construct their theories.

Rise of Industrial and Bureaucratic Organizations

As the Industrial Revolution spread through developing countries, and as each innovation in production became common knowledge, economic survival depended upon steadily increasing productivity by workers. The success and survival of factories and states depended upon a hard-working and efficient work force. Inevitably, workers came to be seen in terms of their economic value rather than their human value as taught by the church.

In Great Britain, in 1833, scandalous abuses of labor occurred and were vividly documented to Parliament in the Saddler Report (1954). Industry employed young children and worked them unmercifully, inflicting irreversible health and psychological damage. The justification for using children was simple and straightforward—they could be paid less than adults. Ultimately, employees were valued only for the economic worth of the role they played in the economic survival of the enterprise.

Clearly, the social and political atmosphere was conducive to change and revolution. The abuses and injustices of unfettered capitalism were addressed by two systems theorists, Max Weber and Karl Marx. Weber attempted an evolutionary change in the functioning of organizations, which maintained its faith in capitalism, while Marx proposed that capitalism would inevitably self-destruct and that a revolutionary method for instituting change was required.

Weber

Max Weber (whose theory is described in a 1947 translation by Hernderson and Parsons) attempted to create the ultimately efficient organization by proposing a rational bureaucracy of integrated activities and positions with inherent duties. Employees occupied roles that were assigned on the basis of technical qualifications that, in turn, were determined by formalized impersonal procedures. Rules and regulations were developed for each position regardless of the person who occupied it. The concept of role became paramount in Weber's system, with employees being conceived almost as preprogrammed interchangeable robots.

Weber left untouched the basic premise of capitalism: Employees are to be valued according to their economic utility. Of course, certain protections for the individual were built into his ideal organizations. Prejudices were reduced by hiring according to the qualifications ascribed to a particular position. Once in the organization, people of low social status were able to climb a career ladder as far as their talents, skills, and experience allowed. Employees also had the power to refuse unauthorized work or to correct specific injustices. In fact, Weber's impersonal bureaucracy seemed to outlaw the development of personal relationships in legitimate organizational activities. Weber has been criticized for ignoring the impact of personal relationships and informal structure upon organizational life (Tausky, 1976).

Marx

In contrast, Karl Marx and Friedrich Engels (as described in a publication appearing in 1961) addressed the impact of social structure and social psychology upon organizational behavior. Marx discussed the internal systems dynamics of organizations. He identified the social relations of production as the critical institutional system of a society leading to its class stratification, its conflicts, both internal and external, and their resolution (Katz & Kahn, 1978). Employees having similar production roles developed ideology as a weapon to handle common role interests. Where Weber ignored the feelings of workers, or at least tried to minimize their impact, Marx identified a major institutional force—class consciousness resulting from shared experience. The impact of Marx's revolutionary systems theory and the related rise of the labor movement in capitalist countries demanded that future systems theorists include concern for both task accomplishment and worker welfare.

Modern Systems Theorists

Taylor

No description of systems theory would be complete without mention of Frederick Taylor (1923). Although not a true systems theorist, his ideas form a bridge between approaches that valued employees only for their economic utility and later approaches that valued employees as resources to be cared for, nurtured, and developed, as well as instruments of production. Taylor made careful time and motion studies for each job to determine the one best way to do a task. In the process, he studied the variables of temperature and illumination, rest intervals, and other conditions of work. In his conception, while man was still a machine, he was a valued one. His research, however, failed to identify important systems dynamics, since tasks were usually studied in isolation from other tasks (e.g., the best way to shovel coal into a furnace). Taylor borrowed heavily from models developed in physics and biology and was reductionistic rather than holistic or systemic in approach. His ideas dominated the field of organizational studies in the early twentieth century.

Mayo

Elton Mayo (1933) initiated a series of studies at Western Electric Company's Hawthorne Plant that were intended to contribute to the concepts of scientific management but that ultimately demonstrated the impact of small group dynamics upon production. Small groups of women and men were selected for intensive study of the impact on productivity of physical conditions of work and psychological capacity of the worker, coupled with monetary incentives. The simple relationships found by Taylor among employees working in isolation from one another did not apply when small groups were studied. Physical comfort and pay had less impact upon productivity than the way workers related to each other socially and economically (i.e., being paid for the group's output rather than individual output). Some complex interactions were noted; for example, male workers resisted efforts at increasing production by increasing incentives, apparently because they feared that would violate norms concerning a "fair day's work."

A number of important principles developed from these studies formed the ground-work for a truly social systems management theory. Tausky (1976) has summarized these principles:

1. An organization must be viewed as a social system, an entity with interdependent parts. A change in one part inevitably ripples out and influences other parts which in turn affect yet more removed parts.
2. An organization performs two functions: a) creating a service or product, and b) distributing satisfactions among its members. Therefore, two classes of problems must be continuously dealt with: 1) surviving as an economic unit by performing adequately in the production and marketing process, or, what we have earlier referred to as effectiveness—and 2) maintaining the allocations of satisfactions at a level which induces cooperation and sustains morale—previously referred to as efficiency.
3. In the organization, as in any social system, the process of social evaluations is a constant feature. Distinctions of superior and inferior emerge on the basis of organization members' values.
4. Every person in the organization, whether in a high or low position, regards those real or imagined occurrences which tend to reduce his status as unjust. Every conceivable object or event thus provides a basis for invidious comparisons. Material surroundings, physical events, wages and hours, or work cannot be considered in isolation from their "value" in relating a person to the status hierarchy of the workplace. No person's behavior in an organization from top to bottom, should be viewed as motivated strictly by economic or rational considerations. Values, beliefs, and emotions are inextricably involved in each member's behavior.
5. An organization is in part formally organized—this includes the policies, rules, and regulations which define what the relations between persons are supposed to be—and informally organized. People in associating with one another spontaneously develop personal relationships. Informal groups form which are the carriers of values, beliefs, and norms. Thus, because membership in such groups is valued, they exert powerful influences on behavior.

From Tausky, C. Theories of organization. In Walter R. Nord (Ed.). *Concepts and Controversy in Organizational Behavior.* Copyright © 1976 Scott, Foresman & Company. Reprinted by permission.

These conclusions, based upon lengthy scientific experimentation and observation, represent tremendous advances in the understanding of how humans must be treated differently from their machine counterparts, how important social and psychological dynamics are to organizational behavior, and how research methodology must be planned to measure the psychological as well as physiologic aspects of the work environment.

General Systems Theory

In the 1950s, von Bertalanffy (1950, 1956) described a general systems theory that provided a consistent operational model for studying systems at all levels of science from a single cell to complex social systems such as business firms, political states, and societies. Although theories specific to certain levels of systems is not disputed, general systems theorists focused upon principles common to all levels of systems.

Open Versus Closed Systems
General systems theory differentiates between open and closed systems. Open systems allow for the interchange of inputs and outputs between a system and its environment.

The social sciences inherited a closed-system perspective from Newtonian physics, which had dominated the physical sciences until the early twentieth century. According to the *law of conservation of energy and matter*, the total amount of energy or matter in a system is constant. The application of this principle to practical problems, such as hydraulics, led to significant advances in technology. This principle was intended to describe energy and matter transformation within a hypothetically closed system, such as a carefully controlled laboratory environment with relatively impermeable boundaries between the system and its environment.

Social scientists, such as Freud (1961), however, regarded this principle as a literal description of naturally existing human systems that have relatively permeable boundaries between the systems under study and the environment. For Freud, energy used to repress a disturbing memory was unavailable for other purposes. Since, according to the law of conservation of energy and matter, no new energy was available to the system, the person had less available energy to use for other mental activities.

General systems theory correctly noted that all living systems are open rather than closed systems, and described principles characteristic of all open systems.

Allport

General systems theory was proposed to supplant the mechanistic theories based upon Newtonian physics. Each new theory, however, is in danger of being characterized primarily by the metaphors and analogies it uses to broaden its appeal. Early general systems theorists used examples from biology in developing their theories, resulting in the overreliance upon biologic concepts in extensions of the theory to social systems.

F. H. Allport (1954, 1962, 1967) believed that patterns of human activity were inadequately described in biologic metaphors. For example, groups do not have separate anatomic structures that parallel their functions in the same way that parts of the body parallel the functions of the body. The physical arrangement of a building does not describe the structure of the social organization (Katz & Kahn, 1978).

The analog to biologic structures for Allport is observable events. If events in a social system are planned and anticipated, they become part of the formal structure. Formal structures of this sort dictate who reports to whom, how communications will occur, what will be in these communications, and where and when employees will work. Conceptualizing structure as events rather than as palpable entities has other advantages. Informal structure is easily conceived of as those events that are not formally planned or anticipated by managers and administrators in the system.

Cycles of events define typical social structures. In most, if not all, social systems, certain typical patterns of behavior occur among members of the system. Events are nodal points in these patterns. Allport rejected the traditional linear model of causation, that is, event A causes event B, that, in turn, causes event C (ad infinitum), in favor of a cyclical model. Event A influences event B, that influences event C, that in turn, influences a recurring event A.

Allport's views of the social system made several important contributions to the theory of social and organizational systems. Instead of looking for analogous anatomic structures, theorists began looking at the interaction of actors in the system, the human members of the system. The functioning of the actors was seen as the structure. Social systems were also viewed as more contrived than biologic systems and frequently having no dependable life cycle. Cycles of events continue as long as humans who are willing to function and interact in the system can be found.

The cyclical view of causation in social systems suggests that change efforts cannot isolate a single cause for an unwanted event. Since each event has an impact on every other event in a particular cycle, attempts to change that pattern must make a contextual analysis of the problem. Many unanticipated results of planned change occurred when this advice was not heeded.

HUMANISTIC APPROACHES TO SOCIAL AND ORGANIZATIONAL CHANGE

Kurt Lewin and Abraham Maslow are best known for their contributions in separate areas of social and organizational psychology; however, both have been embraced by a significantly large number of organizational and management science theorists to warrant inclusion in this discussion. Preeminent figures, such as McGregor (1960), Likert (1967), Blake and Mouton (1964), and Rogers (1961) were greatly influenced by both of these men.

Lewin

Kurt Lewin is clearly recognized as a systems theorist although his field theory of social systems (1951), with its mathematical complexity, has been embraced totally by only a few organizational theorists. A number of important Lewinian concepts, however, have been incorporated into current theories of social systems based upon open systems theory. The characteristics of boundaries (e.g., permeable or impermeable) between an organism and its environment were identified as key concepts in understanding social events. The need for contextual analysis was also stressed. Analysis begins with the situation as a whole from which the component parts are differentiated. Lewin (1936) also argued that system behavior can only be understood in terms of the events in the system at any given time. Approaches that looked to the past (e.g., Freud) or the future (e.g., Jung) were rejected for practical as well as epistemological reasons.

The concept of dynamic equilibrium was considered key in attempting to change systems. Lewin recognized that all systems tend to establish equilibrium states between forces attempting to change the system and forces attempting to keep the system the way it is. Lewin explored, through theory (1951) and applied research, strategies for changing the level of equilibrium states involving behaviors (eating habits, 1943) and attitudes (racial attitudes, 1946). In fact, his interest in applied behavioral science led to the forming of the National Training Laboratories (NTL) in Bethel, Maine, for the purpose of supporting and developing theories and methods for social change.

Maslow

Abraham Maslow is well known for his theory of a hierarchy of needs (1954). According to Maslow, the first-level needs are physiologic (hunger, thirst, sex, elimination, sleep/ rest). Safety needs are the second-level needs (protection from physiologic and psychological harm). Next are the needs for love and belonging, followed by the needs for self-esteem. The highest level need is that for self-actualization. Successively higher level needs become salient motivating factors once more basic needs have been satisfied. Once fully satisfied, a need is no longer a motivating factor.

Maslow (1968) viewed a person's hierarchy of needs to be intrinsic to his or her psychic and biologic state, that is, a part of his or her inner nature. Since these needs are intrinsic and natural, Maslow views them as neither good nor evil. Organizational and management theories that ignore the human being's intrinsic nature are detrimental to the psychic and physical health and well-being of employees. Although these needs, especially higher-level ones, may be suppressed, ignoring basic human needs will contribute to lower productivity, high absenteeism, high turnover, low morale, and job dissatisfaction.

POSTINDUSTRIAL ORGANIZATIONS AND SOCIETY

Many economically advanced countries, such as the United States, are moving into a postindustrial era that is service oriented yet technology intensive. The exponential growth of knowledge and the development of ultra-advanced technologies for information processing are having profound effects. In computer companies, employees devote a quarter of their time to training activities in order to keep up with current trends. The turbulence of the environment in which organizations find themselves—with quickly appearing scarcities or gluts, fluctuating political climates, and unstable economic climates—have changed the character, pace, and stress level of organizational life. Survival and growth require adaptive organizational goals, structures, and processes.

The nurse leader, manager, or supervisor faces some of the same changes and problems today as those with which managers in both health care and non-health care organizations must cope. More nursing information is available to the nurse as a result of an increased emphasis on nursing research and theory development. Medical technology and information that have an impact on the nursing profession are increasing at astounding rates. Consumers are not only more informed about health care today, they are demanding even more information about promoting their own health, about understanding any illness experienced, and about understanding their nursing and medical care more fully. Nursing staff and faculty find it increasingly important to engage in continued self-development through formal advanced degree programs, continuing education, or in-service training in order to keep current.

Other changes and trends are also occurring. Intraprofessional and interprofessional interfacing are becoming common terms. Conflicts at these boundaries arise and must be resolved. Motivational patterns of employees are changing. Nursing staff and faculty are demanding work environments conducive to quality patient care or sound educational programs. Nurses search for organizations that permit them opportunities for continuing education. Flexible work hours—flexitime and compressed time—as well as adequate salaries that are compatible with other personal commitments are sought.

Political, economic, and professional forces demand that nurse leaders, managers, and supervisors give serious consideration to issues of quality control, accountability, and cost containment. Organizational processes and structures that maximize quality patient care yet are cost effective are being sought.

Social systems theory offers a contextual approach that encourages the consideration of the system-wide impact of such problems and changes. Social systems theory acknowledges the interactive effect of human characteristics and technology. Its use is conducive to the development of humanistic work atmospheres in which there is blended an emphasis on methods to improve productivity, a mix essential for organizational goal achievement.

SUMMARY

This chapter briefly described the changing environment and systems confronting nurse leaders, managers, and supervisors. Processes and strategies needed to manage effectively a system's input, throughput, output, and feedback processes in such a milieu were identified. The authors' approach and orientation were outlined and a central theme was identified: Attempts at increasing productivity and goal achievement must consider human factors and system maintenance. Nurse leadership, management, and supervision were defined.

The chapter also traced the evolution of social systems theory from the early church and military concepts, through the theories of Weber, Marx, Taylor, and Mayo, to the more recent social systems theories of general systems theory, for example, Allport, Maslow, and Lewin. Current and future trends in postindustrial organizations and society were also discussed.

Most contemporary theories of social systems employ the open systems model described first in general systems theory. Allport extended open systems theory to describe the organizational system. Avoiding biologic metaphors, Allport described organizational structure as cycles of events. This approach emphasized circular, nonlinear views of causation in social systems. Lewin's and Maslow's theories heavily influenced major organization writers such as McGregor, Likert, and Blake and Mouton. Lewin's concepts of boundaries, contextual analysis, and present orientation and Maslow's theory of hierarchy of needs have widely influenced management theory and practice.

The implications of concepts from social systems and other relevant theories for nurse leadership, management, or supervision in health care or educational organizations are numerous. Among these implications are (1) an understanding of the (a) input, throughput, output, and feedback processes, (b) importation, transformation, and exportation of energy in systems, (c) organization of life cycles, and (d) processes within subsystems; (2) the importance of common goals, values, and norms to gain the commitment and support of nurse employees; (3) the need for professional development to ensure continued quality system output; (4) the clarification of roles and authority so that teams and interdisciplinary staff work effectively in crisis states or under time pressure; and (5) the need to ensure employee welfare as well as maximum productivity.

The authors contend that a humanistic management atmosphere, with an emphasis on methods to improve productivity, is essential for effective organizational goal achievement. A clear definition of organizational problems that impede goal attainment, an assessment of the consequences of proposed alternative intervention strategies, the selection and implementation of intervention strategies, along with an evaluation of their results, will continue to foster the development of a sound scientific base for leadership, management, and supervision.

REFERENCES

Allport, F. The structuring of events: Outline of a general theory with application to psychology. *Psychological Review*, 1954, *61*, 281–303.

Allport, F. A structuronomic conception of behavior: Individual and collective. I. Structural theory and the master problem of social psychology. *Journal of Abnormal and Social Psychology*, 1962, *64*, 3–30

Allport, F. A theory of enestruence (event structure theory): Report of progress. *American Psychologist*, 1967, *22*, 1–24.

Blake, R., & Mouton, J. *The managerial grid*. Houston: Gulf, 1964.

Freud, S. [*The interpretation of dreams*] (J. Strachey, trans. & ed.). New York: Science Editions, 1961. (Originally published, in German, 1900.)

Katz, D., & Kahn, R. *The social psychology of organizations* (2nd ed.). New York: Wiley, 1978.

Lewin, K. *Principles of topological psychology*. New York: McGraw-Hill, 1936.

Lewin, K. Forces behind food habits and methods of change. *Bulletin of the National Research Council*, 1943, *108*, 35–65.

Lewin, K. Action research and minority problems. *Journal of Social Issues*, 1946, 2, 34–46.

Lewin, K. *Field theory in social science*. New York: Harper, 1951.

Likert, R. *The human organization*. New York: McGraw-Hill, 1967.

McGregor, D. *The human side of enterprise*. New York: McGraw-Hill, 1960.

Marx, K., & Engels, F. The manifesto of the Communist party (1948). In *The essential left*. New York: Barnes & Noble, 1961.

Maslow, A. *Motivation and personality*. New York: Harper, 1954.

Maslow, A. *Toward a psychology of being* (2nd ed.). New York: Van Nostrand, 1968.

Mayo, E. *The human problems of an industrial civilization*. New York: Macmillan, 1933.

Rogers, C. *On becoming a person*. Boston: Houghton Mifflin, 1961.

Saddler Report. Great Britain, Sessional Papers, 1833, vol. *123*, ed. 706. In B. Knowles, & R. Snyder (Eds.), *Readings in western civilization*. Philadelphia: Lippincott, 1954.

Tausky, C. Theories of organization. In W. Nord (Ed.), *Concepts and controversy in organizational behavior*, (2nd ed.). Santa Monica, Calif.: Goodyear Publishing Co., 1976.

Taylor, F. *The principles of scientific management*. New York: Harper, 1923.

von Bertalanffy, L. The theory of open systems in physics and biology. *Science*, 1950, *111*, 23–28.

von Bertalanffy, L. General systems theory. *General Systems*, 1956, *1*, 1–10.

Weber, M. [*The theory of social and economic organization*] (A. Hernderson, & T. Parsons, trans. & T. Parsons ed.). New York: Free Press, 1947.

CHAPTER 2
THE NATURE
OF SOCIAL SYSTEMS

THE ORGANIZATION AS AN OPEN SYSTEM

Early Organizational Theorists tended to view organizations as closed systems. In a closed system, there is no exchange of energy between the system under study and the environment in which it is embedded. This principle, known as the *law of conservation of energy and matter*, was popular among most social scientists, who envied the precision and mathematical rigor of the physical sciences.

Meanwhile, the "pure" sciences, such as theoretical physics, moved away from viewing phenomena in an absolute Newtonian framework toward a probabilistic and relative Einsteinian view. For example, the possibility of being able to predict perfectly the precise parabolic trajectory of an electron shot from an ideal atomic gun was demonstrated to be impossible because the very act of measurement and observation, which requires photons or other sources of energy, distorted the path of the electron. Heisenberg (1930) argued that the moment that we attempt to measure a phenomenon, we distort it.

These revolutionary changes in theoretical perspective, however, were not rapidly integrated into the social sciences. Taylor (1923) and advocates of scientific management conducted time and motion studies as if they were laboratory experiments, with little regard for the organizational context in which a particular job was located. Even studies that involved work groups, such as the Hawthorne studies of the 1930s (Mayo, 1933), assumed that each such subgroup was relatively independent and autonomous. The emergence of work norms (e.g., "a fair day's work") that transcended the study boundaries were seen by many as confounding variables that muddied the "ideal" work environment. These variables were not considered as important factors in all organizational systems, ideal or otherwise.

Theorists of the human relations school often made the same closed systems assumptions implicitly if not explicitly. Their strategies for organizational improvement often involved sending employees, frequently management, to human relations training seminars or workshops, which were openly viewed as "cultural islands" (e.g., encounter groups, sensitivity groups), unconfounded by the politics or normative resistances of on-the-job behavior. As evidence supporting this approach, dramatic changes were reported in these workshops that were attended by members who were virtual strangers to each other. When these workers returned to their jobs, however, it was frequently noted that these changes disappeared, since there was no supportive organizational climate.

On the other hand, attempts to replicate the T-group and sensitivity group in the work setting itself were, at the very least, ineffective and were often experienced as disruptive and dangerous by management and rank-and-file alike. It began to sink in that these "confounding" factors must be acknowledged and included in any organizational change strategy.

By the 1950s, social and physical scientists alike had dispensed with the assumption that the systems they studied and tried to change were closed systems. Closed systems occur only hypothetically since at the present we are not able to totally isolate any system from its environment. Further integration of the social and physical sciences began to occur in the development of general systems theory. Von Bertalanffy (1950), a biologist, joined with Boulding (1960), an economist, Ashby (1958), a bacteriologist, J. G. Miller (1955), a psychiatrist, Rapoport (1956), a mathematician, and Emery and Trist (1960), organizational theorists, in developing a theory that described and explained behavior in open systems of all types. This theory has been designated as *open systems theory*.

COMMON CHARACTERISTICS OF OPEN SYSTEMS

A System Defined

A *system* is a unitary whole composed of two or more elements in interaction, differentiated by an identifiable boundary from its environment, and characterized by input→ throughput→output energy cycles (see Figure 2-1).

Importation, Transformation, and Exportation of Energy

All open systems have input→throughput→output energy cycles. A simple example from cellular biology would be the human cell's importation of oxygen and nutrients from the bloodstream, the transformation of these inputs into cellular material and metabolic processes, and the export of energy in the form of necessary body functioning (i.e., muscle activity, digestive processes, mental processes) and "waste." As will be seen later, waste from one system or subsystem may be useful input for another system or subsystem.

In a social system, such as a school of nursing in a university, *inputs* include student nurses; faculty and other personnel, including consultants; tuition, grants, contracts, and other forms of funding; information inputs from consultants, faculty, students, professional colleagues in clinical facilities, advisory groups, interested community citizens, nursing conferences, nursing research, books, and journals, and from other

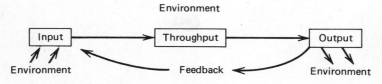

FIGURE 2-1. OPEN SYSTEM

related disciplines; facilities, equipment, and supplies, such as classrooms, learning laboratories, clinical facilities, and audiovisual hardware and software; and support services, such as the student health and counseling services, financial aid office, and the library. *Throughput*, or transformation processes, involves the implementation of the designed nursing curriculum, including the philosophy, conceptual framework, terminal objectives, course objectives, teaching methodology (lectures, seminars, independent study, group discussions, laboratory study and practice, supervised clinical practice), and the evaluation plan; university administration; faculty and student research; and other student and faculty professional activities. *Outputs* from this system are educated nurses; reports of new knowledge in journals, books, and presentations; direct services through university or school of nursing sponsored clinics and health programs; consultation to other nursing schools or to health care agencies; and other direct services, all ultimately contributing to improved patient care.

Energy can be observed in the form of useful work (muscle action, clinical nursing practice, or teaching) or in the potential to perform useful work. Since information enables a system to increase its capacity to perform useful work, it is considered equivalent to potential energy. Management activities make use of this characteristic of information to provide effective control and coordination of system activities. Living systems require both matter–energy and information to survive and function effectively (Miller, 1965).

Systems as Cycles of Events

Typically, systems demonstrate repetitive cycles of energy input→throughput→output. One can count on nursing schools to graduate nurses, General Motors to build cars, and human beings to breathe and carry out complex but predictable patterns of behavior in order to put food on the table. The outputs in all of these systems are means for sustaining the system. If the environment does not value a system's output and provide reciprocal input energy, the system will die.

Each system has a primary task that it must perform in order to survive. When this primary task is improperly identified, or ignored, the output of the system is considered waste by other systems in the environment. They, in turn, withhold inputs for the system. When a system gets out of touch with its environment, it fails to modify its product to suit the needs of importers of the system's output.

It can be argued, for instance, that U.S. auto producers in the mid-1970s incorrectly identified their primary task and built large, comfortable, but energy-inefficient and poorly built cars when the environment wanted high-quality and energy-efficient automobiles. The primary task was not simply to build cars in the traditional way, but to build cars that reflected the rapidly changing attitudes and needs of potential consumers. The fact that the environment changes over time provides the basis for adaptation and evolution in the cycles of events in a system. Successful systems will modify their characteristic cycles of events to prevent death or to ensure growth.

In organizations, the cycles of events themselves constitute the structure of the system (Allport, 1962). In our nursing school example, the pattern of activities inherent in implementing the academic curriculum describes its structural functioning far better than merely considering the formal table of organization of the school of nursing or the physical layout of university buildings. Accrediting agencies base their acceptance or rejection of an educational program upon the degree to which the curriculum accomplishes the terminal objectives of the program and the established standards for the nursing profession. Tables of organization and building use must support the curriculum and contribute toward the achievement of terminal objectives. To recap, the basic method for identifying social and organizational structures is to follow the energy in the chain of events through the input→throughput→output cycles.

Negative Entropy

The universal *law of entropy* states that all systems move toward disorganization, decay, and death. This process is reversed (negative entropy) while a system is in its "life cycle." Systems require the constant importation of energy or energy storage capacity to carry them through lean energy periods. Death occurs when the system loses its sources of energy inputs, its capacity to transform energy, or its market for exports.

To provide a buffer from environmental turmoil, systems will attempt to maximize the ratio of imported versus expended energy. Companies retain profits, states pass laws to ensure budget balances or surpluses, and countries stockpile fuel and scarce materials. Educational nonprofit organizations build up special areas of academic and research expertise along with highly qualified faculty in order to ensure a steady flow of students and to attract sources of funding. These processes serve to ensure evolutionary rather than revolutionary changes in a system's cycle of events (its structure).

In discussing the relationship between a system and its environment, it is useful to identify the boundary region separating the two. In general, boundaries are identified by a discontinuity or modification in the quality, quantity, or phase of energy. Boundaries vary in the degree of their permeability to energy and information. A hypothetically closed system would allow no energy or information to enter or leave the system. Under such conditions, the universal law of entropy assures that over time such a system's internal organization would disintegrate into random particles of matter of nonproductive activities and would experience depletion of energy. Living systems, therefore, must have permeable boundaries. The boundary must also have coding capabilities. The boundary region must be able to identify the appropriate inputs for the system and allow them to pass through while denying entry to other irrelevant or disruptive inputs.

Once inputs have been allowed to enter the boundary region, they must be reorganized or decoded into forms and patterns familiar to the system. For example, the eye performs a coding operation by being sensitive to certain forms of energy (light as opposed to sound) and performs a decoding operation by transforming this energy into impulses that are acceptable to the neural subsystem. Information inputs into a school of nursing are analyzed for their relevance to the current operational program and for improvement of the program.

Suprasystems and Subsystems

Any system under study is located within a larger system (the suprasystem) and at the same time is composed of smaller systems (subsystems). The suprasystem is commonly called the environment or ecosystem. Subsystems are component parts of a system that are separated by boundaries and have an internal consistency with respect to quantity, quality, frequency, or phase of energy utilization. Just as body organs transform energy in a consistent way to provide a needed output for system functioning, social systems have departments to provide coordination and production functions necessary for total system functioning.

Systems are nested in hierarchical ways so that a given system will be a suprasystem for smaller related systems and a subsystem for a larger related system. The food chain represents an analogy to this hierarchical arrangement. A small fish is a predator to smaller fish and a food source to larger fish and so on, up and down the food chain. For a school of nursing, the suprasystem is the university in which the school is located. Subsystems, for example, the graduate department, the undergraduate department, and the department of continuing education, are the major component parts of the school of nursing. For a nursing service, the suprasystem is the hospital. The subsystems, for example, the medical-surgical division, pediatric division, obstetrical division, in-service training division, and psychiatric division, are the major parts of the nursing service department.

Information Input and Negative Feedback

One type of information input for a system is negative feedback. The message delivered by negative feedback is "continuation of current behavior without modifications threatens the stability and survival of the system." The subsystems or individuals primarily concerned with regulation of the system then know to act to correct the problem. The critical nature of negative feedback is expressed in a statement by Miller (1955): "When a system's negative feedback discontinues, its steady state vanishes, and at the same time its boundary disappears and the system terminates" (p. 529).

Many examples of regulatory functions in systems responding to negative feedback exist. When the temperature drops below or exceeds certain critical levels, the sensing mechanisms in a thermostat are activated, sending instructions through electrical impulses to heating or cooling devices to bring the temperature back within acceptable limits. In the human body, the hypothalamus provides much the same kind of regulatory functions and depends upon negative feedback from sensory organs. In a well-functioning school of nursing or nursing service department in a health care organization (both being social systems), nurse administrators, leaders, managers, and supervisors analyze negative and positive feedback for its relevance to the system's optimal functioning. Based on the analysis, appropriate changes are initiated to maintain system viability. Declining or decaying social systems may no longer attend to negative feedback and thus will no longer institute necessary and appropriate change.

The Steady State of Dynamic Equilibrium

The input→throughput→output energy conversion cycles operate best if the system behaves in a relatively consistent manner over time. This so-called steady state of dynamic equilibrium allows for the most efficient ratio of energy to be expended for production versus coordination and provides a reliable and predictable output for other systems in the environment. Nations prefer to trade with other stable nations even if they do not approve of their political practices. Nursing schools that are accredited and have a history of producing quality graduates and contributing to the development of new nursing knowledge attract qualified nursing applicants, well-prepared faculty, and often a variety of funding. Accredited health care organizations with a history of providing excellent medical and nursing care and sound administrative policies tend to attract qualified nurses who want to work there. Among the citizens of the community, it is common knowledge that this is a good place to obtain assistance with health problems and disease prevention.

This steady state, however, is not a true motionless equilibrium. A certain amount of variability or flux is tolerated so long as the overall character of the system is maintained. For example, the catabolic and anabolic processes of tissue breakdown and restoration operate to produce an organism that is slightly different from moment to moment. Humans, however, do not normally grow a third eye, ear, or leg. The characteristic relation of subsystems will remain the same over time.

In dynamic equilibrium, systems reflexively resist any internal or external pressures to change the characteristic ways of functioning (Lewin, 1947; Bradley & Calvin, 1956). This homeostatic characteristic must be considered when system change is contemplated. Because of the complex interrelationship of a system with its environment and its subsystems, there are functional reasons for homeostatic and conservative mechanisms to resist major changes in the character of a system. Nurse leaders, managers, and supervisors must consider the homeostatic principle of open systems when change strategies are introduced.

System-threatening circumstances or the introduction of planned change strategies will override these homeostatic mechanisms. Even apparently invariant system characteristics, such as normal body temperature, can be modified through efforts to survive in hostile environments. Australian aborigines have developed the capacity to lower body temperature at night as a way of surviving in the cold desert. Psychotherapists use the anxiety, pain, and depression experienced in crisis situations to bring about personality changes that are frequently impossible to make in calmer times. Driving forces that move the social system in the desired direction are augmented during constructive planned change.

Growth and Expansion

In another respect, the system's steady state is not motionless. Since environments vary in the rate at which they provide needed energy inputs, systems learn that they must generate energy-material reserves to buffer the system in energy-matter lean times.

One way to do this is to expand (to make larger profits), diversify (to provide a greater variety of energy-matter inputs/outputs), or create monopolies (to control critical parts of the environment). Although successful systems attempt to maintain their essential character, they also acknowledge their need to gain greater control over their environment through growth and expansion.

Differentiation

Open systems develop through differentiation and elaboration. Early in the life of a system there frequently is little to distinguish one component of the system from another. Animal life generally begins with the fertilization of one cell (the egg) by another (sperm). The growth of the embryo through successive cell division leads to an increase in cell specialization until separate organs become established.

In social systems, members of an infant organization frequently are involved with all phases of operations. As the organization grows, members focus their activities on areas of interest, skill, and necessity. New members are added to provide functions that become required and for which older members have no time, interest, or skills.

A reason for this trend in increased differentiation with growth is that specialization allows for increased efficiency and, therefore, greater survivability. As a consequence of specialization, there is a shift from the varied dynamic interactions of early organizational life to the fixed and highly regulated interactions of more mature social systems. Increased efficiency is gained at the expense of adaptability of the component parts of the system.

Integration and Coordination

The trend toward growth, expansion, and differentiation places greater demands upon the system to integrate and coordinate its component subsystems. In early life, an organization survives because of the vigor and adaptability of its founding members. Since the small number of members is continually in interaction because of spatial and functional overlaps, integration and coordination occur informally, albeit inefficiently.

Growth brings in members who may not have the same commitment to the organizational goals as founding members. More space is required, limiting informal contact. Specialization decreases the extent of functional overlap in member activities. For these reasons, integration and coordination subsystems (management) are created.

In social systems, coordination and integration serve somewhat different purposes (Katz & Kahn, 1978). Coordination assures that tasks and roles mesh properly. For example, curriculum activities are sequenced and occur in a timely manner, allowing for the planned progression of students through the program. Integration, on the other hand, ensures that members share the same norms and values. Orientation programs for new nursing staff, staff luncheons or retreats, and faculty or nursing staff handbooks provide an integration function for the system.

Equifinality   *equifinality*

The principle of *equifinality* (van Bertalanffy, 1940) states that a system can reach the same final state from differing initial conditions and by a variety of paths. Simple and primitive systems demonstrate this principle most dramatically. Normal sea urchins, for example, can develop from a complete ovum, from each half of a divided ovum, or from the fusion product of two whole ova. The increase in regulatory activity in open systems, however, inhibits the process of equifinality (Katz & Kahn, 1978). However, although fixed arrangements of regulation activities certainly limit the range of alternative methods for accomplishing a task, the principle of equifinality disputes the doctrine that there is one best way to do a job.

SUMMARY

This chapter presented the essential characteristics of all open systems, biologic, social, organizational, or otherwise. The most important characteristic of open systems is the importation→transformation→exportation of energy, matter, information, and products, and the interaction of the system with its environment. In this process, open systems have recurring cycles of events that correspond to structure in social organizations. Boundary regions provide regulation of input and output of energy–matter and information as well as coding and decoding functions with regard to information. At any given time, each system has a primary task that it must perform in order to survive as a viable system.

Each system fights against negative entropy by trying to import more energy–matter than it exports and by storing the excess energy–matter to serve as a buffer against environmental change. Each system is embedded in a hierarchy of systems so that it is a subsystem for a larger system and a suprasystem for smaller systems.

Systems require information input and negative feedback to adapt to changing environmental conditions. In doing so, systems try to maintain a steady state of dynamic equilibrium. However, growth and expansion are required to build reserves and exert more control over the environment. In this process, the steady state changes without radically changing the essential character of the system. Growth is accomplished by differentiation, which makes the system more efficient while restricting its flexibility. Growth also requires the development of regulatory subsystems that ensure coordination and integration of subsystem activities.

Finally, open systems are characterized by equifinality that allows a final state to be accomplished from differing initial states and developmental paths. A description of the characteristics of open systems provides the essential ingredients for understanding any social or organizational system.

REFERENCES

Allport, F. A structuronomic conception of behavior: Individual and collective. I. Structural theory and the master problem of social psychology. *Journal of Abnormal and Social Psychology*, 1962, *64*, 3–30.

Ashby, W. General systems theory as a new discipline. *General Systems Yearbook*, 1958, *3*, 1–6.

Boulding, K. Towards a general theory as a new discipline. *General Systems Yearbook*, 1960, *5*, 66–75.

Bradley, D., & Calvin, M. Behavior: Imbalance in a network of chemical transformations. *General Systems Yearbook*, 1956, *1*, 56–65.

Emery, F., & Trist, E. Socio-technical systems. In *Management science models and techniques* (Vol. 2). London: Pergamon, 1960.

Heisenberg, L. *The physical principles of the quantum theory*. (C. Eckart, & F. Hoyt, trans.). New York: Dover, 1930.

Katz, D., & Kahn, R. *The social psychology of organizations* (2nd ed.). New York: Wiley, 1978.

Lewin, K. Frontiers in group dynamics. *Human relations*, 1947, *1*, 2–38.

Mayo, E. *The human problem of an industrial civilization*. New York: Macmillan, 1933.

Miller, J. Toward a general theory for the behavioral sciences. *American Psychologist*, 1955, *10*, 513–531.

Miller, J. Living systems: Basic concepts. *Behavioral Science*, 1965, *10*, 193–237.

Rapoport, A. The diffusion problem in mass behavior. *General Systems Yearbook*, 1956, *1*, 6.

Taylor, F. *The principles of scientific management*. New York: Harper, 1923.

von Bertalanffy, L. Der organismus als physikalisches system betrachtet. *Naturwissenschaften*, 1940, *28*, 521 ff.

von Bertalanffy, L. The theory of open systems in physics and biology. *Science*, 1950, *111*, 23–28.

CHAPTER 3
THE ORGANIZATION
OF SOCIAL SYSTEMS

ORGANIZATIONS DEFINED

A *system* is a unitary whole composed of two or more elements in interaction and differentiated from its environment by an identifiable boundary. Although this is a very simple and parsimonious definition, it is inadequate for an exposition of the kinds of social systems in which nurse managers, leaders, and supervisors work. Modern health care systems function quite differently from social clubs, neighborhoods, and other informally organized social systems.

What distinguishes the modern health care organization from a club, street gang, or lecture audience is the degree to which (a) cycles of events are formalized and routinized; (b) elements are interdependent upon one another; (c) individuals within the system are differentiated from one another in terms of function, status, and power; and (d) information derived from within and without the organization is used for regulation and decision making. Simple social systems can survive and function with a minimum of formal organization, interdependency, differentiation, and information feedback. Larger, more mature organizations, performing complex tasks in competitive environments, almost inevitably develop in these directions in order to survive. Modern health care systems are not exceptions to this rule.

TASK ACCOMPLISHMENT AND SYSTEM MAINTENANCE

General systems theorists have recognized the existence of separate processes to ensure the production of marketable products and to ensure the maintenance of the system itself. Berrien (1968) referred to the former processes as signal inputs (recognizing the equivalence between energy and information) and to the latter processes as maintenance inputs. Cattell, Saunders, and Stice (1953), in discussing social groups, defined effective synergy as energy used to carry out the "purposes for which the group explicitly exists," while maintenance synergy was defined as the energy used in operating the "internal machinery" of the group.

Before the formal development of general systems theory, astute observers and researchers studying human systems had come to the same conclusion. The Parliamentary Committee set up in 1833 to study working conditions in British industry (Saddler Report, 1954), noted that slaves in the West Indies were treated more humanely and intelligently than factory workers in Great Britain. A testifying physician noted the necessity and value of maintenance processes as follows:

> I think that twelve hours labour is too much for a large majority of human beings. If I am to state the precise quantity, in my experience, as tending to give the longest and the most vigorous life, I should take it, even in the adult, at eight active exertion, eight hours sleep, and eight hours allowed for recreation and meals. Those are the divisions of the day which would procure the *happiest* and most *vigorous* life, and which would, I think, *yield the greatest sum of labour*; but the child requires a greater proportion of sleep than adults; for *sleep is not simply repose, but it is a restorative process.* (pp. 9–13; italics added)

The economic advantage of attending to the maintenance processes in human biologic systems was emphasized in another quote from the Saddler Report (1954):

> So that you consider that the limitation of the length and degree of the labour of the children and young persons in Barbados is imminently advantageous to the planter himself, with a view merely to his own interest and fortune advantage?—Certainly; it is necessary. In English factories, every thing which is valuable in manhood is sacrificed to an inferior advantage in childhood. *You purchase your advantage at the price of infanticide*; the *profit thus gained is death to the child*. Looking at its effects, I should suppose it was a *system directly intended to diminish the population.* (pp. 9–13, italics added).

In this passage, failure to be concerned with maintenance processes is linked to diminution and death of the system itself. The Saddler Report provided the negative feedback required to pass the Factory Act of 1833, which mandated proper treatment for child and adult factory workers. Economic as well as humane motives were clearly evident in the passage of this law.

In the early twentieth century, Frederick Taylor attempted to identify, through scientific study, the most effective production and maintenance processes in doing any job. It proved more difficult, however, to identify maintenance needs in social systems than in biologic or mechanical systems. It is a far simpler problem to determine the necessary nutritive and caloric intake to maintain a biologic system than to determine what inputs will attract, sustain, motivate, and satisfy employees in organizations. The temptation is great to assume a direct analogy between biologic and social systems in developing maintenance processes. Mayo (1933) reasoned that employees would produce best in environments that best suited the physical characteristics of humans. Better lighting, therefore, should increase productivity. It was quite disturbing to discover that, under certain circumstances, *less* illumination produced greater productivity.

With somewhat similar reasoning, organizations have experimented with varying pay systems, rest and work schedules, employee benefit schemes, and labor-management relationships in order to attract and retain valued employees and get maximum productivity from their work forces. These efforts, however, have sometimes been ineffective. Labor-management disputes and strikes have not disappeared, as was predicted by Taylor (1923). Low motivation for task accomplishment and low job satisfaction continue to plague industry, government, universities, and health care organizations, at times.

It will be recalled that Tausky (1976), in summarizing the findings of Mayo's work, noted:

> An organization performs two functions: a) creating a service or product, and b) distributing satisfactions among its members. Therefore, two classes of problems must be continuously

dealt with: 1) surviving as an economic unit by performing adequately in the production and marketing process, or, what we earlier referred to as effectiveness . . . and 2) maintaining the allocations of satisfactions at a level which induces cooperation and sustains morale . . . which we previously referred to as efficiency. (pp. 292–293)

Task accomplishment and system maintenance are emphasized throughout this book in discussions of motivation, job satisfaction, leadership style, organizational dynamics, planning and goal setting, and strategies for dealing with organizational problems. The recognition of the special problems of providing maintenance functions in organizational life, while at the same time valuing and rewarding task accomplishment, has led to the greatest advances in the theoretical underpinnings for leadership, management, and supervisory practices.

ROLES

Open systems develop and grow through processes of differentiation and elaboration. In social systems, roles are developed both formally and informally in an effort to gain efficiency and remain competitive in their environment. Many studies have reported the natural or spontaneous development of roles in groups organized around concrete as well as more abstract tasks. Guetzkow (1960) reported that certain roles evolved naturally and reliably when five-man groups were asked to solve a puzzle. These roles, which he labeled end men, relayers, and key men, evolved and stabilized after a relatively brief period of work.

One would expect, therefore, that roles would develop to ensure that a group's task was accomplished while maintaining necessary social relationships. Bales (1950), in fact, presented convincing data to establish that in groups without designated roles (therapy groups, leaderless groups, and groups organized to study group dynamics), individuals will take on roles that will ensure task accomplishment (task-oriented leadership) and group maintenance (social/emotional leadership). Although different group members may take on these roles, there is generally at least one person taking responsibility for these processes at all times.

Role development in formal organizations is a good deal more complex. Katz and Kahn (1978) have defined roles in organizations as ''standardized patterns of behavior required of all persons playing a part in a given functional relationship, regardless of personal wishes or interpersonal obligations irrelevant to the functional relationship'' (p. 43). The manner in which organizational roles become depersonalized can have benefits and drawbacks for both the organization and the individual occupying the role. The organization gains a measure of control over an employee's behavior, which facilitates coordination and integration of activities and cuts down on the variability and consequent unpredictability of employee behavior. Organizations, in creating job descriptions, are able to specify the primary and secondary tasks for a position, which then specify how an employee's behavior is to be evaluated. Roles stabilize and routinize an organization's cycle of events, thus making the organization more efficient and reducing conflict between employees and subsystems.

Roles can be used as protection against supervisors' attempts to reward or punish employee behavior on the basis of prejudice or non-job-related feelings toward the employee. On the other hand, role-prescribed standards of behavior can serve as the basis for firing an employee who may be quite popular with other employees or has the support of a local union.

On the negative side, the regimented aspect of roles leaves many employees feeling dehumanized. Personal freedom is limited and many conflicts can develop between behavior required in a role and an individual's personal feelings. Examples of conflicts between role requirements and personal feelings and the stress that results abound. For example, newly graduated nurses may experience conflicts between their internal professional values and the reality based expectations of their staff nurse roles.

The depersonalizing aspect of roles presents problems for organizations as well. Communication becomes more difficult as employees restrict their behavior and become less spontaneous. The nonverbal cues upon which humans rely so heavily to fully communicate feelings and nuances in meaning are lost as the memorandum replaces the informal discussion over coffee. Argyris (1960) argued that the development of depersonalized roles in organizations encourages regression and discourages personal growth and maturation. The personal satisfactions that are necessary in a job become more difficult to achieve. Attempts to "humanize the workplace" often miss the boat by creating more depersonalized roles (Director of Employee Development) or adding more system maintenance responsibilities to existing depersonalized roles. The gold watches given at retirement parties are frequently the object of scorn because employees do not attribute feelings of generosity or appreciation to ritualized ceremonies given for everyone.

Informal roles that often serve system maintenance functions do develop, however. A staff member remembers to tell his or her boss whose birthday is coming up or serves as an information source concerning effective ways to deal with crucial or difficult persons in the organization. Some employees band together for social lunches or organize after-hours events that serve to maintain harmonious interpersonal relationships. During staff meetings, certain individuals will consistently play the role of harmonizer, defuser of conflicts, or distractor, with the purpose of keeping everyone talking and working with each other. These roles are often covertly established with the silent agreement of the entire system or subsystem.

Some leaders, managers, or supervisors will view these activities as wasteful, while others will encourage constructive system-maintenance roles. An organization in which conflict cannot be expressed openly is invariably uncreative and sterile and can be unproductive because it fails to be adaptive. The continual smoothing over of legitimate conflicts encourages organizational members to express their disagreement in passive–aggressive ways, thereby eroding support for decisions reached by the organization and driving silent wedges between individuals, inhibiting their ability to work together. The wise nurse leader, manager, or supervisor will tolerate and, at times support, the open critic in the system, or the staff member who brings conflict to the surface, by referring to the obvious but unspoken issues facing the organization.

Our view of roles is that they are necessary and inevitable in the development of an organization. They serve to restrict the range of behaviors of employees, thus increasing coordination and integration of system behavior and increasing the efficient accomplishment of a system's primary task. When roles have been effectively developed, peoples' overall performances can be enhanced because they are asked to do what they do best and restricted from doing tasks for which they have no skill, talent, experience, or authority.

Roles can also limit an employees' ability to fully contribute by either making them feel depersonalized and alienated from their peers or by locking them into a role that uses a small fraction of their talents. This latter problem is referred to as role-lock and will be addressed in more detail when we examine the decision-making process. It is important that organizations maintain the ability to fill important roles with the most competent people *at any given time* and that they not lose vital skills through neglect and disuse. Problem-solving capabilities, system adaptability, and achievement of organizational goals are enhanced in this process.

NORMS

Social psychologists frequently refer to *norms* as rules of behavior and proper ways of acting that have been accepted as legitimate for all members of a group or system (Berrien, 1968). Norms are frequently used to define appropriate behavior for particular roles and become an essential part of job descriptions. More generally, system-wide norms are found in employee handbooks and negotiated labor contracts.

Another way of looking at the interrelationship between roles and norms is to see them as boundary phenomena. It will be recalled that boundaries were described as creating a discontinuity or modification in the quality, quantity, or phase of energy utilization. Boundaries may, therefore, be seen as filters that control the flow of inputs and outputs to and from the system or subsystem.

Figure 3-1 represents the interrelationship among norms, roles, and boundaries in systems terms. The arrows indicate alternative employee behaviors. Only some behaviors are allowed by the norm and role boundary filters. Fewer behaviors are allowed through both filters. Ideally, norm and role filters will match up so that required behaviors are allowed by norms developed by the organization and the employee work group. It is not unusual, however, for work group norms (e.g., covering for each other when away from the job) to clash with prescribed roles (keeping accurate track of time on and off the job) and vice versa.

Norms provide rules that define how employees should behave while they are within the boundaries of an organization. When employees leave their job they are fairly free to do as they please as long as they behave according to the norms of the community, state,

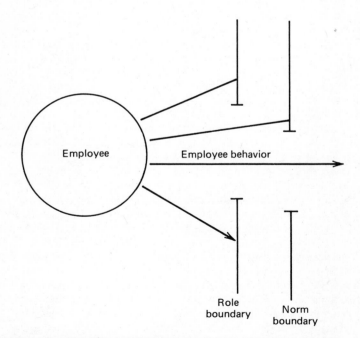

FIGURE 3-1. THE RELATIONSHIP AMONG NORMS, ROLES, AND BOUNDARIES.

Adapted from Berrien, K.F. *General and social systems.* Copyright © 1968 by Rutgers, The State University of New Jersey (p. 112).

or country in which they reside. We say "fairly free" because the filtering function of norms is not as precise as, for example, an electronic filter. The appropriate norms for company executives frequently overlap with family and community norms. They are expected to have harmonious marriages, well-behaved children, and to chair important community charities.

Like roles, norms can be formal or informal. Contractual agreements specify formal norms. Informal norms, however, are probably more numerous than formal norms. Even if the employee handbook specifies working hours as 9 to 5, employees learn informally how their supervisor enforces this norm. Nurse managers and supervisors will often communicate in informal and nonverbal ways about what extra nursing professional activities, if any, their nurses should engage in to gain the most approval. An informal norm often exists on psychiatric units in hospitals that nurses may wear "street clothes" instead of standard nursing uniforms. In the Hawthorne studies of the 1930s, it was discovered that male employees had developed strong norms around "a fair day's work" specifying what the rate of production should be. These norms persisted despite strong economic incentives to increase production.

Norms develop naturally for several reasons. The presence of norms cuts down on time-consuming decision making. If norms are well thought out and consistently applied, employees know with some certainty whether they are performing as expected. Much organizational conflict and tension can be avoided in this way.

One danger is that norms will be too behavior specific and will not be related to principles and values that the employee can understand and respect. When this happens, norms are created for every conceivable contingency, and countless loopholes are exploited. Many bureaucracies have volumes of policies and procedures for their employees that create the company parliamentarian and yet leave other employees ignorant of important norms for their behavior. New employees are often advised to "keep a low profile" until they "learn the ropes." This advice points to the importance of both formal and informal norms.

VALUES

Values can be seen as the ideological justification for roles and norms, and as expressing the aspirations for required organizational activities (Katz & Kahn, 1978). For-profit businesses justify many activities by referring to the profit value or "the bottom line." Health care organizations value quality of care, the use of drugs and procedures whose safety and effectiveness are based on research, and a high degree of integrity and accountability among professional staff. Private for-profit hospitals also are in business to make a profit, which results in inevitable conflicts in values, norms, and role systems. The most economic procedure may not provide the highest quality, lowest risk, or most humane service.

Of the three systems, values may be the most abstract, may not be formally stated, and may be least understood by employees at various levels of the organization. Marx and Engels (1961, pp. 7–14) understood that different organizational roles developed role-specific ideology that, in turn, created much class stratification and conflict. Boardroom executives are concerned with pleasing stockholders while production line workers care to please their co-workers and give scant concern for stockholders' feelings. Conflict may arise between those new nurse graduates whose role behavior is governed by professional values and those long-term employees whose role behavior is influenced instead by bureaucratic values.

HIERARCHIES

One obvious characteristic of organizations is the presence of hierarchies among system membership based upon power, status, and prestige and reflected in salary, responsibility, and privilege. The tendency for living systems to evolve into hierarchical arrangements seems to be nearly universal as countless biologic, anthropological, and sociological studies indicate (Caplow, 1968; Henley, 1977). Haley (1978) states emphatically:

> If there is any generalization that implies to men and other animals, it is that all creatures capable of learning are compelled to organize. To be organized means to follow patterned, redundant ways of behaving and to exist in a hierarchy. Creatures that organize together form a status, or power, ladder with someone below him. . . . We may dream of a society in which all creatures are equal, but on this earth there is status and precedence and inequality among all creatures. (p. 101)

Henley's (1977) research is supportive of Haley's observation that, like it or not, hierarchies of power, status, and prestige do exist rather universally. In discussing inequality of power between men and women she notes that "the distribution of power in our society is very unevenly patterned"(p. 184). Henley does not address the question of the inevitability of these inequalities, but expresses confidence that men and women can learn to treat each other more equitably. Her arguments may be more appropriate in addressing inappropriate hierarchies rather than eliminating hierarchies altogether.

Henley (1977) is not alone in expressing discontent with hierarchies. There are frequent calls for their elimination and the institution of truly democratic structures. There are several explanations for the incongruity between social behavior and social ideals. Hierarchies in many systems are based upon tradition and social status rather than competency. The established order becomes the object of scorn and ridicule when incompetent and unqualified people occupy critical roles in the system. Since compensation for work is generally pegged to hierarchical level, much discontent can result from such an arrangement.

In many rigid hierarchies, differences in status and power between levels of a hierarchy become so pronounced that communication up and down the hierarchy becomes strained and difficult. Not only do language differences emerge, but fearful lower-echelon members edit their communications to superiors, denying them important information. It is commonly assumed that rigid hierarchies interfere with communication and morale. Rigid hierarchies also tend to maintain the same order in chains of command for all problems. Nursing assistants may be ignored when discussions occur concerning the effects of medication upon the patient. Nurse supervisors may not grant requests by staff nurses for more input in making decisions and policies.

In American culture, at least, the value of personal freedom creates resentment toward hierarchies since their existence creates dependency inequalities whereby employees are dependent upon, and therefore controlled by, system members above them. On the other side of the coin, some individuals also feel uncomfortable controlling the lives of others who are below them in the hierarchy. Some employees, in time, adopt bureaucratic values as their own, without question or modification, and become quite comfortable with the status quo, including rigid control.

In general, the advantages of hierarchies in facilitating coordination, integration, and control outweigh their problems. Efforts need to be made, however, to achieve congruency amoung status, power, and competency. Allowances that permit changes in the hierarchy also need to be built into the structure of a system for situations in which a problem calls for a competency held by an employee who normally would not have such status (e.g., when entering crowded harbors, the command of large ships passes from the captain to a tug boat pilot).

Attempts also need to be made to keep the differences in power and status between levels of hierarchies to a minimum. This is frequently referred to as "flattening the hierarchy." It does not mean eliminating hierarchy altogether. That may not be possible or desirable. It does mean, however, permitting members at all levels of the organization to use their creative and professional abilities as much as possible in contributing to the achievement of organizational goals.

SUMMARY

This chapter has extended open systems theory to social systems in general, and health care organizations in particular. Two processes, task accomplishment and system maintenance, were identified as being critical to system survival and productivity. Concentration on one process to the exclusion of the other leads to system breakdown. Most contemporary management theories recognize the need to allocate energy and material for both processes.

Definitions were offered for the three related concepts of roles, norms, and values. Roles are developed as organizations differentiate and elaborate and are seen as efforts to maintain control and coordination over employees. Role development is almost inevitable and leads to benefits and disadvantages to both organizations and employees. In general, advantages to role development seem to outweigh disadvantages.

The rules by which employees operate, or norms, have both a formal and informal basis. Norms are also essential to organizational survival. A crucial problem with norms is that they often are too behavior-specific and may not be related to general principles and values. In this instance, norms must be developed for each behavior needing control. Informal norms often have great impact upon organizational functioning but are often ignored in formal organizational analyses.

Values are the ideological justification for roles and norms, expressing the aspirations of employees of all levels of organization. The values at each level (hospital administrators, directors of nursing, head nurses, and staff nurses) may be somewhat different from each other, giving rise to important differences in formal and informal norm development as well as role behavior. Conflicts may also arise between those new baccalaureate nurse graduates with highly developed professional values and those long-term nursing personnel who have adopted bureaucratic values.

Hierarchies are a fact of organizational life whether we like it or not. Informal hierarchies of power and dominance develop even if not formally recognized. Several problems are associated with hierarchies: (a) incongruity between location in a hierarchy and competency, (b) communication difficulties between levels of hierarchies, and (c) inflexibilities in hierarchy arrangement that prevent the organization from using its most competent members for certain activities.

REFERENCES

Argyris, C. Personal vs. organizational goals. *Yale Scientific*, February 1960, 40–50.

Bales, F. *Interaction process: A method for the study of small groups.* Cambridge, Mass.: Addison-Wesley, 1950.

Berrien, K. *General and social systems*. New Brunswick, N.J.: Rutgers University Press, 1968.

Caplow, T. *Two against one: Coalitions in triads*. Englewood Cliffs, N.J.: Prentice-Hall, 1968.

Cattell, R., Saunders, D., & Stice, G. Dimensions of syntality in small groups. *Human Relations*, 1953, *6*, 331–356.

Guetzkow, H. Differentiation of roles in task-oriented groups. In D. Cartwright, and A. Zander, (Eds.), *Group dynamics*. Evanston, Ill.: Row, Peterson, 1960.

Haley, J. *Problem-solving therapy*. San Francisco, Calif.: Jossey-Bass, 1978.

Henley, N. *Body politics*. Englewood Cliffs, N.J.: Prentice-Hall, 1977.

Katz, D., & Kahn, R. *The social psychology of organizations* (2nd ed.). New York: Wiley, 1978.

Marx, K., & Engels, F. The manifesto of the Communist party (1848). In *The essential left*. New York: Barnes and Noble, 1961.

Mayo, E. *The human problems of an industrial civilization*. New York: Macmillan, 1933.

Saddler Report. Great Britain, Sessional Papers, 1833, vol. *123*, ed. 706. In G. Knowles, & R. Snyder (Eds.), *Readings in Western Civilization*. New York: Lippincott, 1954.

Tausky, C. Theories of organization. In W. Nord, (Ed.), *Concepts and controversy in organizational behavior*. Santa Monica, Calif.: Goodyear, 1976.

Taylor, F. *The principles of scientific management*. New York: Harper, 1923.

CHAPTER 4
ORGANIZATION LIFE CYCLES: GROWTH, MATURATION, AND DECLINE

THE BIRTH OF AN ORGANIZATION

As with any living or nonliving system, organizations have distinctive life cycles that include birth, growth, maturation, decline, and death phases. Organizations are most vulnerable during the early stages of their life cycle. It is estimated that 55% of business failures occur during the first 5 years of existence. If an organization can remain alive past its infancy, it has a very high chance of survival. Between 1924 and 1973, only 57 of 10,000 businesses failed per year (Kaufman, 1976). The assumption in this description of organization life cycles is that an organization's input→throughput→output process has been established and that the environment values the product or service enough to provide energy inputs to the infant system. In other words, the organization has proved it can sell its products for a profit on the open market or that its services are valued enough so that the environment provides the essential needed inputs. For example, the input for a hospital would consist of patients. For schools of nursing, the input would be reflected in an adequate supply of students. The fledgling organization can then consider whether it wants to expand. If this critical point has been reached, the organization can generally look forward to a long future.

THE DECISION TO EXPAND

There are a number of reasons why a small business, health care agency, or other organization decides to grow: (a) to increase profits, (b) to become more stable, (c) to remain competitive with similar organizations, and (d) to provide new services. The promise of greater profits is a frequent reason for expansion. Many businesses with new and superior products find that they can sell as much of their product as they can produce. Management frequently decides that the organization should expand as quickly as possible while competition is small.

Many organizations believe that they will remain too vulnerable to environmental fluctuations if they depend on a small number of products and/or services or if they rely upon a small number of key employees. Diversification becomes a major goal for organizations seeking greater stability. New or additional services or new products will be developed to add to or replace older services or products that have lost their attractiveness in the environment. Management will also attempt to find services or products that will be popular in various economic situations. These methods are attempts to smooth out the impact of environmental forces upon the organization, and they require growth in structure, resources, and personnel.

In many organizations there is a marked advantage to growth in terms of efficiency. This simple principle was really the basis for the Industrial Revolution. Before the advent of mass production, individual artisans were organized into simple guilds. The individual craftsperson had all the skills and tools necessary to make a product. By organizing work and employees, human and technological resources were pooled resulting in more efficient production.

The young organization frequently strives to grow quickly in order to remain competitive with other organizations offering similar products and services. The early advantage of innovation may be lost if the new organization does not grow fast enough to take advantage of economies of scale. A recent example of the risk in slow growth is the Gablinger Beer Company. After being the first to market a low-calorie beer, the company was unable to expand rapidly enough to capture the market before other larger companies entered the market with similar products. Gablinger Beer remains a small company because it failed to solidify its marked initial advantage in this market.

Methods of Growth in Health Care and Other Organizations

Most organizations, including health care organizations, decide to grow. Medical practice groups are quite popular today for economic, personal, and professional reasons. Small, inefficient, and outmoded hospitals are replaced by more modern, efficient, and frequently larger facilities. Although lucrative, the medical market is very competitive in certain regions. A surplus of hospital beds is currently being reported in certain urban areas.

There are four basic methods of growth available to health care organizations: increase the size of existing units without other structural change; increase the number of units doing identical work; differentiate and specialize functions within the organization; and merge existing organizations.

The first method, increasing the size of existing units without other structural change, is frequently employed by smaller medical practice groups which are known for a particular service and receive more referrals for work than can be handled with existing personnel. At some point, however, the integration and coordination of organizational members becomes too difficult and the addition of new personnel *decreases* rather the *increases* efficiency, and effectiveness. In traditional organizational terms, the optimum span of control has been surpassed.

The second method of growth, increasing the number of units doing identical work, is then a frequent result. A subgroup of the original organization will split off and form a smaller, more efficient and effective group with the same essential structure. Another example of this form of growth is a hospital establishing additional surgical facilities and forming new surgical teams when demand outstrips its current surgical capacity.

The third method of growth, differentiating and specializing functions within the organization, occurs when small homogeneous health care or other organizations decide to add to the variety of services requiring the creation of new departments. Some hospitals, for example, are adding community and professional education programs in response to the needs of the community and the hospital's need for self-promotion. In recent years, specialized psychiatric units have emerged in general hospitals throughout the country. As growth occurs in young schools of nursing, new departments or units are formed whose functions center on specific responsibilities, for example, continuing education.

The fourth method of growth, merging existing organizations, is also prevalent today in health care and other organizations. In cases where the supply of hospital beds outstrips the supply of patients, older, less-efficient facilities are frequently closed down. The staff and, frequently, the name of the hospital, is then merged with the staff and building of a newer hospital. With increasing pressure from within the profession to place all nursing education programs in academic institutions, some diploma school of nursing programs have sought mergers with academic institutions rather than ceasing to exist entirely. Until recently, legislation governing the federal Nursing Special Project Grants Program supported mergers of diploma nursing programs and academic institutions with grant monies.

MATURATION OF THE ORGANIZATION

Health care organizations and new schools of nursing, following the typical trend of organizations with complicated throughput processes requiring many specialized skills and procedures, choose to expand. With successful expansion, the organization enters a maturation phase of development.

An interesting outcome of growth is that it frequently is not accompanied by increases in productivity (Parkinson, 1957). Sometimes a decrease in productivity occurs when personnel are increased and new departments are created.

Many times management feels compelled to expand rapidly, despite a loss in efficiency, in order to increase the amount or scope of service, to make the organization less dependent upon an unstable environment, or even as an attempt to resolve internal conflict. As Katz and Kahn (1978) pointed out, an internal conflict sometimes will be resolved by adding additional subsystems or departments rather than fundamentally changing either of the two systems in conflict. For example, when two departments are in conflict in hospital staff meetings, a frequent compromise is to create another committee to study the problem. The likely recommendation is for the creation of a new department to circumvent the conflict.

Problems Resulting from Increased Size

Katz and Kahn (1978) identified four types of problems resulting from increased size:

> (1) The loss of the primary group in motivating people to achieve organizational goals; (2) inadequacies and errors in communication among organizational members of subgroups; (3) weaknesses in integration, that is, in utilizing skills, knowledge, and experience of organizational members; and (4) problems of social traffic and congestion. (pp. 107–108).

Most, if not all, of these problems are related to processes that inevitably occur as an organization grows and matures: differentiation, and coordination efforts. Differentiation refers to categorizing personnel according to such characteristics as role, authority, power, and professional expertise, and the creation of homogeneous subsystems with distinct primary tasks and boundaries. Some of the advantages and disadvantages of differentiation have been discussed in the sections discussing roles and hierarchies.

Members of the primary group, whose professional expertise, energy, and creativity are responsible for the birth of the organization, frequently consider themselves to be peers or partners. There often is a corresponding lack of distinction among them in terms of specific activities, authority, pay, power, and status. Small nuclear groups at this stage view themselves as being homogeneous and provide each other with nurturance, encouragement, and support as well as performing the primary task-related activities. Differentiation and increased compartmentalization create physical and psychological boundaries among organizational members, which destroys that "homogeneous feeling." Although organizational efficiency may improve, system maintenance needs are less well satisfied. The spontaneous drive and enthusiasm associated with the "good old days" disappears and "motivation" problems begin to emerge as new employees, who have not experienced the excitement and promise of personal and professional gain associated with the early years, are added. Frequently, new employees are employed on salary without being able to share directly in the profits or other benefits of the organization. Likewise, employees may not experience the fears and instabilities of an infant organization, and they treat their position as "just a job."

Coordination and integration functions emerge in growing organizations in order to solve the problems associated with specialization and compartmentalization. Formal lines of communication are established, departmental meetings are created, uniform policy and procedure manuals are developed, and training programs for "better communications" are established. Formalization of structure becomes realized. Cycles of events become routinized, codified, inspected, and regulated. The mature organization has arrived!

Maturation in Health Care Organizations

There are additional problems resulting from the natural maturation process for health care organizations. Since a large part of the throughput process in health care involves the provision of health care services, the development of rigid and specialized roles, the erection of barriers between disciplines and departments, the loss of personal feelings between employees, and the loss of commitment to organizational improvement can have a negative impact on the quality of patient care.

Nursing and medicine, more than other professional fields, must develop policies and structures that will satisfy the human and emotional needs of both staff and patients. If any part or subsystem in a health care organization feels dehumanized, unmotivated, or devalued, patients will begin feeling the same way, as their human needs are ignored by a disgruntled and alienated staff. The quality of patient care will inevitably decrease.

DECLINE AND DEATH OF THE ORGANIZATION

Few health care organizations fail if they have reached the mature phase. However, declining health care systems can become prime targets for mergers. Old and obsolete facilities may be abandoned since they have limited useful life remaining. The professional and nonprofessional staff are easily assimilated into newer and more modern facilities. The main concern during this phase is that patient care may suffer because little investment is being made in equipment or staff development. Ethical considerations do not permit the same kind of slow decline characteristic of other business enterprises. The organization cannot afford to relax once it reaches the mature phase. In order to meet production goals, continuous efforts need to be made to maintain and improve (a) facilities and equipment, (b) the professional skills of staff, and (c) professional and personal satisfactions of the staff. When profits are no longer an outcome and the future does not look promising, drastic measures may be taken in an attempt to remedy the problems and again create financial stability. If unsuccessful, the business may be purchased by a larger successful firm, or it may even declare bankruptcy.

SUBSYSTEMS DEVELOPMENT

By the time an organization has entered the mature phase of development, it has well-developed subsystems with discernible boundaries, differences in throughput processes and primary tasks, and, frequently, subtle differences in norms and values. In fact, many subsystems act as if they were autonomous systems within the organization with no need to be coordinated with other subsystems.

Typical subsystems as found in health care organizations have been described by Katz and Kahn (1978) as generic subsystems since they apply to virtually all organizational systems. The subsystems described here are somewhat arbitrarily organized. Each subsystem described has identifiable boundaries and primary tasks, but other classifications are possible. For instance, physicians and nurses may be organized as systems if one is interested in studying interdisciplinary phenomena. Since the major concern here is with a broader analysis of organizational behavior, the classification system does not focus upon disciplinary differences. The point being made is that subsystems are identified according to the purposes of the analysis. Any classification is correct as long as the criteria mentioned above are met.

Product or Technical Subsystems

Product or technical subsystems are concerned with the throughput process itself: converting energy, information, and material into a useful product or service. In health care organizations, this subsystem applies treatment knowledge through nursing intervention, medicine, surgery, rehabilitation, and other methods in order to cure or improve the health condition of patients. The patient enters in a "sick" condition and hopefully leaves in a "cured" or "improved" condition. In order to survive, a health care organization must demonstrate that this throughput process produces a better condition than if treatment had not been provided, and meets professional standards as well.

Supportive Subsystems

Supportive subsystems ensure that the product or technical subsystems receive inputs and can dispose of their products or services. In hospitals, for instance, a subsystem needs to be responsible for publicity so that doctors join its staff and admit their patients to that hospital. Nurses in the community are informed, by means of this subsystem, of the quality and scope of patient care services provided and nursing career opportunities and benefits available in order for a hospital to attain adequate nurse staffing. When dealing with patients with chronic conditions, the hospital must ensure that its patients will be properly cared for once released. In general, this subsystem informs the environment of its services, promotes the advantages of its organization against competitors, and maintains favorable relations with the environment.

Maintenance Subsystems

Maintenance subsystems have as their primary task the maintenance of equipment, facilities, and human resources. Although maintenance of equipment and facilities is frequently straightforward and amenable to routinization, maintenance of human resources, the organization's investment in personnel, is often vexing. Much controversy still exists concerning the best ways to motivate personnel, increase job satisfaction, select the right personnel, develop necessary leadership, and attain constructive working relationships.

In health care organizations, maintenance functions are typically carried out through a system of rewards and punishments (pay and promotion), in-service and preservice training programs, encouraging and supporting participation in continuing education programs outside of the hospital or facility, vacation and leave policies, programs to mold attitudes and beliefs, and special assignments.

Adaptive Subsystems

Adaptive subsystems ensure that a system's products or services remain viable and attractive to the environment. An automobile company producing a quality "gas-guzzler" will find few customers for its products. The adaptive subsystem assists the organization in finding a new clientele or in redesigning its products or services to be in keeping with current customer needs. Adaptive subsystems bear names such as product research, market research, long-range planning, research and development, division of experimental programs, or special projects unit.

In health care organizations, these subsystems tend to be somewhat underdeveloped. Patient needs are obvious and relatively stable over time. Medical and nursing schools that are already operational rely, to some extent, upon self-selection processes and market demand to help determine how many pediatricians, psychiatric nurses, radiologists, intensive care nurses, or surgeons will enter the field following their training. However, in establishing satellite programs of existing schools, in making significant program and curriculum changes, or in establishing new medical or nursing schools, sophisticated needs assessment studies are usually conducted.

Managerial Subsystems

Managerial subsystems are of major interest and importance to many nurses who assume leadership, managerial, or supervisory roles in health care organizations. These subsystems are concerned with controlling, coordinating, and directing the many subsystems of an organization. They are different from most other subsystems in that their cycles of events are linked vertically rather than horizontally through the hierarchy of the system. Although other subsystems are primarily concerned with energy and material exchange, managerial subsystems rely heavily upon information transformation and exchange. Directives, policy, and general information are typical forms of information exchanged up and down the managerial hierarchy.

The managerial subsystem has two main functions vis-à-vis the larger organization: regulation of the throughput process based upon valid information from internal and external sources, and establishment of an authority structure for deciding who has the right and responsibility to make certain decisions and carry out work functions. Regulation of work activities and determination of authority relationships are of critical importance to nursing leadership, management, and supervision.

LEADING SUBSYSTEMS

All five of the previously identified subsystems are crucial for successful organizational functioning; however, one subsystem may become prominent over the others as a result of internal or environmental conditions. Thalen described such a prominent subsystem as the "leading subsystem" and defined it as "a component system whose output exerts the greatest influence on the inputs of other component systems, and through this, controls the interactions of the suprasystem" (cited in Katz & Kahn, 1978, p. 60).

The United States automobile industry provides a good illustration of this point. Prior to 1973, the production and adaptive subsystems of major automobile manufacturers took a back seat to the supportive subsystems that developed innovative marketing and advertising methods to sell a product that changed little from year to year except for cosmetic design refinements. Engineering and quality control departments were viewed to be less important by the organization than the sales and marketing subsystems, which dictated price and exterior design. With the oil embargo of 1973, however, environmental conditions changed dramatically and required the organization to change its production and design methods radically. The adaptive subsystem represented by the engineering and quality control departments suddenly became the leading subsystem. Consequently, exterior design changes were reduced and radical engineering innovations, such as front-wheel drive, were adopted.

ORGANIZATION LIFE CYCLES AND THE ENVIRONMENT

Any system is embedded within a hierarchy of larger and smaller systems (suprasystems and subsystems). Open systems theory offers a logic for analysis of this hierarchy which is useful to nurse managers in their efforts to understand health care organizations or universities.

Unlike reductionist theories of organizations, which encourage managers to break down their operations into component parts for further analysis, open systems theory recommends that the first analysis be focused upon the next higher level of system organization. The reason for this strategy is straightforward: generally, the organization or subsystem is dependent upon the next higher level of organization for its survival and the understanding of system functioning is greatly enhanced if one fully understands the requirement for survival dictated by an organization's environment.

SUMMARY

In most cases, organizations, including health care organizations, choose to expand. In most cases, organizations feel compelled to expand to remain competitive with similar organizations, increase profits by capturing markets for products or services, and increase stability.

Four basic methods of growth are available to health care organizations: (1) increasing the size of existing units without other structural change; (2) increasing the number of units doing identical work; (3) differentiating and specializing functions within the organization; and (4) merging with one or more existing organizations.

With growth and expansion, the organization enters the mature phase of its life cycle. While organizations expand, productivity may sometimes decrease rather than increase as a result of the development of new problems and challenges to the system. The zeal and motivation of the original members is diluted. Communication problems emerge with the development of specialized roles, increased physical distance, and broadening of the hierarchical structure. Communication difficulties, interdepartmental rivalries, and role-lock prevent the organization from best utilizing employee skills, knowledge, and experience. Finally, increased size inevitably leads to logistical problems, traffic, and congestion. A simple problem must find its way through a labyrinth of bureaucratic channels, each contributing to the probability of error and misinterpretation.

Health care organizations experience special challenges during this phase. Increasing the structure and stability of health care systems (creating a bureaucracy) can have serious detrimental effects upon patient care, which relies heavily upon direct services from nursing and other health care staff. Medical and nursing staff cannot provide adequate personal care to patients if their human, emotional, and professional needs are not met.

Because of the nature of medical and nursing services, every effort must be made to keep the system from declining and placing patients at risk. To this end, health care organizations must maintain and improve facilities and equipment, the professional skills of the staff, and professional and personal job satisfaction of the staff.

Five generic subsystems were identified for health care organizations: (1) product or technical subsystems, (2) supportive subsystems, (3) maintenance subsystems, (4) adaptive subsystems, and (5) managerial subsystems. At any given time, one of these subsystems, the leading subsystem, is likely to achieve prominence over the others because of the nature of environmental demands. As environmental demands change, so will the subsystem designated as leading.

Analysis of system dynamics best begins with the demands made by the next higher level of organization, frequently the environment in which the system exists. The system under analysis inevitably has a dependent relationship with the next higher level in the hierarchy of subsystems, systems, and suprasystems.

REFERENCES

Kaufman, H. *Are government organizations immortal?* Washington, D.C.: The Brookings Institute, 1976.

Katz, D., & Kahn, R. *The social psychology of organizations* (2nd ed.). New York: Wiley, 1978.

Parkinson, C. *Parkinson's law.* Boston: Houghton Mifflin, 1957.

CHAPTER 5
PROCESSES
WITHIN SUBSYSTEMS

It is essential that nurse managers and supervisors understand the structure and dynamics of the larger organization and organizational environment in which they work. However, a large portion of the nursing managers/supervisors' time will be occupied with initiating or reacting to processes that occur within their subsystem. This chapter describes the important processes or structures of communications, trust, reward systems, and covert processes that occur within subsystems. Other subsystem processes such as power and authority, leadership and followership, decision-making processes, and goal setting are considered in following chapters.

MODES OF COMMUNICATIONS

A general systems theory approach to the topic of communications will be used. The concern here is not with communicative behavior of one person, but the interactive process involving at least one other party and inevitably impacting upon every member of a subsystem, group, or team, directly or indirectly.

The process of communication will be examined from a pragmatic perspective (Watzlawick, Beavin, & Jackson, 1967). For this reason, the emphasis is upon nonverbal behavior and contexts as well as with words and written communication. From a systems perspective, a piece of behavior alone is meaningless unless it elicits behavior in another person. It can be seen, therefore, that the present discussion involves a much broader range of phenomena than simply discussions, conversations, memoranda, reports, and signs.

Behavior has no opposite—there is no such thing as *non*behavior. It is an assumption that all behavior in a social situation has meaning (i.e., has some purpose). It then follows that since communication is a form of behavior, it is impossible *not* to communicate something by one's actions (Watzlawick et al., 1967). This simple proposition defines a most basic property of behavior: The behavior has occurred for some reason and, therefore, has some message value.

The certainty that others will read messages into any behavior results from the usual efforts made by people to make sense out of what they perceive. Kelly (1955) describes people as behaving *as if they are scientists*, constantly sampling and experimenting with their environment, developing minitheories, and making predictions to help give them some control over their lives. People attempt to develop a social reality (Festinger, 1954) and will "make something of" activity or inactivity, words or silence, presence or absence. Interpretations will be made of a staff member's absence at a staff meeting.

Unless a staff member's absence is openly and fully discussed (not a usual occurrence), it is likely that individual staff members will make different interpretations concerning that behavior. These interpretations may not be what is intended by the absent staff member. It is difficult to communicate successfully what we want, perceive, and feel when others are constantly receiving messages from us based upon what we do or do not do, say or do not say. The message received may or may not be what we intend, consciously or unconsciously.

It is even more difficult to avoid communicating or to disguise our intentions, feelings, and attitudes in our communications. By the time we arrive at adulthood, we have had many years of experience in experimenting with communication and have developed sophisticated models for deciphering human communication.

Content and Relationship Levels of Communication

Imbedded in every communication there is a content aspect (the "data" of the communication) and a relationship aspect (how this communication is to be taken). For instance, "John, take this letter to room 3B," not only instructs John to deliver a letter, but also defines the relationship as a superior giving orders to a subordinate (John). The relationship aspect of a communication is frequently delivered by nonverbal behavior or contextual indicators while the content aspect is usually delivered either verbally or in written form. The addition of a pointing finger to the above directive strengthens the relationship interpretation of superior to subordinate.

In most cases, understanding the relationship message takes precedence over understanding the content message. Most people attach a higher level of importance to the relationship message because it tells them what to do with the content. Since relationship messages are frequently delivered through nonverbal and contextual cues, careful attention is directed to these aspects. When there is a contradiction between relationship and content messages, the relationship message is perceived as more valid. What would you believe if your supervisor said, "Now, don't take this as a criticism ..." with a raised eyebrow, a frown and folded arms?

The Punctuation of the Sequence of Events

The cyclical nature of organizational and system behavior has been discussed previously. This characteristic makes a nonlinear perspective for communication most suitable for social systems. For instance, in the communication "John, deliver this letter to room 3B," a linear view would consider the direction of causality as moving from the supervisor to the subordinate in a straightforward, stimulus-response manner.

This is a limited view of this interaction, however, and does not consider how John's behavior will impact upon the supervisor. He may deliver the letter properly or may "accidentally" lose the letter in transit. It would be a mistake to assume that the supervisor does not receive feedback of one sort or another as a result of his or her own behavior. In one hospital, lower-echelon staff reminded senior-level staff of this fact through the expression, "What goes around comes around!"

The reason why patterns of behavior are seen in a linear manner is that a person chooses to "punctuate" the behavior so as to obscure the feedback links that are present (Whorf, 1956). In the above example, by starting with the supervisor's behavior and ending with John's presumed response of delivering the letter, we only see a simple linear pattern of interaction. If, however, we had started our analysis with John's failure to deliver the letter and ended with the negative impact this action had upon the supervisor, we would have a different view of the causative process. In a popular cartoon that gives another humorous example of the effects of punctuation, a rat says, "I have got my experimenter trained. Each time I press the lever he gives me food."

Punctuation, like roles, is neither good nor bad. It is a reality in the communication process since one must find some way to organize the never-ending flow of communication. Disagreement about how to punctuate a sequence of events is at the heart of many conflicts within organizations. Consider the follow exchange: (1) (team leader) "If I don't check on your work constantly you goof off"; (2) (team member) "I take time off when I can because you're always peering over my shoulder." Figure 5-1 graphically presents this monotonous and disagreeable sequence.

The team leader perceives only the causative sequences of 2→3→4, and 4→5→6 while the team member perceives the causative sequences of 1→2→3, and 3→4→5. As long as each party holds to his or her particular punctuation of this sequence, obscuring the larger circular pattern, it will be difficult to begin discussion of the larger issue determining this pattern—mutual distrust. Linear punctuations of this sort inevitably lead to blaming behaviors and a frustration of efforts to find a collaborative framework to resolve the conflict.

Digital and Analogic Communication

Separate forms of communications, digital and analogic, have been present since humans began to communicate in verbal and written form. Jaynes (1976) argues that preverbal man communicated primarily in *analogic* forms—conveyance of a likeness of what one is trying to express. Analogic communications are "thinglike" and consist of drawings, figures, sculpture, music, gestures, sign language, and so on. Analogic communication involves a 1:1 correspondence between the communication and what the communication symbolizes.

Because an analog communication must closely match what it stands for in order to be effective, it has only a positive value. There is no way to express negation in analogic communication. It is impossible to draw, for instance, not-a-house and make it interpretable. Similarly, it is not possible to express logical relationships such as "if-then" and "either-or" in analogic communication. Analogic representations can only be approximations of the things to which they refer.

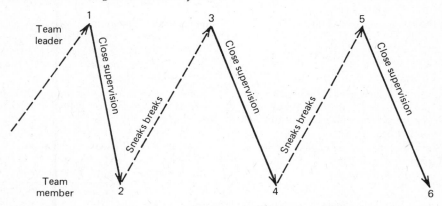

FIGURE 5-1. PUNCTUATION OF A TYPICAL LEADER/SUBORDINATE INTERACTION.

It was a great advance for civilization when man learned how to substitute arbitrary signs or symbols to represent concepts as well as things. There is nothing intrinsically friendly about the letters f-r-i-e-n-d. By freeing symbols from the need to be an analogy of the thing they represent, logical operators that have no palpable existence could be added to the syntax of communication.

Each arbitrary symbol has an exact reference and, thus, this form of communication is termed *digital*. The term was taken from the field of cybernetics in which digital computers manipulate arbitrary binary switches using a similar logical syntax.

A comparison of human physiology and neuroanatomy yields some remarkable parallels. For instance, it is well-known that the central nervous system functions in a digital, all-or-none fashion, while the endocrine system is based upon the release of varying amounts of hormones into the bloodstream. The left hemisphere of the cortex normally controls language, which is a digital form of communication, while the right cerebral cortex is known to be largely language-free, relying primarily upon analogic processes such as visual images, tones, and spacial representations for communication (Gazzaniga, 1972). The human brain normally utilizes both forms of communication in a complementary and highly complex manner. Table 5-1 presents the characteristics of "left-brain" digital communication and "right-brain" analogic communication.

TABLE 5-1. COMPARISON OF LEFT BRAIN AND RIGHT BRAIN CHARACTERISTICS

Left Brain	Right Brain
Verbal: Using words to name, describe, define	**Nonverbal:** Awareness of things, but minimal connection with words
Analytic: Figuring things out step-by-step and part-by-part	**Synthetic:** Putting things together to form wholes
Symbolic: Using a symbol to stand for something. For example, the sign + stands for the process of addition	**Concrete:** Relating to things as they are at the present moment
Abstract: Taking out a small bit of information and using it to represent something	**Analogic:** Seeing likenesses between things, understanding metaphoric relationships
Temporal: Keeping track of time, sequencing one thing after another: doing first things first, second things second	**Nontemporal:** Without a sense of time
Rational: Drawing conclusions based on *reason* and *facts*	**Nonrational:** Not requiring a basis of *reason* or *facts*: willingness to suspend judgment
Digital: Using numbers as in counting	**Spatial:** Seeing where things are in relation to other things, and how parts go together to form a whole
Logical: Drawing conclusions based on logic: one thing following another in logical order. For example, a mathematical theorem or well-stated argument	**Intuitive:** Making leaps of insight. Insight is often based on incomplete patterns, hunches, feelings, or visual images
Linear: Thinking in terms of linked ideas, one thought following another, often leading to a convergent conclusion	**Holistic:** Seeing whole things all at once; perceiving the overall patterns and structures, often leading to divergent conclusions

SOURCE: Adapted from Edwards, B. *Drawing on the Right Side of the Brain.* Copyright © 1979 by Betty Edwards. Reprinted by permission of Houghton Mifflin Company.

Jaynes (1976) and Watzlawick, et al. (1967) speculate that since early man primarily utilized right-brain and nonverbal communication, analogic communication has more general validity than the more developed left-brain digital forms of communication.

Analogic communication includes virtually all nonverbal behavior: posture, gesture, facial expression, voice inflection, and the sequence, rhythm, and cadence of the words themselves (Watzlawick, et al. 1967). It follows from the earlier discussion, therefore, that the relationship aspect of any communication is conveyed through analogic modes, while the content aspect is transmitted via digital modes. In fact, most people find it very difficult to describe relationships using rational discourse. Lovers choose nonverbal expressions of affection, metaphors or poetry, rather than cool and logical digital language. In choosing political leaders, it has been suggested that the public listens to debates but votes on gut feelings about how trustworthy, competent, and courageous, the candidates appear. Richard Nixon is said to have lost a debate and the ensuing 1960 presidential election to John Kennedy because of his "five o'clock shadow"!

Digital communication has great advantages over analogic communication in conveying the content (what to do) aspects of a communication, such as greater precision, versatility, abstraction, speed, and the ability to utilize temporal dimensions and negatives.

Implications for Management Science

The existence of the parallel digital/content and analogic/relationship aspects of communication complicate the process of conveying thoughts, ideas, commands, feelings, and attitudes to one another. Frequently, a message sender believes that careful attention to the words of a communication will ensure receipt of an unambiguous and clear message. One can now see that this will occur only when the digital/content aspects are congruent with the analogic/relationship aspects. In a conflict, the receiver will generally judge the analogic/relationship aspects to have greater validity.

In dealing with relationship difficulties, it is often useful to employ analogic and nonverbal methods as well as digital and verbal methods. A number of team-building strategies include analogic communication methods. Finally, analogic thought, which is more holistic, intuitive, and synthetic than digital thought, is of great value in creative problem solving. Any organization that requires creativity, adaptation, and healthy interpersonal relationships should encourage analogic as well as digital communication and feedback.

TRUST

Trust is included as an essential ingredient in contemporary management theory (Blake & Mouton, 1964; Ouchi, 1981; Zand, 1976). Earlier studies of trust (Gibb, 1961) found that low levels of trust resulted in a "defensive climate" that produced difficulties in concentrating on messages; distorted perceptions of motives, values, and emotions of others; and increased distortion of the meaning of messages. Disruptions and distortions in the communication process because of low trust levels can destroy the effectiveness of any team, group, or organization.

Those who do not trust will conceal or distort relevant information. They will avoid stating facts, ideas, conclusions, and feelings, or they will disguise them. In the process, the information provided will be low in accuracy, comprehensiveness, timeliness, and will have low congruence with reality. There will be a high level of suspicion that devious attempts to control or influence exist, so that there will be general resistance to direction. Those who do not trust will try to minimize their dependence upon others. These behaviors will interfere with the exchange of information, will reduce the reciprocity of influence and the exercise of self-control, and will diminish the effectiveness of joint problem-solving behaviors (Zand, 1976).

The Dynamics of Trust

Following Deutsch (1962), Zand (1976) defines trust as

> consisting of actions that (a) increase one's vulnerability, (b) to another whose behavior is not under one's control, (c) in a situation in which the penalty (disutility) one suffers if the other abuses that vulnerability is greater than the utility one gains if the other does not abuse that vulnerability. (p. 567)

In other words, trust is not developed unless people take risks with each other. Without risk, interpersonal trust is not required. Trust is not a global feeling of warmth or affection, but rather, involves the conscious regulation of one's dependence on one another and an awareness of the interdependent nature of human relationships (Zand, 1976).

Another implication of this definition is that trust must be built from zero, that is, trust is not an initial characteristic of relationships. There is a common misconception that trusting someone we do not know (directly or indirectly) is a desirable or healthy behavior (confidence men and women play on this fallacy with the line "don't worry, just trust me!"). Productive relationships must build trust from the ground up with first one party taking a risk, not being taken advantage of, and gaining some benefit from risking behavior, and then the other party taking a risk, not being taken advantage of, and gaining some benefit that leads the first party to take another risk, and so on. Trust, therefore, has the characteristics of a feedback loop in which trust spirals up or down. Following Gibb (1964), Zand (1976) suggests the model shown in Figure 5-2 for understanding the development of trust.

Successful application of these principles for building trust will result in information exchange that is relevant, comprehensive, accurate, and timely. Team members will have less fear that exposure of vulnerability will be abused, and will be more receptive to influence from one another. They will accept interdependence because they feel confident that agreements will be kept and they will have less need to control others. Perception of the intentions of others will be more accurate, leading to a decrease in social uncertainty. Underlying problems are more likely to be identified and solutions will be more appropriate, creative, and long range (Zand, 1976).

REWARD STRUCTURES

Decades of research in the fields of human motivation and learning emphasize the advantages of positive reinforcement (rewards) over punishment (Morgan & King, 1966). Punishment may be used to suppress an undesirable behavior temporarily but is no more effective than withholding reward in extinguishing a behavior when punishment is not constantly applied (Estes, 1944). Furthermore, punishment is largely ineffective in teaching new behaviors, while the use of positive reinforcement is effective (Skinner, 1953). The use of punishment also generates fears and anxieties that can have dysfunctional consequences for individual and team functioning.

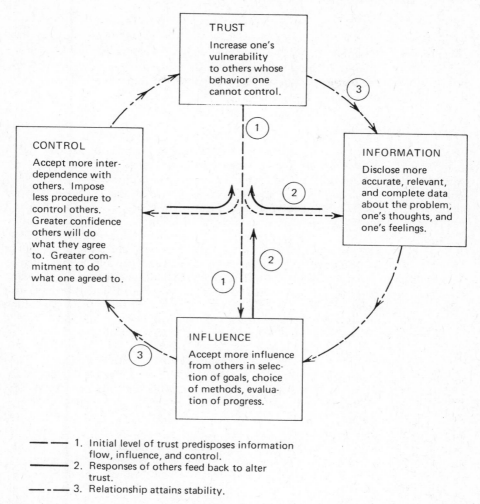

FIGURE 5-2. A MODEL OF THE RELATIONSHIP OF TRUST TO INFORMATION, INFLUENCE, AND CONTROL.

From Zand, D. Trust and managerial problem solving. In W. Nord (Ed.), *Concepts and controversy in organizational behavior.* Copyright © 1976 by Scott, Foresman & Company, Reprinted by permission.

Management science has been heavily influenced by this persuasive research and has greatly encouraged the use of rewards rather than punishments in their employee motivation strategies (Katz & Kahn, 1978). Punishments and sanctions have been restricted in use to preventing specific behaviors that threaten the integrity or profitability of the organization (i.e., stealing, tardiness, flagrant disregard for policy and procedure). In many cases, the only punishment available to the supervisor or organization is termination of employment, since other parameters of punishment (cutting pay, increasing the unpleasantness of the environment, etc.) are prohibited by contract and monitored by unions. Of course, supervisors and organizations have legal and subtle methods for punishing employees, but the ultimate goal of such strategies often is to force the individual to quit or resign so as to avoid firing the employee.

Types of Rewards

It has been traditional to distinguish between *extrinsic* rewards (pay and benefits, advancement, pleasant working conditions) and *intrinsic* rewards (interest level of the job, challenge, professional recognition, contribution of work to human welfare). While both extrinsic and intrinsic rewards may be utilized, their effectiveness will vary under different conditions.

Reward Effectiveness

The effectiveness of any reward is a function of three factors: (1) the desirability of goal-object or condition, (2) the connectedness of a reward to the behavior the superior or organization wants enacted, and (3) the amount of reward in relation to the effort expended (Katz & Kahn, 1978). Following Atkinson's (1958) model of achievement motivation, Katz and Kahn suggest that an estimate of the effect of various rewards can be obtained by assigning positive values for each of the three dimensions and multi-plying these three values together. For example, if one assigns values of 1 for desirability of a goal, 2 for the connectedness of a behavior to the reward, and 3 to the amount of reward gained as a result of one's effort, a rewarding power of 6 would be computed by multiplying the three dimensions. Another reinforcement would have a rewarding power of 2 if the first two dimensions had values of 1 and the third dimension a value of 2. If any of the dimensions has a value of 0, then the model predicts that a rewarding power of 0 would result. Since the model is multiplicative, in order for a reward to be strongly positive in reward power, all three dimensions have to be highly evaluated by the individual.

This model and others (Herzberg, 1966; Holland, 1966; Lofquist & Dawis, 1969) propose that the motivating capability of a given reward is an interactive function of the individual's needs, values, interests, and the characteristics of the reward. As Maslow (1954) predicts, job interest and work recognition have little rewarding power if someone is trying to feed a large family on minimum wage. Basic needs have to be satisfied before higher needs become motivators. Also, offering more money to an employee who wants to move from a cold climate to southern California for the weather and lifestyle may be an exercise in futility. Since positive job satisfaction has been related to productivity and job dissatisfaction to job absenteeism and turnover, the consideration of appropriate rewards for desired behaviors and specific employees is extremely important.

COVERT PROCESSES

In every interpersonal interchange in a subsystem there are two levels of interaction: the overt and the covert (Schutz, 1958). The *overt level* refers to what is publicly advertised to be going on in an interaction and is similar to the content aspect of a communication. The *covert level* refers to processes that are going on in addition to or instead of what is publicly advertised, and is similar to the relationship aspect of a communication. Schutz refers to covert processes as the "interpersonal underworld."

Hidden Agendas

For example, at the overt level, a nursing team leader may hold a team meeting to discuss changes in safety procedures for patients. During the meeting, many "hidden agendas" will be revealed, often without a word concerning them being spoken. The team leader may be bringing up the topic because one of the team members may have violated a safety rule. The rule may have been violated by a team member to express resentment for not receiving a positive performance evaluation the previous week. One member may strongly support the team leader's position to curry favor for future evaluations. Another member may withhold her dissent for fear of going against the team's views. Finally, an innocent team member may silently be blamed for the safety violation because he is considered the rebellious one on the team. Each of these behaviors is related to a personal or group agenda that has not been acknowledged openly in the meeting. Given the various motives and perceptions that operate, it will be difficult for the group to stay on task and a great deal of time and energy will be wasted trying to decipher what is really going on.

The leader needs to set an example by being as open and explicit about his or her agenda in such situations and must encourage others on the team to divulge their agendas. Conflicts and problems cannot be resolved and needs cannot be met if the issues involved are not clearly and openly expressed. Nursing leaders may also promote more productive team process by emphasizing the need to consider the relationship aspect of team member communications. In the chapter on formal nursing meetings (Chapter 18), it is suggested that one member of a meeting take the role of "process observer" to assist in surfacing hidden agendas and covert processes.

Basic Assumption Behavior

Bion (1961) observed that groups often behave as if there were a reason for their meeting other than the reasons publicly stated. He identified three typical recurring states that he termed *basic assumption states*. The group-as-a-whole seemed to be behaving "as if" members were making basic assumptions that (a) the leader was the only member able to provide direction, information, skilled behavior, and so forth, in the group (*basic assumption state dependency*); (b) the group-as-a-whole had met to fight or flee someone or something (*basic assumption state fight/flight*); or (c) that the group-as-a-whole was waiting for a messiah to emerge from group interaction to deliver the group from its internal difficulties and incompetency (*basic assumption state pairing*).

These basic assumption states are part of the normal covert processes of any group or team. The team leader, with help from other perceptive team members or an outside consultant, can help the team to repudiate these basic and erroneous assumptions and thus enable the team to get back on task.

Splitting

The phenomenon of splitting is very common in health care organizations. Klein (1948) relates this process to the difficulty human infants have in accepting that their mothers are both good (nurturant) and bad (restrictive/punishing). Rather than experience the ambivalence and anxiety of accepting that mother is both good and bad, one of the attributes (usually the good) is retained while the other attribute is projected onto someone else in the infant's life. The result is to divide mommy into good and bad parts and to expel the bad part from consciousness. This simple method for dealing with complex feelings is used thereafter whenever the person has difficulty accepting the good and bad aspects of important people in her or his life.

Because nursing is stereotypically viewed as having a strong nurturant component, patients and staff may have difficulty perceiving and accepting that nurses have faults as well as virtues. Instead, their anger and disappointment with the nurse will be projected onto others.

This process also has undesirable effects upon the nurse's self-concept. Nurses often have difficulty accepting their own imperfections: angry feelings toward patients, dislike of certain patients, or their inability to improve the health of every patient. The resulting splitting of complex feelings contributes to low self-esteem because of a lack of open communication about personal inadequacies and vulnerabilities (I am the only bad nurse here—everyone else seems so good!). This process also leads to difficulty in receiving and accepting negative feedback.

Manipulative patients are expert in using splitting behavior to circumvent rules and policies on a unit or to control a staff member. One staff member (the good mother) is identified as supporting a patient's wish so that the nurse who is attempting to enforce a rule will look and feel like the "bad guy" (bad mother) and capitulate to the patient's request. In reality, the "good mother" does not realize that she or he is covertly being pitted against another staff member's authority. The antidote for this maneuver is close communication, trust, and respect among staff members. Teamwork is especially important in these situations.

Scapegoating

The phenomenon of scapegoating is closely related to splitting. From prehistoric times, humans have tried to expel unacceptable feelings and suffering experiences from their tribes and societies (Frazer, 1922; Kahn, 1980). One method for expelling pain and evil from a group or society is to load all the malignant forces onto some person, animal, or object, which is then beaten, burned, buried, or otherwise driven off, thus carrying away the pain and evil of the community (Kahn, 1980). In this way, the bad aspects of society are split off from the good or healthy aspects that are retained.

This, of course, is magical thinking since everyone and every society, group, team, organization, or tribe has good and bad characteristics and is capable of nurturant, productive, competent behavior as well as cruel, inefficient, and incompetent behavior. The discomfort resulting from acceptance of this reality is reduced if a convenient scapegoat—the supervisor, the Democrats, the Republicans, the Communists, the doctor—can be found.

In work settings, many behaviors and feelings are considered unacceptable: competition, hostility, rebellion, seduction, open expression of sexuality, and so on. Each group's culture defines what is unacceptable. Group forces that will attempt to identify likely receptacles for these malignant aspects will emerge.

Scapegoating does not occur in a random manner. The target of scapegoating will demonstrate some evidence of the undesirable characteristic being split off from or expelled from the group. For instance, if a team or group sees itself as conflict-free, totally harmonious in interpersonal relationships, and composed only of "nice" people, one team member (usually young, impatient, brash, and unconventional) will be seen as the only person on the team who is not "nice" and as having a personality defect which prevents him or her from getting along with others on the team. If the "troublemaker" accepts this perception and the resulting role, he or she will be forced out of the team, thus maintaining the team's previous perception of itself and the homeostasis.

There are several antidotes to this unhealthy system dynamic. First, the team must be made aware of their magical thinking in this regard. The team leader or outside consultant can educate and confront the team concerning the dynamics of scapegoating and its appearance in the team's dynamics. Second, the scapegoated individual or subgroup can refuse to accept that they are the only ones having these feelings or characteristics. Usually this dynamic is so powerful that most individuals are unable to cast off the labels and many ultimately accept the characterization placed upon them if they choose to stay in the system. Resolution of this problem requires intervention at the group level, since individuals will be unable to extricate themselves from the scapegoat role without the other group members reowning their unacceptable projections.

SUMMARY

This chapter explores four basic processes that occur in organizational subsystems: (1) modes of communication, (2) trust, (3) reward structures, and (4) covert processes. Communication is an interactive behavior for which there is no opposite, that is, it is impossible *not* to communicate something through any behavior. Communicative behavior has two aspects: the *content* of the message, and the *relationship* between parties that is implied by the behavior. The content of a communication is frequently expressed through verbal media while the relationship aspect is usually expressed through nonverbal and contextual cues. If there is a contradiction between content and relationship aspects, people tend to place more validity upon the relationship aspect (nonverbal cues).

A nonlinear perspective is most appropriate for social systems. In most social interactions, it is not possible to establish that A caused B which caused C, and so on. Nevertheless, most people tend to view causation from a linear and egocentric perspective. The resulting punctuation of causation is at the root of much interpersonal conflict. Circular perspectives to interpersonal behavior must be gained if successful collaboration and problem solving are to be achieved.

Two forms of communication, digital and analogic, have been present since man began to speak and write. Analogic communication conveys a likeness of what is being represented and consists of drawings, figures, sculpture, music, gestures, and sign language. Digital communication uses arbitrary symbols for representation and consists of language and mathematics. Each form of communication has advantages and disadvantages. Analogic communication is very useful in establishing the relationship aspect of a communication while digital communication is very useful in expressing the complex and abstract ideas that are the basis of civilization.

Trust is essential for productive organizational behavior. Trust is not a given but must be built through a reciprocal process of taking a risk (and not being burned) for the sake of a relationship.

Reward is more useful than punishment in building motivation and promoting learning. The effectiveness of a given reward, however, will be different for each person and situation. The desirability of a reward, the connectedness of a reward to a behavior, and the amount of reward in relation to the effort expended must be considered in evaluating the effectiveness of a reward.

There are overt and covert aspects to behavior in organizations. Hidden agendas exist that are different from the agendas that are publically advertised. These hidden agendas can consume a great deal of energy and time if they are not made explicit. Subsystems also behave "as if" they were making basic assumptions about their task. These basic assumptions invariably interfere with work and must be confronted by the subsystem. Splitting dynamics also occur as an attempt to deal with the good and bad elements in any system or person. Scapegoating is a form of splitting behavior in which the subsystem attempts to assign all the malignancy, pain, incompetency, and evil to one person or subgroup. These irrational forces are ubiquitous and prevent subsystems from growing and being adaptive.

REFERENCES

Atkinson, J. Toward experimental analysis of human motivation in terms of motives, expectancies and incentives. In J. Atkinson (Ed.), *Motives in fantasy, action and society*. Princeton, N.J.: Van Nostrand, 1958.

Bion, W. *Experiences in groups*. New York: Basic Books, 1961.

Blake, R., & Mouton, J. *The managerial grid*. Houston: Gulf Publications, 1964.

Deutsch, M. Cooperation and trust: Some theoretical notes. In M. Jones (Ed.), *Nebraska Symposium of Motivation*. Lincoln: University of Nebraska Press, 1962.

Edwards, B. *Drawing on the right side of the brain*. Los Angeles, Calif.: J.P. Tarcher, 1979.

Estes, W. Experimental study of punishment. *Psychological Monographs*, 1944, *57* (Whole No. 263).

Festinger, L. A theory of social comparison processes. *Human Relations*, 1954, *7*, 117–140.

Frazer, J. *The golden bough*. New York: Macmillan, 1922.

Gazzaniga, M. The split brain in man. In R. Held & W. Richards (Eds.), *Perception: Mechanisms and models*. San Francisco: W.H. Freeman, 1972.

Gibb, J. Defense level and influence potential in small groups. In L. Petrillo and B. Bass (Eds.), *Leadership and interpersonal behavior*. New York: Holt, Rinehart & Winston, 1961.

Gibb, J. Climate for trust formation. In L. Bradford, J. Gibb and K. Benne (Eds.), *T-group theory and laboratory method*. New York: Wiley, 1964.

Herzberg, F. *Work and the nature of man*. Cleveland: World, 1966.

Holland, J. *The psychology of vocational choice*. Waltham, Mass.: Blaisdell, 1966.

Jaynes, J. *The origin of consciousness and the breakdown of the bicameral mind*. Boston: Houghton Mifflin, 1976.

Kahn, L. The dynamics of scapegoating: The expulsion of evil. *Psychotherapy: Theory and Practice*, 1980, *17*(1), 79–84.

Katz, D., & Kahn, R. *The social psychology of organizations* (2nd ed.). New York: Wiley, 1978.

Kelly, G. *The psychology of personal constructs*. New York: Norton, 1955.

Klein, M. *Contributions to psycho-analysis: 1921–1945*. London: Hogarth, 1948.

Lofquist, L., & Dawis, R. *Adjustment to work: A psychological view of man's problems in a work-oriented society*. New York: Appleton-Century-Crofts, 1969.

Maslow, A. *Motivation and personality*. New York: Harper, 1954.

Morgan, C., & King, R. *Introduction to psychology*. New York: McGraw-Hill, 1966.

Ouchi, W. *Theory Z: How American business can meet the Japanese challenge*. New York: Avon Books, 1981.

Schutz, W. Interpersonal underworld. *Harvard Business Review*, 1958, *36*, 123–135.

Skinner, B. *Science and human behavior*. New York: Macmillan, 1953.

Watzlawick, P., Beavin, J., & Jackson, D. *Pragmatics of human communications: A study of interactive patterns, pathologies, and paradoxes*. New York: Norton, 1967.

Whorf, B. Science and linguistics. In J. Carroll (Ed.), *Language, thought, and reality: Selected writings of Benjamin Lee Whorf*. New York: Wiley, 1956.

Zand, D. Trust and managerial problem solving. In W. Nord (Ed.), *Concepts and Controversy in Organizational Behavior* (2nd ed.). Santa Monica, Calif.: Scott, Foresman & Company, 1976.

CHAPTER 6
TEAM AND GROUP DYNAMICS IN NURSING

Teamwork in nursing and interdisciplinary health care has received increased attention in recent years. The increasing specialization in all the health care professions has heightened the opportunity for highly skilled and comprehensive care but, at the same time, has created problems of communication, role definition, value conflicts, and highly complex group dynamics. The need for effective teamwork is self-evident, yet the problems of cooperation, collaboration, coordination, and communication in nursing and interdisciplinary health care teams require a sophisticated knowledge of both the dynamics of task groups and effective strategies for managing teams and task-directed groups.

The development of effective teamwork and group work needs to be an important objective for a nurse manager/supervisor. Therefore, we will present the conceptual foundations for teams and groups in nursing that are necessary for the implementation of management strategies. These concepts apply whether the team or group is composed entirely of nurses or from a number of disparate disciplines, or whether teams and groups are stable and routine or special and temporary, as in task forces.

TEAMS DEFINED

For a concept so widely touted as essential to organizational effectiveness, relatively few definitions of a team are available that differentiate a team from other kinds of groups of people or that offer a classification or taxonomy of the various kinds of teams. Several recent and well-known texts on team building omit any definition of a team (French & Bell, 1978; Patten, 1981). Some authors describe the characteristics of an effective team (French & Bell, 1978; Francis & Young, 1979). Analogies to sports teams and organizational health are offered to describe how people learn to be team members (Anundsen, 1979) and how to move teams from unhealthy states of "disease" to more healthy modes of functioning (Patten, 1981). Apparently these authors assume there is consensus on what constitutes a team and that we all "know one when we see one."

It is more likely, however, that precise definitions have been avoided because of the confusion and complexity of the concept. Concepts such as "intact work group" (Friedlander, 1972) or tasks groups (Shaw, 1976) are neither necessary nor sufficient elements in an adequate definition of a team. With the advent of technologically sophisticated information/communication systems, teams can be created which neither see nor meet each other and in which team members may not have a comprehensive knowledge of the team's mission. Specialists, expert resources, and technicians may be invited to be temporary members of teams, but they may have little appreciation of the team, its history, or its efforts.

Task groups vary widely in the degree to which teamwork is necessary. Football, basketball, and volleyball teams require high levels of teamwork. Practice sessions devote large segments of time to integrating and coordinating the activities of team members. At the other extreme, tennis teams, ski teams, and track teams spend most of their time on the individual's skill development and relatively little time on coordinating team members' efforts. Baseball teams require a blend of individual effort and team-work.

The existence of a jointly held mission does not define which groups do and do not require teamwork. In sports such as skiing, all teams members will be doing their best to score points for their team, but little of each team members's activities would be described by most people as teamwork.

An adequate definition of a team must include a description of how each member relates to the mission of the team and how each member of the team is required to work with other team members. Dyer (1977, p. 4) defines teams as "collections of people who must rely upon group collaboration if each member is to experience the optimum of success and goal achievement." Patten (1979, p. 12) identifies a "singleness of mission and a willingness to cooperate" as critical characteristics of teams.

Groups need to develop teamwork when members have the same overall goal and when they have to work cooperatively and creatively in a skilled manner in order to be effective. Many so-called teams do not have these characteristics and are not considered true teams under this definition.

Group Task Dimensions

Shaw (1973) has presented empirical evidence that group tasks can be described best by 6 primary dimensions out of a possible 104 task dimensions. The dimensions may be briefly described as follows:

Difficulty—the amount of effort required to complete the task.

Solution multiplicity—the degree to which there is more than one solution to a task.

Intrinsic interest—the degree to which the task is interesting, motivating, or attractive to the group members.

Cooperation requirements—the degree to which integrated action of group members is required to complete the task.

Intellectual/manipulative requirements—the ratio of mental to motor requirements of the group task.

Population familiarity—the degree to which members of the larger society have experience with the task. (Adapted from Shaw, 1973, pp. 311–312.)

These six dimensions may be combined when describing teams so that a three-dimensional model of task groups, which differentiates teams from other task groups and provides a taxonomy of teams, results.

A THREE DIMENSIONAL MODEL DEFINING TEAMS

The primary characteristic distinguishing teams from other groups of people is that all members of the team share a common mission (task) and have developed a consensual perception of their goals in pursuing the mission. All teams share this feature whether or not they require a large degree of what has been popularly described as "teamwork."

As we have demonstrated, however, not all teams require much teamwork and therefore do not stress team practice and are not greatly concerned that team members like, care, or respect each other. Some executives, in fact, such as George Steinbrenner, owner of the New York Yankees in the 1970s and early 1980s, believe that their teams function best with a certain degree of tension and conflict among team members. Steinbrenner remarked at a news conference announcing the rehiring of the bellicose manager, Billy Martin, in January 1983, that "a sailboat without wind goes nowhere." Baseball, apparently, does not require a high degree of cooperation among all team members. The consequences of a lack of coordination, cooperation, liking, caring, and mutual respect for team members on a psychiatric team, however, would be potentially disasterous.

Since Shaw (1973) apparently assumes that group tasks are concensually accepted by group members, none of the six task group dimensions relates to the shared mission characteristic of teams.

The second dimension of the model defining teams, the extent to which a group requires and expects cooperation, is clearly related to Shaw's group task dimensions (cooperation requirement).

Teams that require or expect team members to cooperate with each other in order to be maximally successful are identified as *true* teams. True teams recognize the importance of teamwork and devote valuable training time to the development of team coordination, collaboration, and positive personal relations. Examples of true teams include interdisciplinary health care teams, psychiatric teams, nursing teams, project teams in engineering task forces, boards of directors, football teams, and volleyball teams.

A distinguishing feature of true teams is the existence or potential existence of a "weak link." Since everyone on a true team needs to work effectively in order for the team to be successful, any one member working ineffectively can cause the entire team to fail. This is not necessarily true of *quasi* teams that have a shared mission but whose members work more or less independently of each other. On tennis teams or baseball teams, the team may be successful with one or two ineffective members if the skills of the other members can compensate for a weak team member.

Team members are less interchangeable or replaceable on true teams than on quasi teams. Since their effectiveness depends as much upon practice and positive interpersonal relationships as upon job skills, the orientation time for new members on a true team is greater than on a quasi team. Ineffective team members on production assembly lines can easily be replaced with new members who have the task-specific skills required for the job.

A third dimension facilitating the classification of teams and groups is the degree to which the work can be routinized and organized into familiar patterns in terms of work content and task process. This third dimension is a synthesis of the task difficulty, solution multiplicity, intrinsic interest, and familiarity dimensions in Shaw's group task taxonomy.

Many, if not most, teams face the same cycles of problems and required tasks every day, and need only minor adjustments in routine from time to time to remain effective. For these teams, keeping team members challenged and alert is as important as providing the necessary teamwork training.

When a team's task is routine and organized into familiar patterns, the work tends to be simplified, standardized, broken down into discrete steps, repetitive, and, consequently, increasingly dull and uninteresting. Management science has developed the strategies of job enrichment, enlargement, and quality circles to solve these problems.

Some team tasks, on the other hand, are quite difficult, require skills and knowledge, and have many possible paths to accomplishment. The required tasks may be unfamiliar to team members at the outset, but tend to become interesting, motivating, and personally rewarding. These teams with complex tasks call for a high degree of problem-solving ability, as well as cooperation, collaboration, and positive interpersonal relations. Some teams, such as highly theoretical scientific teams, may be required to develop new processes for solving problems in completely new content areas. Other teams, such as most task forces, may rely on familiar problem-solving methods to solve problems in new content areas. Still other teams, such as surgical teams, may operate in fairly routinized patterns until an unexpected emergency occurs requiring well-rehearsed problem-solving skills.

The three-dimensional model for classifying teams and groups is presented pictorially in Figure 6-1. By dichotomizing each of these variables, Table 6-1 can be constructed. This discussion will be concerned mostly with Type A and Type B teams given in Table 6-1 since they describe the two kinds of teams most often encountered in nursing.

The surgical team, and some nursing teams practicing functional nursing, come closest to a description of nursing teams that have a shared mission or task (highest quality care for team's patients), require and expect cooperation between team members to perform their duties effectively, and whose tasks are relatively routinized, known, and understood. Because of the complex health care needs of many patients, however, nursing care is not devoid of the need for good problem-solving skills. Each member must be able to respond creatively and professionally. Nurse leaders must know how to engage the team effectively when varying efforts and skills are necessary.

Teams that have a shared mission, require and expect cooperation, and whose tasks are relatively routinized will be termed *Type A* teams. Team-building strategies for Type A teams typically focus upon team member role definition and clarification, issues of

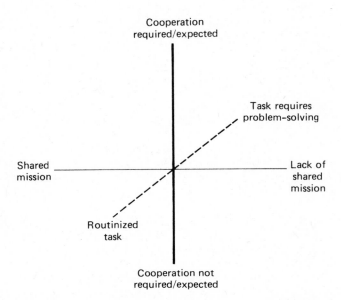

FIGURE 6-1. A THREE-DIMENSIONAL MODEL OF TEAMS AND GROUPS.

TABLE 6-1. TYPES OF TEAMS FROM THE THREE-DIMENSIONAL MODEL OF TEAMS AND GROUPS

Type A Teams

Shared mission
Cooperation needed/
  expected
Routinized task

Example: Surgical team

Type C Teams

Shared mission
Little cooperation required/
  expected
Routinized task

Example: Assembly line

TEAMS

Type B Teams

Shared mission
Cooperation needed/
  expected
Problem solving required

Example: Task forces

Type D Teams

Shared mission
Little cooperation required/
  expected
Problem solving required

Example: Research team
  working independently
  to avoid bias

supervision and authority, effective communication, interpersonal conflict management, goal setting, time management, team health and stress management, socialization and team culture, and measurement and evaluation of team effectiveness.

In recent years, problem-solving skills have begun to be appreciated even for teams involved in the most routine tasks such as industrial production teams. The Japanese systematically teach employees at all levels how to conduct applied research and how to make effective decisions through *quality circle programs* (Franklin, 1981; Ross, 1982). The Japanese management model supports the open systems theory assumption that every healthy adaptive team requires internal feedback and problem-solving skills to remain effective. To stand pat is to invite decline and entropy. Successful team functioning requires continuous training and team-building activities.

Type B teams require problem-solving skills as well as sharing a common mission and requiring and expecting cooperation from team members. Temporary task forces, committees, team nursing, faculty teams, interdisciplinary psychiatric teams, boards of directors, and political cabinets represent Type B teams.

In these teams, effective problem solving, decision making, and follow-through processes are emphasized in team-building programs. Within the context of these processes are interwoven issues involving communication, conflict resolution, creativity and innovation, time management, leadership and power, and goal setting and evaluation. The development by the team itself of the appropriate structure for carrying out the team's mission also has a high priority, whereas structure may be a given from above in Type A teams. Roles may be intentionally blurred to limit role-lock and to tap as much creativity as possible from team members.

The colleague status of team members is emphasized, which places everyone formally on an equal basis with regard to status and power except, perhaps, the task force leader, committee chair, or president of a board of directors. Informal distinctions in status and power, of course, will emerge among members as the team develops. Type A teams may attempt to diminish differences in power and status that result in hierarchies, but frequently will maintain formal distinctions on these dimensions.

TEAM DEVELOPMENT

Very little direct empirical research has been reported concerning the stages or phases of team development. Evidence from two related areas of research, however, has been applied to the problem of identifying typical patterns of team development: (1) studies examining problem-solving behavior in short-term, temporary task groups (Bales & Strodtbeck, 1951) and (2) descriptions of group development in experiential or self-study groups such as T-groups, encounter and sensitivity groups, human relations courses, and Tavistock Conferences (Babad & Amir, 1978; Bennis & Shepard, 1956; Bion, 1961; Caple, 1978; Gibbard, Hartman & Mann, 1974; Near, 1978; Schutz, 1966; Slater, 1966; Tuckman, 1965).

Problem-Solving Behavior in Small, Short-Term Groups

Bales and Strodtbeck (1951) reported that the behavior of groups working toward a group decision on a specific problem could be divided into three phases. In the *orientation* phase, information possessed by individual members that is relevant to group decision is made available to the group and is coordinated in relation to the group problem. Members try to understand the problem and the information relevant to it. In this process, it is inevitable that differences in values and interests regarding judgments of the facts, as well as proposed courses of action, occur. When the group focuses upon these differences, the *evaluation* phase occurs. When alternative perceptions and solutions have been explored by the group, there is a shift to the *control* phase in which there is an attempt to regulate member behavior and the common environment to facilitate a group decision. In this phase it is common for members to give and ask for direction so that the task may be accomplished.

While this early classic research on group development is well accepted and is consistent with other research concerning group development in long-term groups, the results are not easily generalizable to team development. The problem-solving groups met typically for one short experimental session, had members who were strangers, had no designated authority structure, and were comprised of college students. The data are best applied in describing the behavior of problem-solving groups and teams working within limited time boundaries (i.e., task forces, brainstorming groups, short-term project teams).

Experiential and Self-Study Group Development

Considerable descriptive and empirical research has been presented concerning small group development in T-groups and encounter groups (Babad & Amir, 1978; Bennis & Shepard, 1956; Caple, 1978; Near, 1978; Schutz, 1966; Tuckman, 1965), semester-length experiential human relations courses in universities (Dunphy, 1964; Gibbard, Hartman, & Mann, 1974; Mann, 1967; Mills, 1964; Slater, 1966), and Bion or Tavistock groups (Bion 1961; Rice, 1963).

All of these types of groups share important features. The group members typically do not know each other at the outset and do not expect to have significant interaction with each other after the group terminates. Initially, there are few distinctions made among group members other than sex, age, personal appearance, and so on. The task of each group member is to learn from their own and the other members' behavior in this "microcosm" and to relate this learning to the life in groups outside of the self-study group. The groups are educational rather than therapeutic in nature. Members are assumed to be normal adults and typically attend the groups to learn how to be more effective leaders and members. In many cases, the groups are conducted away from normal work locations at "retreat" sites (such as resorts, or isolated or rural locations). When conducted away from work and home, group sessions are held 8–12 hours per day for 3–10 days.

There is considerable variation among types of groups in the manner in which leadership is exercised. T-group leaders, known as "trainers" or "facilitators," are nondirective and encourage members to examine and learn from the group's efforts to accomplish its task, to become more effective as a group, and to become more effective as group members. Since the trainer does not define the specific goals for the group, leadership is expected to emerge from the group membership itself. While a role boundary between the trainer and the members is evident, the trainer will interact with members; share feelings, thoughts, and personal reactions with group members; will make didactic presentations; and will encourage the flattening of hierarchical differences between himself or herself and group members, as the group experience progresses. The personal learning orientation is shared by trainer and members.

Leaders or "consultants" in self-study, Tavistock, and Bion groups, on the other hand, are nondirective and will interact with the group as a whole when they believe its behavior is not "on task." While the task is clearly stated (the group is to study its own behavior), in reality it is quite perplexing and paradoxical. The consultant does not tell group members what they are supposed to do. The consultant does point out that the group is avoiding work when it is talking, analyzing, not behaving, or when it is behaving and acting out and not studying its behavior. Since the focus of attention is upon learning about *group* dynamics, the consultants avoid making comments about the behavior of specific individuals, except as that behavior relates to the behavior of the entire group. Consultants make little attempt to decrease hierarchical distance between themselves and the group, and often interpret attempts to become more personally involved with the consultant as efforts to gain more power in the group or to seduce the consultant into doing the work of the group.

Membership in all of these groups usually results in an intense emotional experience and significant personal learning experiences concerning behavior in small groups. As a device for learning about team development and how to become more effective team leaders and members, however, these groups have serious limitations. (1) Leadership in teams is generally not emergent—superiors are selected from above and are not elected or approved by the team itself. (2) Members are not strangers, as they often know each other before joining the team and will maintain a relationship when they leave the team. (3) Roles for team members are frequently formally defined by the organization when they enter a team. (4) Leader and team members are more clearly interdependent than in experiential self-study groups—leaders cannot allow a group to fail for the sake of a "learning experience." For this reason, team leaders are directive and will encourage personal relationships with members to increase her or his influence with the team. (5) The life span of teams is measured in months, years, and decades rather than days and weeks; the ramifications of one's behavior on a team is far greater and longer-lasting than on an experiential self-study group. (6) Finally, the task of a team is to produce a valued service or product, not to promote learning, understanding, and individual or group change. These differences must be considered when extrapolating results from small and experiential groups to actual work teams.

Linear, Cyclical, and Pendular Models of Group Development

While there is general agreement concerning the basic processes, phases, or stages that describe experiential groups, there is dispute about the order, if any, in which these phases occur. Linear or sequential models that specify which phases occur first, in the middle, and last have been proposed by Bennis and Shepard (1956), Mills (1964), Tuckman (1965), Mann (1966), Slater (1966), and Dunphy (1974).

There is general agreement by all of these authors that the nature of experiential and self-analytic groups with nondirective leadership by trainers and consultants, non-explicit and problematic group tasks, and expectations of "heavy" inter- and intra-personal experiences ensures that new members in these groups will experience a mixture of anxiety, fear, and bewilderment.

The beginning phase, which corresponds to Bales and Strodtbeck's orientation phase, is characterized by Tuckman (1965) in his review of small group development theories as a "forming" one in which members test the boundaries of the group, its leaders, and other group members. They seek answers from the leader and members concerning their tasks, how they should relate to each other, and why they and others in the group act and feel the way they do. Group members look to the identified leader, trainer, facilitator, or consultant for the answers to the problems facing themselves and the group acts *as if* the group is unable to carry out these functions itself. Bion (1961) describes this phenomenon as a basic assumption state of dependency, that is, the group appears to be making a basic assumption that it is helpless and totally dependent upon the leader to provide answers and direction.

When the trainer or consultant disappoints the group by failing to meet the groups' dependent expectations, some members will ignore or attack the leader for being weak, incompetent, insincere, and manipulative. This subgroup rejects its dependence upon the leader (becoming counterdependent) and resists any efforts by the leader to assist the group in its task. Typically, another subgroup maintains its unrealistic dependent relationship with the leader and defends the leader when the counterdependent sub-group attacks him or her. The resulting behavior is an oscillation between submitting to or attacking authority. Considerable conflict occurs among group members and between the group and the identified leader (the trainer or consultant) or anyone else who attempts to exercise leadership. In effect, the group appears to be behaving *as if* the reason it meets is either to fight someone or flee from someone. Bion referred to this as a basic assumption state of fight/flight. As a consequence, the group lacks cohesiveness, is resistant to any attempts at leadership, and is completely unable to accomplish its task. Tuckman (1965) has summarized this phase as "storming" (intragroup conflict and member–leader hostility). This phase parallels roughly Bales and Strodtbeck's (1951) evaluation phase.

Some groups never resolve their problems with authority, remain in perpetual conflict, and are never able to establish consensus for an agenda for its activities. Bennis and Shepard (1956) and Slater (1966) described a typical method that groups employ to resolve their authority problems. In a move toward solidarity, the group supports a revolt against the trainer or consultant. Hierarchical power issues among members are put on the back burner for the sake of expelling the "bad" leader under the assumption that he or she is repressing or preventing "good" leadership from emerging from the group itself. The actual behavior ranges from completely ignoring to physically removing the leader from the group's meeting place. In the process, the group hopes that its feelings of anger, anxiety, and disappointment will be expelled with the "bad" leader.

A period of "enchantment" (Bennis & Shepard, 1956) follows, in which the group has a heightened sense of accomplishment and cohesiveness resulting from the revolt and expulsion. The revolt is the first cooperative effort by the group that leads to the consensual adoption of its first set of norms, "equality, fraternity, and autonomy." Tuckman (1965) refers to this phase as "norming."

This pure democracy, however, breaks down when the group returns to resolving their own differences and accepting leadership from within its membership. Nevertheless, the quieting effect of the revolt and suppression of intragroup conflict allows for a shift in emotional attachment from the deposed leader to each other. In heterosexual groups, sexual attachments begin to emerge. Slater (1966) describes this phenomenon as "sexual liberation through revolt." The revolt also demonstrates that it is possible for the group to unite and act together. The results encourage making further efforts to resolve the group's authority and intimacy problems.

Many groups utilize the new-found sexual liberation in tackling both the authority and intimacy problems. The group pins its hopes for "good" leadership upon a pair of individuals (usually heterosexual) whom they perceive as being intimately involved with each other. It is *as if* the group hoped and expected future leadership that will solve the group's problems to be "born" to this couple. This is referred to by Bion (1961) as a basic assumption state of pairing. When the "messiah" does not emerge and their problems are not magically solved, the group is forced to deal more realistically with its problems.

This stage of "disenchantment" (Bennis & Shepard, 1956) ushers in a phase termed "performing" by Tuckman (1965). Members recognize that they must all participate in leadership and followership and are more spontaneous in their expressions of intimacy and anger. The group recognizes the need for some structure and appreciates the necessary, if flawed, efforts of the designated leader, the trainer or consultant, to assist them in their task. A much greater percentage of group time and activity are devoted to work rather than "basic assumption" activity.

While there is some variation in the order of stages or phases, theorists supporting the linear or sequential view of group development are in agreement that groups confront issues of inclusion, authority, and power before focusing upon issues of intimacy and affection. Other theorists, however, note that while the pattern of group development is consistent, it is not linear, but rather, cyclical or pendular.

Bion (1961), in a very early account of group development, stated that there was no developmental pattern in the occurrence of basic assumption activity; that is, basic assumption dependency did not necessarily occur before fight/flight or pairing basic assumption states. Rather, the group shifted from one basic assumption state to another in avoidance of its work, depending upon the participation patterns of group members and their predisposition (or valency) to favor one basic assumption state over another. Thus, each group tends to have dependency leaders, fight/flight leaders, and pairing leaders who are "enlisted" by the group to lead them when issues of authority, power, affection, and so forth, arise.

Schutz (1958) proposed that group phases occurred recurrently in the order of (a) inclusion (issues of contact, interaction, and belonging), (b) control (issues of power, competition, and authority), and (c) affection (issues of emotional closeness) until the groups terminated. At termination, the order of phases reversed. Schutz's model predicts a cyclical patterning of group interaction such as ICAICAICA . . . ACI.

Slater's (1966) model is a pendular one that incorporates a discussion of group and individual boundaries to describe group development. In Slater's view, a member who has voluntarily joined a group is faced with a wish/fear dilemma that shapes his or her behavior. Presumably, new group members want to be included psychologically in the new entity, the group. To do so, however, they must give up some individual autonomy. The price one pays for acceptance as a group member, therefore, is a loss of individual freedom.

In our Western/American society, this sets up an intense intrapersonal conflict enacted as approach/avoidance activity. The conflict, expressed in a general systems theory perspective, occurs as individual boundaries are threatened when a member begins to merge into the group in the early stages of group development and a fear of fusion with the group develops. This results in flight from the group (basic assumption state fight/flight) and anarchical revolt against authority. Paradoxically, the group has unified in its attempts to demonstrate its independence and a movement back toward group cohesion occurs. Slater suggests that each individual and the group will struggle with the wish/fear dilemma of fusion into the group and independence from the group throughout the group's life, resulting in a cyclical or pendular pattern of group development.

The Slater model became the precursor of the most recent conceptions of small group development that have included family and life-cycle elements. While earlier theorists had been intrigued with the similarities between group and individual development (Bennis & Shepard, 1956; Dunphy, 1964; Mann, 1967; Mills, 1964), Gibbard and Hartman (1973) offered a model explicitly comparing individual and small group development.

In a simplification of this elaborate psychoanalytic model, these authors believe that the group recapitulates the conditions that group members experienced in their nuclear family. The derivative father in a male-led group is easily identified. In female-led groups, however, members may have difficulty acknowledging her authority in the way that our culture routinely acknowledges male authority (Kahn, 1977). If the group perceives the leader to be the father in the group, members will respond in the typical dependent/rebellious, affectionate/hostile manner with which they responded to their fathers as they grew up. Males will perceive the leader as a threat to their relations with other women in the group and to their autonomy as males competent in their own right. The leader will struggle with his own impulses to suppress the rebellion and threat to his authority and masculinity.

Conflict and rebellion are likely sequelae. Females (and the leader) will struggle with their sexual feelings toward a male leader and will experience difficulty establishing close relationships that are not highly sexually charged. Establishment of a comfortable distance between female members and the male leader will be difficult.

Males will have difficulty accepting the authority of a female leader and will often attempt to take an inappropriate dominant role in their relationship with the leader based upon sex-role stereotypes. Female leaders will have a hard time shaking the perception of male subordinates that they are behaving seductively or maternally toward them. Some female subordinates, believing that leadership is traditionally a male role, may covertly behave to subvert the authority of their female leader. Other female subordinates may unrealistically support every action of a female leader for the sake of female solidarity. As it can be seen, separating appropriate leadership/followership behavior from the family and societal perceptions and expectations is a very difficult process.

Gibbard and Hartman (1973) speculate further (with some data from group experiences) that the group itself takes on a maternal identity and that group members respond to it in the primitive way that infants respond to their mothers. Borrowing heavily from Klein's work (1948), Gibbard and Hartman interpret member movement cyclically toward and away from the group as developmentally similar to the child's difficulty accepting mother as having both good and bad attributes.

By "splitting" the feelings into "good" and "bad" elements and investing these feelings in the leader or other group members, the group attempts to resolve its basic ambivalent feelings toward the group-as-mother. Attempts to split the leadership (if it is multiple), to separate the leader from the group, or scapegoating actions against individual group members are explained in this fashion.

Whether or not one chooses to accept this highly elaborate and psychoanalytic view of groups, the trend in current thinking in small groups and management science is toward concepts that include family dynamics. Ouchi (1981), in a recent comparison of Japanese and American management science philosophy, points to the importance of the organization as family or clan in explaining Japanese successes. Coming back to the primary theme in this book, these theories emphasize the importance of the maintenance functions of teams and small groups in providing personal satisfactions for employees and not just production advantages for the organization.

The various models of small group development (linear, cyclical, pendular, and life cycle), with some exceptions, are not in disagreement with each other. Most theorists are in agreement concerning the typical phenomena in groups and disagree chiefly concerning the best way to describe the dynamics of these phenomena. Bion (1961) alone is positing that no predictable pattern exists for the occurrence of basic assumption states. He was also one of the first to write systematically concerning group process. Linear models evolved into cyclical and pendular ones as theorists integrated observation of group events with psychoanalytic theory, general systems theory, and family systems concepts. What at first seemed to be linear process, under greater analysis turned out to be repetitive and cyclical in keeping with most processes in open systems. The reader will find many useful observations and explanations in all of these models regardless of his or her acceptance of any one model.

IMPLICATIONS FOR NURSING TEAMS AND GROUPS

From the authors' perspective, a synthesis of a general systems theory of teams, small groups, and family systems concepts seems most appropriate for nursing teams and groups. The profession of nursing places emphasis upon caring for the biopsychosocial needs of their patients. It is not surprising, then, that nurses themselves expect their jobs to be both physically and psychologically rewarding. Grandjean, Aiken, and Bonjean (1976) report that nursing faculties at four major state universities in the midwest, south, and southwest rank supportive colleagues as second behind quality teaching as sources of job satisfaction. Effective teamwork, therefore, must combine concern for both productivity and the human needs of the team members.

In some nursing roles, especially within hospitals and large health care agencies where functional assignments are made, the individual nurse will find herself or himself working within a Type A team: All team members have a shared mission, are required and expected to work cooperatively, and the typical tasks of the team are well rehearsed and fairly routine. Problem-solving demands will occur frequently but not on a predictable basis. The nursing manager/supervisor should focus her or his team-building activities upon role definition and clarification, issues of supervision and authority, effective communications, interpersonal conflict management, goal setting, time management, team health and stress management, socialization and team culture, and measurement and evaluation of team effectiveness. Team members should also be trained in effective problem-solving methods.

Many nurses today find themselves working in or with Type B teams. In addition to a shared mission and expectations and requirements of cooperation, team members spend a significant portion of their time in problem-solving activities. As part of public or community health teams, nurses may be called upon to come up with creative solutions for chronic problems, to perform complicated diagnostic functions, and to solve complex problems for which he or she may need continuing education. Nursing educators are required to develop innovative curricula for their students and nursing departments. In addition, high percentage of nurses who normally perform their duties in Type A teams will occasionally be invited or called upon to be part of task forces, special problem-solving committees, and brain-storming sessions, that is, become members of Type B teams. Leaders, managers, and supervisors of these teams should emphasize effective problem-solving, decision-making, and follow-through processes in their team-building programs.

When starting new teams, nursing leaders and managers can expect team dynamics to follow the forming, storming, norming, and performing progression identified by Tuckman (1965). Leaders should keep in mind that authority and power issues, including the conflict between personal and group boundaries, will generally occur before the group can deal with intimacy problems. In keeping with Hersey and Blanchard's model of leadership (1976), new teams require more attention to structure that will facilitate resolution of authority and power issues.

As the work group matures, the leader should encourage the team to attend to the interpersonal issues of conflict and intimacy. Premature focusing upon these "process" issues before dealing with the team's need for structure and satisfaction of dependency concerns will often result in a floundering team that lacks respect for itself and the team leader.

Highly advanced teams will be self-regulating, will be able to create and modify their structure to match the task, and attend to their interteam process issues as they occur. While the team leader who manages highly mature work teams has worked hard to achieve this state, it may seem that she or he is hardly working and that the team could manage itself. The impact of the effective team leader may only be felt some time after he or she leaves the team. As has been pointed out, all social systems will slowly become disorganized if energy is not expended to keep them functioning effectively. This is precisely the reason for continuing team-building activities *even if* the team is currently functioning effectively.

When nurse leaders, managers, or supervisors join an already established team they must be able to assess the maturity of the work group in order to know how much structure to initiate. Any change in leadership will almost certainly result in some regression in team effectiveness. The team members must necessarily divert some attention from their primary tasks in efforts to assess the new leader's expectations, values, power, and idiosyncracies. The mature team, however, will have the team skills that are necessary to solve the problem of leadership transition and will soon return to previous levels of performance given appropriate leadership.

At the start, the new team leader should expect a temporary return to dependent and boundary testing phases of group development. When the group has resolved its authority and power issues with the new leader and has adjusted to any new hierarchical relationships among group members resulting from the change in leadership, it will return its attention to task accomplishment and maintenance of group harmony.

Women as Team Leaders

Female leadership is quite prevalent in nursing today. In the discussion of group development reference was made to the impact of sex differences in group leadership.

The works of Gibbard and Hartman (1973), Kahn (1977), Beauvais (1976, 1977), Wright (1976), and Bayes and Newton (1978) are consistent in reporting that groups have difficulty accepting women leaders who attempt to be task-oriented, instrumental and nonemotionally expressive rather than tension reducing, expressive, and relationship-oriented. Apparently, task leadership is seen as a masculine role while team maintenance is viewed as a feminine role. Beauvais (1976, 1977) reported that, if anything, female members were more disturbed by female leaders who were task-oriented than were male members.

Reactions to female leadership in nursing teams are confounded by the existence of an even higher authority (usually male) in the person of a medical doctor. Much dissatisfaction and hostility felt toward the often female team leader is projected upon the often male doctor who returns the hostility and scrupulously protects his authority.

Much of this conflict and tension could be resolved if all team members could openly discuss their feelings toward both male and female leadership. Identifying task leadership as solely a masculine/paternal role and relationship leadership as solely a feminine/maternal role is an example of how role-lock can result in ineffectiveness and prejudice. Since this process has its genesis in a common cultural and familial experience, all team members, male and female, must struggle with sex-role bias in this respect.

SUMMARY

The importance of effective teamwork has been stressed in recent years as nursing has become more specialized and professional. A team is defined as a group of individuals who share a common mission or task and who have developed a consensual perception of their goals in pursuing the mission. Many "teams" that satisfy this definition, however, do not require much teamwork.

In our three-dimensional model of teams, "true" teams expect or require their members to work cooperatively together. Teamwork and team-building activities will vary depending upon whether the primary task of the team is routine and organized into familiar patterns (Type A) or requires creativity and problem solving (Type B).

Team development is discussed, generalizing from research in problem-solving groups and experiential small groups. Linear-sequential, cyclical and pendular, and life-cycle perspectives are used to explain how group members deal with problems of inclusion, power and control, authority, intimacy/sexuality in the life of a team. The special problem of feminine leadership was addressed from a historical perspective of nursing and cultural and familial sex-role expectations.

REFERENCES

Anundsen, K. Keys to developing managerial women. *Management Review*, February 1979, *68*, 55–58.

Babad, E., & Amir, L. Bennis and Shepard's theory of group development: An empirical examination. *Small Group Behavior*, 1978, *9*(4), 447–492.

Bales, R., & Strodtbeck, F. Phases in group problem-solving. *Journal of Abnormal and Social Psychology*, 1951, *46*, 485–495.

Bayes, M., & Newton, P. Women in authority: Sociopsychological analysis. *Journal of Applied Behavioral Science*, 1978, *14*(2), 7–20.

Beauvais, C. The family and the workgroup: Dilemmas for women in authority (Doctoral dissertation, CUNY, 1976). *Dissertation Abstracts International*, 1977, *37*(7), 3595–B.

Beauvais, C. *Dilemmas for women in authority*. Paper presented at the U.S. Commission on Civil Rights, Washington, D.C., September 1977.

Bennis, W., & Shepard, H. A theory of group development. *Human Relations*, 1956, *9*, 415–457.

Bion, W. *Experiences in groups*. New York: Basic Books, 1961.

Caple, R. The sequential stages of group development. *Small Group Behavior*, 1978, *9*(4), 470–476.

Dunphy, D. Social change in self-analytic groups. (Doctoral dissertation, Harvard University, 1964). *Dissertation Abstracts*, 1964.

Dunphy, D. Phases, roles, and myths in self-analytic groups. In G. Gibbard, J. Hartman, & R. Mann. (Eds.), *Analysis of Groups*. San Francisco: Jossey-Bass Publishers, 1974.

Dyer, W. *Team building: Issues and alternatives*. Reading, Mass.: Addison-Wesley, 1977.

Francis, D., & Young, D. *Improving work groups: A practical manual for team building*. La Jolla, Calif.: University Associates, 1979.

Franklin, W. What Japanese managers know that American managers don't. *Administrative Management*, September 1981, *42*, 36–39.

French, W., & Bell, C. *Organization development* (2nd ed.). Englewood Cliffs, N.J.: Prentice-Hall, 1978.

Friedlander, F. The impact of organizational training laboratories upon the effectiveness and interaction of ongoing work groups. In W. Burke & H. Hornstein, (Eds.), *The social technology of organization development*. Fairfax, Va.: NTL Learning Resources, 1972.

Gibbard, G., & Hartman, J. The oedipal paradigm in group development: A clinical and empirical study. *Small Group Behavior*, 1973, *23*, 305–354.

Gibbard, G., Hartman, J., & Mann, R. (Eds.). *Analysis of groups*. San Francisco: Jossey-Bass, 1974.

Grandjean, B., Aiken, L., & Bonjean, C. Professional autonomy and the work satisfaction of nursing educators. *Nursing Research*, 1976, *25*, 216–221.

Hersey, P., & Blanchard, K. Leadership effectiveness and adaptability description (LEAD). In J. Pfeiffer, & J. Jones, (Eds.), *The 1976 annual handbook for group facilitators*. La Jolla, Calif.: University Associates, 1976.

Kahn, L. Theme and role development in same-sex, self-analytic groups (Doctoral dissertation, American University, 1977). *Dissertation Abstracts International*, 1977, *38*(2), 905–B.

Klein, M. *Contributions to psycho-analysis: 1921–1945*. London: Hogarth, 1948.

Mann, R. The development of the member-trainer relationship in self-analytic groups. *Human Relations*, 1966, *19*, 85–115.

Mann, R. *Interpersonal styles and group development*. New York: Wiley, 1967.

Mills, T. *Group transformation: An analysis of a learning group*. Englewood Cliffs, N.J.: Prentice Hall, 1964.

Near, J. Comparison of developmental pattern in groups. *Small Group Behavior*, 1978, *9*(4), 470–476.

Ouchi, W. *Theory Z: How American business can meet the Japanese challenge*. New York: Avon Books, 1981.

Patten, T. Team building, Part 1: Designing the intervention. *Personnel*, January–February 1979, *56*, 11–21.

Patten, T. *Organizational development through teambuilding*. New York: Wiley, 1981.

Ross, J. *Japanese quality circles and productivity*. Reston, Va.: Reston Publishing, 1982.

Rice, A. *Learning for leadership*. London: Tavistock Publications, 1963.

Schutz, W. *FIRO: A three-dimensional theory of interpersonal behavior*. New York: Holt, 1958.

Schutz, W. *The interpersonal underworld*. Palo Alto, Calif.: Science and Behavior Books, 1966.

Shaw, M. Scaling group tasks: A method for dimensional analysis. *JSAS Catalog of Selected Documents in Psychology*, 1973, *3*, 8. (Ms. No. 294.)

Shaw, M. *Group dynamics: The psychology of small group behavior* (2nd ed.). New York: McGraw-Hill, 1976.

Slater, P. *Microcosm.* New York: Wiley, 1966.

Tuckman, B. Developmental sequences in small groups. *Psychological Bulletin*, 1965, *63*, 384–399.

Wright, F. The effects of style and sex of consultants and sex of members in self-study groups. *Small Group Behavior*, 1976, *7*(4), 433–457.

PART TWO
THE PROCESSES
OF NURSING
LEADERSHIP,
MANAGEMENT,
AND SUPERVISION

CHAPTER 7
THE NURSING LEADERSHIP PROCESS

Earlier the processes of leadership, administration, management, and supervision were differentiated. Leadership was defined as interpersonal influence by which the efforts of a group are directed, through the communication process, toward the achievement of a specified goal or goals in a given situation. It is important to recognize that while nurses in management and supervisory roles are in a position to provide leadership, not all nursing managers or supervisors are leaders. Equally true is that not all nursing leaders are in management or supervisory roles. The process of leadership should be examined carefully to identify what characteristics or activities determine who is "the leader."

THE LEADERSHIP PROCESS

Many of the first attempts to define leadership were confined to the listing of characteristics and personality traits of persons widely recognized as leaders. However, by the 1940s, research was demonstrating that persons with widely varying characteristics were recognized as leaders and the focus had shifted to the interactions among the leader, the followers, and the situation, or the process of leadership. The last 20 years have seen an increase in research and literature dealing with leadership. Several theories have been developed. Among the most prominent are McGregor's *Theory X* and *Theory Y* (1960), the *Immaturity-Maturity Theory* of Argyris (1962), *Motivation Theory* of Herzberg (1959), Likert's *Management Systems Theory* (1967), the *Leadership Contingency Model* of Fiedler (1967), and the *Managerial Grid Theory* of Blake and Mouton (1978). Each of these theories focuses on one or more variables of the leadership process and has proved valuable in identifying significant relationships between the leader and the group as well as the leader and the situation. Hersey and Blanchard (1977) have further developed the interrelationship of leader–group–situation in their *Situational Leadership Theory*, which forms the framework for this chapter.

Variables in the Leadership Process

The definition of leadership identifies five variables that must be considered in any discussion of the process: the leader, the followers (or groups), the situation, the process of communication, and the goals. The characteristics of these five variables and the interactions among them define the boundaries of the system within which the leadership process occurs.

The Leader

The leader as an individual occupies a central position in the process. The unique characteristics of the individual leader are directly related to leadership behavior and to those factors that determine behavior.

Although no single characteristic or combination of traits has been identified as universally present and necessary in leaders, research has produced interesting findings. Studies concerned with physical characteristics such as age, height, weight, activity, gender, and physical appearance found little statistical evidence that any of these were of significance in predicting leaders. Although above-average height and weight for the peer group and appearance may be an advantage to those seeking leadership positions, the major physical characteristics seen in successful leaders are an abundant reserve of energy, stamina, and ability to maintain a high rate of physical activity (Stodgill, 1974). Social factors, such as socioeconomic status and educational level, may influence the emergence of a leader. In his comparison of all surveys of leadership characteristics from 1948 through 1970, Stodgill concluded that

> (1) high socioeconomic status is an advantage in attaining leadership status; (2) leaders who rise to high level positions in industry tend to come from lower socioeconomic strata at present than they did a half century ago, and (3) they tend to be better educated than formerly. (1974, p. 77)

Personality factors that seem to contribute to the emergence of a leader include intelligence, ability, judgment, knowledge, decisiveness, high motivation, originality, personal integrity, and persistence. In summary, Stodgill (1974) characterized the leader as one with

> a strong desire for responsibility and task completion, vigor and persistence in the pursuit of goals, venturesomeness and originality in problem solving, drive to exercise initiative in social situations, self-confidence and sense of personal identity, willingness to accept consequences of decision and action, readiness to absorb interpersonal stress, willingness to tolerate frustration and delay, ability to influence other persons' behavior and capacity to structure social interaction systems to the purpose at hand. (p. 81)

These physical, social, and personality factors, however, are less important than the values, skills, and perceptions of the leader. A person's most distinguishing characteristics spring from the internalized pattern of values. Basic *values* dictate both the choice of actions and the methods. While values determine objectives and the methods appropriate to use in reaching these objectives, *skills and abilities* are the essence of the implementation process. The learned skills and abilities constitute the competencies in terms of performance. With values providing boundaries for goal setting, and with abilities providing the means of implementation, the leader develops a relationship with the followers and the situation. This relationship is necessarily modified by the *perceptions* the leader has of self, the followers, the situation, and the role to be assumed.

The observable behavior of the leader, or *leadership style*, is thus a result of the unique combination of physical, social, and personality characteristics as well as the values, skills, and perceptions that have been developed. In spite of individual differences in leader characteristics, researchers have attempted to define categories of leader behavior in order to predict which behaviors are more likely to be successful. Tannenbaum and Schmidt (1958) developed a continuum of leader behaviors moving from an authoritarian style at one end to a democratic style at the other. *Authoritarian* leaders tend to be task-oriented, to retain decision-making responsibility, and to tell their followers what to do and how to do it. *Democratic* leaders, on the other hand, tend to be oriented toward people or relationships, to share the responsibility for decisions by involving the followers in the planning of both goals and methods of reaching them, and to provide freedom for the members of the group to function without specific directions. A third leadership style, *laissez-faire*, has sometimes been included. This style of behavior permits the members of the group to function in any way they desire with no established policies and procedures and no attempts to influence the goals or methods of achieving them. This style, in reality, represents an absence of formal leadership and suggests that an informally designated leader is functioning or emerging to control the group.

Studies initiated in 1945 by the Bureau of Business Research at Ohio State University found that the dimensions of task behaviors previously identified with an authoritarian leadership style and the dimensions of relationship behaviors previously identified with a democratic leadership style were separate and distinct rather than a continuum (Stodgill & Coons, 1957). Thus, task-oriented behavior and relationship-oriented behavior are not either/or leadership styles, since the effective leader uses a combination of task and relationship behaviors. The mix of these behaviors is a result of the unique characteristics of the leader and the interaction of the leader with the other variables in the leadership process.

The Followers

The expectations and personalities of the followers are a key variable in the leadership process. Too often in the past nursing leaders have set goals for the profession or for a single school or service agency and attempted to lead toward those goals without making sure that anyone was following. Unless the group members, both as individuals and a total group, accept the influence of the designated leader, there is no formal leadership regardless of the competency and behavior of the leader. Therefore, it becomes vital to understand the characteristics of the group or followers.

The *expectations* that the group holds of what makes an effective leader usually stem from their previous experiences. If the staff of a nursing unit has previously worked well under a head nurse who gave specific assignments and expected obedience to directions, they may be concerned about the competence of a new team leader who expects them to make their own decisions. Conversely, a group that has experienced great satisfaction from being involved in the planning and development of their own goals and activities will resent a supervisor who attempts to retain all decisions as a part of his or her role. Nurse leaders should become aware of the expectations of the group. This can sometimes be accomplished by direct questioning, particularly if one is being considered for a new position. More frequently, observation of the results of leader–follower interactions and use of evaluative feedback provide the necessary data to determine the extent of both task behaviors and relationship behaviors expected by the group.

The personality of the group in relation to the goals and tasks of the organization must also be determined. The specific aspects of achievement motivation, willingness, and ability to assume responsibility and education and/or experience, have been found to be significant in determining effective leader–follower relationships (Hersey & Blanchard, 1977). The combination of these factors has been designated as the *maturity* level of the individual or group. It must be noted that these aspects can only be considered in relation to a specific task, not in any total sense. Thus, a staff nurse may be extremely responsible, competent, and motivated to provide high quality direct patient care but very casual about completing charge slips for equipment and supplies used in giving that care. Thus, the maturity level would be different for the two separate tasks.

The Situation
The situation also contains variables that must be understood if the leader is to influence a group toward the attainment of specific goals. Important variables to be considered are the organization, the immediate superiors and associates of the leader, the job demands, time element, and available resources. This list is not all-inclusive, but it does contain the major elements of interest and importance to the leader.

Organization.   Consideration of the organization begins with understanding the written statements provided for employers and consumers. Unlike other industries, most health care agencies have explicit statements of philosophies in addition to policies and procedures that serve as a guide for understanding the expectations and style of the organization. It is extremely useful to study these documents carefully, for they reflect the system of values derived from the history of the organization and the people who have played a vital role in its development. Unnecessary conflict can be avoided if the values and expectations of the organization and the potential leader are congruent. For example, a nurse who perceives himself or herself to be a democratic leader should consider the potential conflicts inherent in accepting a head nurse position in an organization that states that final authority for all patient care decisions rests with the chief medical officer of the unit. While, ideally, an effective nurse leader might influence a change in this aspect of the organization, the reality of conflict during the change must be examined. Although most health care agencies have written statements reflecting the values and expectations of the organization, the potential leader should attempt to determine to what extent these statements are actually implemented. Frequently, informal customs and tradition developed over time will have more influence on the actual work setting than the approved policies.

Most organizations exist as open systems in a nested hierarchy. A nursing unit may be seen as an individual system or a subsystem of the larger organization. Thus, the leader of one system or group, such as a unit, functions as a follower in a suprasystem, such as the nursing service department. Since any change in one subsystem has impact on the total, the effective leader attempts to be aware of changes in other areas and to assess the impact of such changes on his or her group. For example, if the head nurse of a medical unit becomes aware that the hospital is installing computer equipment to handle the inventory in central supply and patient billing, it would seem reasonable to expect that staff development would be needed to understand new forms or procedures required to account for the use of supplies charged to specific patients. One might also anticipate the opportunity to begin exploring the use of computers for nursing records. Awareness of the total organization is essential for the effective leader.

Styles and expectation of one's superiors and associates.   The style and expectations of the persons with whom one works also influence the performance of a leader. If the leadership behavior of the person in charge tends to be extremely task-oriented, it is less likely that relationship behavior in a subordinate will be seen as appropriate. A person wanting to advance in an organization will frequently behave in a manner reflecting the group they wish to join rather than that of their associates or subordinates. Thus, a head nurse who wishes to move to a supervisor position may develop a leadership style in keeping with the expectations of the director of the nursing service and other supervisors, rather than maintaining behaviors consistent with those of the other head nurses. However, people who are satisfied with their present position may be more concerned with the expectations of their associates or those individuals who have similar positions. Faculty in schools of nursing are a good example. Often they are more interested in being viewed as a leader of either their peers, other faculty, or clinical practitioners, than in becoming a leader in the organization. Thus, their behavior reflects the values of their associates rather than the administration.

Job demands.   The job demands are another important element of the situation. Fiedler (1967) defined this variable as the degree of structure in the task that the group has been asked to do. Studies have indicated that task structure and follower maturity are related when determining an appropriate leadership style (Stinson & Johnson, 1975). Thus, a follower who is underqualified for an unstructured task would benefit from task-oriented leader behaviors, but a follower who is highly qualified for the task would benefit more from relationship behaviors on the part of the leader. For example, a student nurse assigned to develop a care plan for a newly admitted patient would require specific directions and identification of specific areas in which to obtain information while developing the plan, but a nurse with several years experience would more likely expect validation and approval from the head nurse on completion of the task.

Time.   Another important element in the situation is the time duration available for decision making. Emergencies tend to require task-oriented behavior. "Code Blue" situations mandate that the leader tell others what to do and how to do it with little or no attention to their feelings. However, if time is not a factor, the leader can consider many other situational variables and utilize a variety of both relationship and task behaviors.

Resources.   The availability of resources is a critical element within the situation. The leader's role in projection of need and resource allocation is vital to system maintenance. Nursing service and nursing education are both personnel-intensive situations. Thus, the available pool of prepared practitioners and/or educators and support personnel may greatly influence the goals and policies of the organization. Among other resources that must be considered are expendable supplies, major equipment purchases and repairs, communication systems, library facilities, and the physical plant. However, since all resources involve some cost, the amount of financial resources available to the nursing unit or educational program may be the greatest determining factor in any situation.

The Communication Process

The definition of leadership identifies the communication process as the means through which the efforts of the group are directed toward goal accomplishment. The communication process is used to provide information as well as to affect attitudes. Analysis of communication includes the following questions (Yura, Ozimek, & Walsh, 1976): Who communicates with whom? How often? For how long? For what purpose? In what manner? Other concerns within the communication process deal with formal communication patterns, informal communications, one-to-one versus group communication, style of communication, pattern of communicating in groups, levels of communication, and the process of filtering communications. The frequency with which "lack of communication" is cited as the reason for ineffective leadership underlines the pervasive nature of this process in all aspects of leadership. For this reason, the authors have devoted other sections of the book to discussing the analysis and application of effective communication.

Goals

Although the discussion of the role of goals in the leadership process is last among the variables, the degree to which both the goals of the organization and the individual goals of the follower are met ultimately determine the perception of leader effectiveness. It thus becomes vital for the leader to have a clear understanding of goals of the organization and to be able to communicate these to his or her followers. It is also essential to help the group identify individual and/or group goals and how these relate to organizational goals.

Organizational goals. Organizational goals are expressed in terms of both task accomplishment and system maintenance. Task accomplishment goals are usually easily identified, can be readily measured, and appear to have a definitive span of time in which to be accomplished. In a hospital, these may include such goals as: to decrease staff turnover, to increase occupancy rate, and to decrease costs per patient day. An educational program may have task accomplishment goals such as: to increase student enrollment, to increase number of faculty publications, and to develop a new course.

System maintenance goals are concerned with the survival and growth of the organization in a changing environment. They tend to be long-range in nature and deal more with values and attitudes requiring an identification of the"ideal" image of what should be in 5 or 10 years. An extended care facility may wish to identify a change in clientele as a means of surviving as a health care agency. Schools of nursing may identify the offering of a specialty program of studies as a means of expanding enrollment. Both hospitals and univerities may engage in expanding computer utilization in order to retain a competitive stance in the current environment.

Group/individual goals. The group and/or individual goals of the followers may also be directed toward task accomplishment or system maintenance. Group goals evolve through group interaction and reflect group decisions (Yura et al., 1976). Examples of group task accomplishment goals are: to complete a test design for a team-taught course and to develop a new staffing pattern. Team-building efforts to reduce interpersonal conflict within a work group may reflect a group system maintenance goal. Individual goals may include: to receive a pay raise or promotion, to complete a research study, and to become a clinical specialist. Individual and group goals coexist with organizational goals and the leader is the individual who can identify the interrelationship among these and influence the direction of the group in order that both task accomplishment and system maintenance goals are met for the organization as well as for the group and individuals within the group.

SITUATIONAL LEADERSHIP THEORY

The results of much research on leader characteristics and behavior during the past 30 years is consistent with the general systems theory proposition of equifinality. This has led to the conclusion that no single style or type of leader behavior is effective in all situations. Hersey and Blanchard (1977) have devised a conceptual framework that helps the practitioner determine the leadership style most likely to be effective in the conditions surrounding a specific situation. This framework is designated as the *situational leadership theory.*

Situational leadership theory attempts to explain the interactions between the leader and followers within a specific situation. The variables of leader, followers, situation, communication processes, and goals are examined to predict the most effective leadership leadership style. *Leadership style* is defined by Hersey and Blanchard (1977) as

> the behavior pattern that a person exhibits when attempting to influence the activities of others as perceived by those others. (p. 103)

A person's leadership style involves some combination of either task behavior or relationship behavior. *Task behavior* is defined by these same authors as

> the extent to which leaders are likely to organize and define the roles of the members of their group (followers); to explain what activities each is to do and when, where, and how tasks are to be accomplished; characterized by endeavoring to establish well-defined patterns of organization, channels of communication, and ways of getting jobs accomplished. (p. 103)

Examples of task behaviors as identified in the Leader Behavior Description Questionnaire (LBDQ) are: makes attitude clear to group; tries out his new ideas with group; rules with an iron hand; assigns subordinates to particular tasks; emphasizes meeting of deadlines; asks that subordinates follow standard rules and regulations; and sees to it that the work of subordinates is coordinated (Halpin, 1959).
Relationship behavior is defined as

> the extent to which leaders are likely to maintain personal relationships between themselves and members of their group (followers) by opening up channels of communication, providing socio-emotional support, "psychological strokes" and facilitating behaviors. (Hersey and Blanchard, 1977, pp. 103–104)

Examples of relationship behaviors of leaders are: does personal favors for subordinates; is easy to understand; finds time to listen to subordinates; explains his actions to subordinates; backs up subordinates in their actions; is willing to make changes; is friendly and approachable; and puts suggestions made by group into action (Halpin, 1959).
Leadership style is thus composed of two dimensions—task behaviors and relationship behaviors. Figure 7-1 shows the combination of the two basic leadership behavior dimensions as four quadrants. Each quadrant represents a leadership style that might be effective or ineffective depending upon the variables in the situation.

Leadership Styles

Four leadership styles have been identified: high-task/low-relationship, or telling; high-task/high-relationship, or selling; high-relationship/low-task, or participating; and low-task/low-relationship, or delegating.

High-Task/Low-Relationship
In a high-task/low-relationship leadership style, the leader defines the tasks and the roles of the followers. It may be referred to as a "telling" style since the leader provides, through one-way communication, the information about what, when, where, and how tasks will be done and who will do them. This style corresponds to the typical "authoritarian" leadership mode. When effective, the leader is perceived to be knowledgeable about the outcomes to be achieved and can impose his or her methods for accomplishing these goals without creating resentment. In other situations, a leader using this style

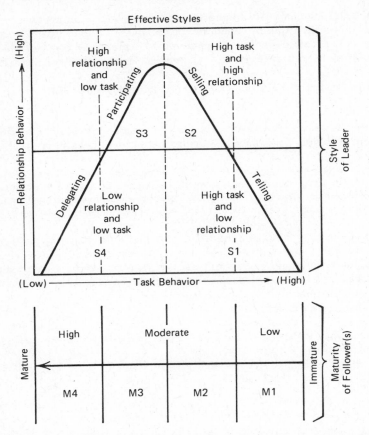

FIGURE 7-1. DESIGNATIONS FOR STYLES OF LEADERSHIP AND MATURITY LEVELS OF FOL-
LOWER(S).

Adapted from Hersey, P. & Blanchard, K.H. *Management of organizational behavior: Utilizing human resources*
(4th ed.). Copyright © 1982, p. 152. Reprinted by permission of Prentice-Hall, Inc., Englewood Cliffs, N.J.

can be perceived as interested only in short-term task completion and appears to
have no confidence in others.

Effective use of this leadership style frequently occurs in emergency or high stress
situations. The person in charge during a major disaster must be able to give clear
directions in order to increase the effectiveness of all persons in accomplishing the
necessary tasks. However, a charge nurse who consistently tells the staff who will take
care of which patients and in which order in all situations is likely to be perceived as
"autocratic" and becomes ineffective.

High-Task/High-Relationship

"Selling" may be applied to a high-task/high-relationship style since most of the direction
is still provided through one-way communication with attempts to aid followers to buy
into decisions through two-way communication that provides socioemotional support.
This style thus satisfies the needs of the group for both task structure and personal
support. However, this style may also be perceived as providing too much structure or
wasting time in personal conversations.

High-task/high-relationship leadership style may be used effectively during the initial stages of a planned change. A team leader who wishes to change the method of patient assignments might combine explaining the new system and requiring the staff to use it (task behavior) with explaining the reasons for the change, asking for evaluation of the new system, and modifying it based on suggestions from the staff (relationship behaviors).

High-Relationship/Low-Task

The leadership style that allows the leaders and followers to "participate" in decision making is a high-relationship/low-task style. This style is characterized by two-way communication and extensive facilitating behavior from the leader. It assumes the followers have the knowledge and ability to accomplish the task. It is often called a "democratic" style. An effective leader using this style appears to have implicit trust in the group and is appropriately concerned with developing their talents. In situations where this style is ineffective, the leader may be perceived as more interested in maintaining harmony than in accomplishing tasks.

Examples of effective use of this style include the clinical area coordinator, in either a nursing program or a patient care agency, who actively seeks suggestions for change from the group and provides sufficient time for the entire group to make the decisions as to when, where, and how a new procedure will be implemented.

Low-Relationship/Low-Task

Low-relationship/low-task behavior reflects a situation in which followers assume responsibilities for their own functioning and the leader offers only general supervision. This style may be referred to as "delegating." A leader who effectively delegates may be seen as appropriately permitting the group to make decisions and rarely plays an important part in social interactions. In other situations, a leader using this style may be seen as having abdicated his or her leadership role, being uninvolved and uncaring about either the group or the task.

Self-Analysis and Development of Leadership Styles

As the central figure in the leadership process, the potential nurse leader must be willing to engage in critical self-analysis to identify his or her potential strengths and limitations. Although many physical, social, and personality characteristics cannot be changed, their impact on leadership effectiveness can be enhanced or minimized through conscious effort. Awareness of one's value system, a realistic appraisal of skills and abilities, and an understanding of one's perceptual set of self, others, and the role is vital to becoming an effective leader. Such analysis is an on-going process, but usually begins in the educational process in professional nursing programs. Faculty members and student peers are excellent initial sources for validation of individual attempts to identify these aspects of one's self and how they relate to total effectiveness. Colleagues and superiors in the work setting continue to be the source of information and feedback most useful in providing input regarding growth and development of leadership skills and abilities. Many organizations are also beginning to provide group training activities which enhance the self-awareness of employees.

The identification of the usual leadership style of the potential leader is also necessary. The extent to which one normally engages in task behaviors and relationship behaviors is a significant factor in determining the range of styles available to the potential leader. Although most people exhibit one basic style of leadership, this range can be extended and may include all four leadership styles previously described. A tool for identifying leadership style based on situational leadership theory is the *LEAD-Self* developed at the Center for Leadership Studies (Hersey & Blanchard, 1977).

The development of leadership skills is a continuing process. Each educational experience provides additional information. Every work setting offers challenges to test new skills. No single leadership style is appropriate for all situations. No leader is effective in every group. The goal is to continue to develop a broad range of leadership behaviors that will enhance the likelihood of becoming effective in a variety of settings.

Task-Relevant Maturity

Since any leadership style may be either effective or ineffective, attention needs to be directed to the other variables in the leadership process. Attempts to identify key variables relating to followers, the situation, the communication process, and goals led to the concept of the task-relevant maturity of the followers as a pivotal variable. It is important to emphasize that maturity as used in situational leadership theory does not refer to either the chronological maturity or to the total maturity of any individual or group. Hersey and Blanchard (1977) state:

> All persons tend to be more or less mature in relation to a specific task, function, or objective that a leader is attempting to accomplish through their efforts. (p. 161)

Task-relevant maturity should be considered only in relation to a specific task to be performed.

Three components of task-relevant maturity have been identified. These are achievement motivation, willingness and ability to assume responsibility, and previous education and/or experience.

Achievement Motivation

Researchers have found that persons with high achievement motivation have the following characteristics:

1. Persons with high achievement motivation prefer to be involved in situations where they can take personal responsibility for the outcomes of their efforts. They want to control their own destinies rather than leaving things to luck, fate, or chance. They like to make independent judgments based on their own evaluation and experiences rather than rely on the opinions of others.

2. Persons with high achievement motivation are interested in excellence for its own sake rather than for the rewards it brings. Money in itself is only a way of "keeping score" and it alone will not make high nAch (need achievement) people work harder. They are interested in working with experts in the field rather than friends. They evaluate roles on the basis of the opportunity to achieve excellence rather than for prestige.

3. Persons with high achievement motivation set challenging but realistic goals. They are moderate risk takers, neither engaging in tasks that are doomed to failure or guaranteed to be successful.

4. Persons with high achievement motivation are more inclined to plan for the future than ones with low achievement motivation. They show greater anticipation for the future. They seldom see themselves as having enough time to get everything done. In order to keep track of their progress toward their goals, they seek, and *use*, immediate, regular, concrete feedback from those they respect (Alschuler, 1973, pp. 24–25).

From the description just given, it can be assumed that many professional nurses possess a fairly high achievement motivation. This is particularly true in nursing education settings and among nursing service personnel who are career-oriented.

Willingness and Ability to Assume Responsibility

Willingness to take responsibility refers to a psychological component of maturity while *ability* to take responsibility refers to the technical competence of the follower in relation to the specific task. The following chart offers some aid in evaluating this dimension (Lyle, 1976, p. 109):

If a Follower Is:	*The Maturity Level Is:*
Unwilling and Unable	Low
Willing but Unable	Low to Moderate
Unwilling but Able	Moderate to High
Willing and Able	High

A faculty member who consistently writes poor test questions (technical competence) and refuses to seek consultation (willingness) is an example of a person with a low maturity level on this component. An example of a person with a moderate to high level would be a staff nurse who is skilled in determining staffing patterns but prefers not to assume that responsibility.

Education and/or Experience

Education and/or experience must be assessed in relation to the specific task. While it could easily be assumed that the person with more education or greater experience would be more mature in any situation, this is not always true. The judgment must be made always in reference to the specific task. One example might be the nursing service coordinator with graduate preparation in psychiatric nursing who may not be skilled in the monitoring of cardiopulmonary functions. On the other hand, advanced education and more experience frequently form the basis for a greater level of maturity in interpersonal relationships and situations requiring judgment based on a variety of experiences.

Assessment of Task-Relevant Maturity

The three components of task-relevant maturity—achievement motivation, willingness and ability to assume responsibility, and previous education and/or experience—have been placed into two categories, job maturity and psychological maturity:

> (1) *job maturity*—ability and technical knowledge to do the task, and (2) *psychological maturity*—feeling of self-confidence and self-respect about oneself as an individual. (Hersey & Blanchard, 1977, p. 163)

Job maturity dimensions include past job experience, job knowledge, understanding of job requirements, problem-solving ability, ability to take responsibility, meeting job deadlines, and follow-through. Psychological maturity dimensions include willingness to take responsibility, achievement motivation, commitment, persistence, work attitude, initiative, and independence (Hambleton, Blanchard, & Hersey, 1977). On the basis of a composite evaluation of the follower(s) within the situation, a judgment can be made on the anticipated level of task-relevant maturity.

Selection of Appropriate Leadership Style

Situational leadership theory proposes that the most effective leadership style will vary depending upon the task-relevant maturity of the followers. Four different leadership styles and four corresponding levels of follower maturity have been identified:

Task-Relevant Maturity	Appropriate Leadership Style
Low	High task and low relationship
Low–Moderate	High task and high relationship
High–Moderate	High relationship and high task
High	Low relationship and low task

This designation of effective leadership styles is based on the suggestion made by Korman (Hersey & Blanchard, 1977) that the relationship between leader behavior and other variables is a curvilinear one. This relationship can be seen in Figure 7-1.

The selection of the appropriate leadership style always begins with the assessment of the task-relevant maturity level of the follower or group in the specific task. It must also be remembered that both the leadership style and follower maturity are not easily definable categories, but shadings along a continuum. It is also necessary to remember that while follower maturity usually increases over a period of time, a variety of reasons may cause a decrease. The leader must be able to change style with appropriate timing as the follower maturity either increases or decreases along the continuum.

In addition, the leader may have to assess the maturity level of the group as a group as well as the maturity level of individuals within the group. This is particularly true when the group interacts frequently within the same area, such as a nursing unit or an educational building. The leader may find that the total faculty or unit staff may be at one level of maturity while individuals within the group are at various maturity levels. For example, a curriculum committee may function at a moderately low maturity level in relation to the writing of program objectives as a group. However, one or more members may have a very high task-relevant maturity level while others are very low. This does not necessarily indicate that the group will function at the average maturity level of members, only that the group level may be different from that of any single individual within the group. Therefore, the leader may need to behave differently within the group as a whole than with individuals in one-on-one situations.

USING SITUATIONAL LEADERSHIP THEORY

The purpose of any theory is to provide a useful framework to explain the phenomena experienced in a situation and to predict potential for success of proposed changes within the situation. Situational leadership theory provides such a framework for determining the outcomes of the leadership process.

Assessment/Input

The initial step in the utilization of any theory is the assessment of the phenomena. In the use of situational leadership theory, this assessment involves identifying the characteristics of the leader, including leadership style(s); characteristics of the followers, specifically the task-relevant maturity level of both the group and individuals within the group; the situation; the usual communication process(es); and the goal(s) of the organization and individuals within the organization. It is often helpful when using the theory initially to complete a written assessment. A sample form is given in Figure 7-2.

FIGURE 7-2. PLANNING SHEET FOR USE OF SITUATIONAL LEADERSHIP THEORY.

IDENTIFIED TASK

I. Assessment
   A. Leader
      1. Individual characteristics
         a. Physical
         b. Social
         c. Personality
         d. Values/perception
      2. Leadership style
         a. Task behaviors
         b. Relationship behaviors
   B. Followers
      1. Expectations
      2. Task relevant maturity
         a. Job maturity dimensions
         b. Psychological maturity dimensions
   C. Situation
      1. Organization
         a. Formal structure
         b. Written philosophy/policies/procedures
         c. Informal structure
      2. Superiors and associates
         a. Expectations
         b. Leadership style(s)
      3. Job demands—structure
      4. Time frame
      5. Resources
   D. Communication process
      1. How do people communicate?
         a. Written
         b. Oral
      2. To whom do people communicate?
         a. Formal chain of communication
         b. Informal chain of communication
      3. When do people communicate?
         a. Routine
         b. Emergency

FIGURE 7-2. (*continued*)

    E. Goals
       1. Organization
         a. Task achievement
         b. System maintenance
       2. Subsystem
         a. Task achievement
         b. System maintenance
       3. Group/individual
         a. Task achievement
         b. System maintenance
II. Implementation
    A. Task-relevant maturity level of group
    B. Appropriate leadership style
       1. Specific task behaviors
       2. Specific relationship behaviors
III. Evaluation
    A. Achievement of goals
       1. Organization
       2. Subsystem
       3. Group/individual
    B. Change in task-relevant maturity level
    C. Evidence of job satisfaction

Implementation of Leadership Style/Throughput

Based on the assessment, the leader can select an appropriate leadership style, that is, a style most likely to be effective in the specific situation with the identified group of followers. Several factors need to be considered in the selection of the leadership style. First, is it a comfortable style for the leader? For instance, many nurses find either of the low relationship styles uncomfortable because of their intensive education in interpersonal relationships. A second factor is the time frame. As mentioned earlier, some situations require immediate action by the group that limits the type of interaction between leader and followers. Third, are the goals primarily task achievement or system maintenance? Goals that are oriented toward task achievement may require more task behaviors in the leadership style, while goals that are primarily system maintenance may require more relationship behaviors. Finally, the task-relevant maturity level of the individuals and group will influence the effectiveness of the style.

When the leadership style that seems most appropriate has been selected, the leader is then able to implement that style through the conscious use of identified task and relationship behaviors. Writing the specific behaviors to be used on a form such as that presented in Figure 7-2 will provide an awareness of how the leadership style is being implemented.

Evaluation/Output

Identification of the results of the interactions between leader and followers is essential. This evaluation should include such factors as: achievement of goals, both organizational and individual; growth of followers; and job satisfaction of both leader and followers. The results of this evaluation then become the new input factors for the assessment of the changed situation.

Case Example of Situational Leadership Theory in a Nursing Setting

The identified *leader* is a registered nurse, (Miss Smith) recently graduated from a baccalaureate program who is assigned to be team leader on one wing of a 60-bed medical unit. Miss Smith has no outstanding physical characteristics, has been perceived as possessing excellent clinical skills by her instructors, and has achieved a high scholastic average in her courses (refer to Fig. 7-3).

The team (*followers*) consists of one registered nurse, Mr. Brown, and one licensed practical nurse, Mrs. Jones. Mr. Brown graduated from an associate degree program several years ago and has been working on the unit consistently since that time. Mrs. Jones has been a licensed practical nurse for 15 years and has worked most of that time in her current position. Both team members are perceived by other staff to be competent in their roles and are used to deciding their own assignments.

The nursing unit (*situation*) is divided into four teams with responsibility for 15 patients, many of whom have acute medical illnesses. The philosophy of the unit speaks vaguely to "providing total nursing care," but the emphasis appears to be on swift completion of tasks. Generally, each team leader assigns an equal number of patients to each member of the team, as well as personally assuming the responsibility for all medications.

Each team receives a brief report from the previous shift and spends approximately 5 minutes reviewing the assignments (*communication*). The team leaders communicate with other members of the team only when a change in orders is received or a problem arises. No formal evaluation of care is conducted and it is assumed that everything is completed by the end of the shift.

The short-range *goals* of the unit seem to be to provide adequate care in the least amount of time. No other unit goals seem identifiable. The hospital has stated a long-range goal of implementing primary nursing in all units within the next 5 years. Miss Smith has identified her own short-range goal as developing competence as both a caregiver and a team leader. Her long-range goals include graduate study.

During her orientation to this unit, Miss Smith spends much of her time identifying the variables and assessing the task-relevant maturity of Mr. Brown and Mrs. Jones. She determines that both of her team members have low to moderate achievement motivation, are technically competent and willing to take responsibility for the direct physical care of their patients, and have both the educational preparation and experience to provide the direct physical care needed by most of the clients on the assigned wing. However, neither Mr. Brown nor Mrs. Jones is able or willing to provide the patient teaching frequently required prior to discharge.

FIGURE 7-3. SAMPLE OF PLANNING SHEET BASED ON CASE STUDY.

IDENTIFIED TASK: Determining patient assignments to allow for patient teaching.

I. Assessment
   A. Leader—Miss Smith
      1. Individual characteristics
         a. Physical—no outstanding characteristics
         b. Social—college graduate, high scholastic average; excellent clinical skills
         c. Personality—?
         d. Values/perceptions—high value placed on patient teaching; fairly positive perception of team members
      2. Leadership style—not given
   B. Followers
      1. Expectations—shared responsibility for team assignments; usually an equal number of patients; team leader to give medications
      2. Task-relevant maturity—moderate
         a. Job maturity dimensions
            (1) Mr. Brown—moderate to high
            (2) Mrs. Jones—moderate to high
            (3) Group—moderate to high
         b. Psychological maturity dimensions
            (1) Mr. Brown—moderate
            (2) Mrs. Jones—low to moderate
            (3) Group—low to moderate
   C. Situation
      1. Organization
         a. Formal structure—team nursing model
         b. Written philosophy/policies/procedures—vague; "total patient care"
         c. Informal structure—cohesive team; emphasis on tasks
      2. Superiors and associates—not known
      3. Job demands—fairly structured; moderate interaction of group
      4. Time frame—presently 5 minutes at beginning of shift; no apparent restriction
      5. Resources—apparently adequate
   D. Communication Process
      1. How do people communicate?
         a. Written—not specified; probably an assignment sheet
         b. Oral—report from previous shift; changes in orders or problems

2. To whom do people communicate?
   a. Formal chain of communication—team leader to members during conference, when orders are changed and when problems arise. Members to leader when problems arise.
   b. Informal chain of communication—not known
3. When do people communicate?
   a. Routine—5 minute conference at beginning of shift
   b. Emergency—when orders are changed; problems

E. Goals
   1. Organization
      a. Task achievement—implementing primary nursing
      b. System maintenance—not specified
   2. Subsystem
      a. Task achievement—provision of adequate care in the least amount of time
      b. System maintenance—none specified
   3. Group/Individual
      a. Task achievement
         (1) Mr. Brown—unknown
         (2) Mrs. Jones—unknown
         (3) Miss Smith—develop competence as a care-giver and team leader; start patient teaching prior to discharge
         (4) Group—unknown
      b. System Maintenance
         (1) Mr. Brown—unknown
         (2) Mrs. Jones—unknown
         (3) Miss Smith—graduate study
         (4) Group—unknown

II. Implementation
   A. Task-relevant maturity level of group—moderate
   B. Appropriate leadership style—low-task/high-relationship
      1. Specific task behaviors
         a. Scheduling longer conferences
         b. Tries out new ideas (changes method of patient assignments)
      2. Specific relationship behaviors
         a. Explains activities to subordinates (discusses rationale)
         b. Puts suggestion made by group into action
         c. Provides positive feedback

FIGURE 7-3. (continued)

  d. Looks out for personal welfare (talks with Mr. Brown about career goals)
  e. Finds time to listen to team members
III. Evaluation
  A. Achievement of goals
    1. Organization—positive movement to meeting this goal
    2. Subsystem—slightly changed
    3. Group/Individual
      a. Miss Smith's are being met
      b. Other members goals are being clarified
  B. Change in task-relevant maturity level—appears to be in moderate to high range
  C. Evidence of job satisfaction—not specified

On the basis of this assessment, Miss Smith determines that a change in the method of assignments should be considered in order for the team leader to have time to implement the necessary patient teaching. However, before such a change can occur, she must establish herself as a competent and effective leader. Having identified that the level of task-relevant maturity of Mr. Brown and Mrs. Jones in relation to direct physical care is in the moderate range (see Fig. 7-1) she decides to use a low-task/high-relationship style in determining work assignments. She lengthens slightly the time used for the morning conference to discuss rationale for the assignment of patients requiring teaching prior to discharge and elicits the suggestion of a slight shift in the number of patients assigned to each of the team members. She also makes a conscious effort to provide feedback to her team members regarding her appreciation of their competence in giving direct care.

As the relationship between team leader and members develops, Miss Smith begins to talk with Mr. Brown about his career goals and to share articles relative to specific clients assigned to the team. When Mr. Brown requests help in developing a teaching plan for one of his clients, Miss Smith decides to use a more task-oriented leadership style and provides very specific directions as well as praise for the interest and effort. Mrs. Jones, meanwhile, is being encouraged to value her contributions in direct patient care to the team without being expected to be involved in patient teaching. Miss Smith spends some time with the licensed practical nurse, helping her to discuss her feelings about the "hard work" versus "just talking to the patients." Eventually, the team begins to discuss daily assignments on the basis of total patient needs, rather than number of patients. Each team member begins to assume sole responsibility for the direct physical care of some patients and shared responsibility for the total care of all patients. Miss Smith has accomplished her goal; the team is one step nearer to understanding the hospital's goal of primary nursing; and each member of the team retains a positive self-image. Miss Smith has acted as an effective leader.

SUMMARY

Research in the field of leadership has focused increasingly on the interactions among the variables in the process. These variables have been defined as: the leader, the followers, the situation, the process of communication, and the goals.

The behavior of the *leader*, his or her leadership style, is a blend of physical, social, and personality factors combined with the values, skills, abilities, and perceptions of the individual. Leadership style is a combination of task behaviors and relationship behaviors. The expectations of the *followers*, as well as their task-relevant maturity, greatly influence the leadership process. Organizational structure, immediate superiors and associates, job demands, time frame, and resources are elements of the *situation* that provide some parameters for the leader. The *process of communication* within the group helps to define the effectiveness of the leadership style. The achievement of *goals* becomes the measure of effectiveness in the leadership process.

Situational leadership theory provides a framework to examine the interactions of the variables and to predict the leadership style most likely to be effective in a given situation. Using task-relevant maturity of the followers as a key concept, this theory suggests a specific leadership style that seems to be most effective with a group at a given task maturity level. However, both leadership style and task maturity are not easily definable categories, but shadings along a continuum.

REFERENCES

Alschuler, A. *Developing achievement motivation in adolescents.* Englewood Cliffs, N.J.: Education Technology Publications, 1973.

Argyris, C. *Interpersonal competence and organizational effectiveness.* Homewood, Ill.: Dorsey Press and Richard D. Irwin, Inc., 1962.

Blake, R., & Mouton, J. *The new managerial grid.* Houston: Gulf, 1978.

Fiedler, F.E. *A theory of leadership effectiveness.* New York: McGraw-Hill, 1967.

Halpin, A. *The leadership behavior of school superintendents.* Chicago: Midwest Administration Center, The University of Chicago, 1959.

Hambleton, R.K., Blanchard, K.H., & Hersey, P. *Maturity scale: Self rating form.* Escondido, Calif.: Center for Leadership Studies, 1977.

Hersey, P., & Blanchard, K.H. *Management of organizational behavior: Utilizing human resources.* (3rd ed.). Englewood Cliffs, N.J.: Prentice-Hall, 1977.

Hersey, P., & Blanchard, K. *Management of organizational behavior: Utilizing human resources* (4th ed.), Englewood Cliffs, N.J.: Prentice-Hall, 1982.

Herzberg, F., Mausner, B., & Snyderman, B. *The motivation for work.* (2nd ed.). New York: Wiley, 1959.

Likert, R. *The human organization.* New York: McGraw-Hill, 1967.

Lyle, B. Leadership and strategic planning for higher education: toward more effective university management (Doctoral Dissertation, University of Massachusetts, 1976). *Dissertation Abstracts International,* 1977, *37,* 5497A. (University Microfilms No. 77-6383.)

McGregor, D. *The human side of enterprise.* New York: McGraw-Hill, 1960.

Stinson, J., & Johnson, T. The path-goal theory of leadership: A partial test and suggested refinement. *Academy of Management Journal,* 1975, *18* (2), 242–252.

Stodgill, R. *Handbook of leadership*. New York: Free Press, 1974.

Stodgill, R., & Coons, E. (Eds.). *Leader behavior: Its description and measurement* (Research Monograph No. 88). Columbus: Bureau of Business Research, The Ohio State University, 1957.

Tannenbaum, R., & Schmidt, W. How to choose a leadership pattern. *Harvard Business Review*, 1958, *36*(2), 95–102.

Yura, H., Ozimek, D., & Walsh, M. *Nursing leadership: Theory and process*. New York: Appleton-Century-Crofts, 1976.

BIBLIOGRAPHY

Anderson, L., & Fiedler, L. The effect of participatory and supervisory leadership on group creativity. *Journal of Applied Psychology*, 1964, *48*, 277–286.

Anderson, R. Activity preferences and leadership behavior of head nurses. *Nursing Research*, 1964, *13*, Part I, 239–243; Part II, 333–337.

Bailey, J., & Claus, K. *Decision making in nursing*. St. Louis: C.V. Mosby Co., 1975.

Bennis, W. Leadership theory and administrative behavior: The problem of authority. *Administration Science Quarterly*, 1959, *5*, 259–301.

Diers, D. Leadership problems and possibilities in nursing. *American Journal of Nursing*, 1972, *72*, 1447.

Douglass, L. and Bevis, E. *Nursing leadership in action* (2nd ed.). St. Louis: C.V. Mosby Co., 1974.

Drucker, P. *The effective executive*. New York: Harper and Row, 1966.

Ingmire, A., & Taylor, C. *The effectiveness of a leadership program in nursing*. Boulder, Colo.: Western Interstate Commission on Higher Education, 1967.

Kelly, W. Psychological prediction of leadership in nursing. *Nursing Research*, 1974, *23*, 38–42.

Leininger, M. The leadership crisis in nursing: A critical problem and challenge. *Journal of Nursing Administration*, March–April 1974, *4*, 28–34.

Pryer, M., & Distefano, M. Perceptions of leadership behavior, job satisfaction and internal-external control across three nursing levels. *Nursing Research*, 1971, *20*, 534–541.

Schurr, M. A comparative study of leadership in industry and the nursing profession, Part 1. *International Nursing Review*, 1969, *16*(1), 16–29.

White, H. Perceptions of leadership styles by nurses in supervisory positions. *Journal of Nursing Administration*, 1971, *1*(2), 44–51.

CHAPTER 8
THE NURSING MANAGEMENT
AND SUPERVISION PROCESSES

Leadership is the process by which an individual influences the behavior of others toward goal achievement. Management and supervision, on the other hand, are administrative processes involved with the execution of policies and regulations of a specific setting. Griffiths (1959) proposed four assumptions:

1. Administration is a generalized type of behavior found in all human organizations.
2. Administration is the process of directing and controlling life in a social organization.
3. The specific function of administration is to develop and regulate the decision-making process in the most effective manner possible.
4. The administration works with groups or with individuals with a group referent, not with individuals as such (pp. 71–74)

One type of hierarchy that exists within organizations is that of *administration*. The roles and functions of administration are identified into hierarchial levels beginning with the Board of Directors and moving downward to the individual employee. This hierarchy is illustrated in Figure 8-1.

Top-level management or executive positions are those that involve responsibility for the functioning of the total organization. Persons in these positions usually interact directly with the controlling body and may have direct influence on policy decisions. In health service agencies, these positions are the hospital administrator, the director of nursing service, and the chief of the medical staff. In larger schools of nursing, the dean or director may function in an executive position.

Administrators or middle-level managers usually direct the activities for several units and are responsible for the implementation of policy and procedures within those units. In hospitals and schools of nursing with traditional organizational structure, persons functioning in this level of administration are usually called supervisors, department chairs, or program directors.

First-level management is concerned with the direct control of the work environment and the supervision of the actual performance of work. In hospital settings, persons at this level may be either a head nurse or a team leader, while in schools of nursing, the persons in charge of single courses may be considered first-level managers.

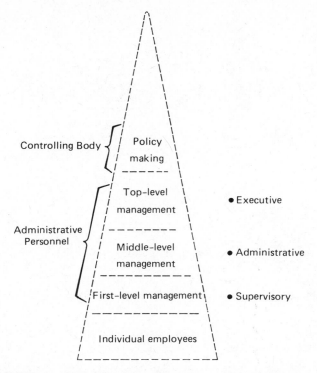

FIGURE 8-1. ADMINISTRATIVE HIERARCHY IN ORGANIZATIONS.

NURSING MANAGEMENT AND SUPERVISION

To many people, the terms *administration, management,* and *supervision* seem synonymous and carry negative connotations. Frequently, employees and management personnel are placed in adversarial positions. It becomes vital, therefore, for professional nurses to understand the responsibilities and functions of persons in management and supervisory positions and the purposes that these levels of administration serve within the organization.

Management

Within the systems theory framework, management operates as the mechanism that regulates and adjusts the system to produce optimum goal achievement (Magula, 1982, p. 30). *Management* is defined as the process by which organizational goals and objectives are accomplished through the use of technical, interpersonal, and conceptual skills to carry out defined functions.

While leadership may be exhibited by many persons within a group, a person may be considered a manager only if he or she has and uses formal authority to organize, direct, and control responsible subordinates (Tannenbaum, Weschler, & Massarik, 1961). Management is viewed as the control of the process of executing given policy. This is differentiated from the functions of administration in formulating and determining policy.

Management requires accomplishing a task delegated by a higher authority and involves processes necessary in working through subordinates. While an integral part of administration, the efforts of the manager are directed to the attainment, rather than the determination, of the goals of the organization.

Supervision

Supervision suggests a dynamic process in which the subordinate is encouraged to participate in activities designed to both meet organizational goals and aid in the development of the subordinate as an employee and a person.

Bowers and Seashore (1969) suggest that a greater emphasis on planning and performing specialized skill tasks in the supervisory role becomes the differentiating characteristic. This emphasis includes behavior that provides communication regarding policy and goals, delegates authority, provides generalized instruction, and supports personal and group growth and achievement. As noted earlier, administration deals with groups and with being the delegated manager of a group. At the supervisory level, one deals with the individual employee. Thus, while the scope of impact of the supervisor may be narrower than that of the manager, the supervisor is more directly involved with the persons performing the tasks. In large agencies, the supervisor role may be designated as a team leader or charge nurse, while in many smaller units the head nurse may function as both supervisor and manager.

Management and Supervision Skills

Three areas of skills—technical, interpersonal, and conceptual (Katz, 1955)—have been identified as necessary in carrying out managerial and supervisory tasks:

Technical skill—use of knowledge, procedures, technique, and equipment to perform specific tasks that can be learned through education, training, and experience.
Interpersonal skill—effective use of leadership and motivation theories to work with and through people.
Conceptual skill—knowledge and understanding of the total organizational system and the interrelationships between various subsystems and the ability to make decisions based on this knowledge.

Managers at each level must possess skills in all three areas, but the appropriate mix differs as the position in the hierarchy changes. Figure 8-2 illustrates this change.

Technical skill is essential in first-level management or supervisory positions since persons in these positions not only oversee the day-to-day work, but frequently are responsible for training new employees. Persons at the executive level, however, may not need to be able to perform all the procedures, but must be able to understand how all the functions are interrelated. Interpersonal skills are essential at all levels.

FUNCTIONS WITHIN NURSING MANAGEMENT AND SUPERVISION PROCESSES

Various components of management and supervision have been delineated by numerous theorists. However, the most common listings include elements of goal setting, planning, organizing, staffing, budgeting, motivating, delegating, directing, control-

Skills needed

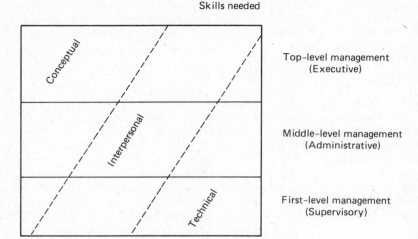

Top-level management
(Executive)

Middle-level management
(Administrative)

First-level management
(Supervisory)

FIGURE 8-2. SKILLS NEEDED AT VARIOUS MANAGEMENT LEVELS.

ling, and evaluation (Donovan, 1975; Hersey & Blanchard, 1977; Longest, 1976; Yura, Ozimek, & Walsh, 1976). Each of these functions will be discussed as it relates to first-level and midlevel managers and supervisors.

Goal Setting

Goals represent a desired aim or condition toward which one is willing to work. Organizational goals are usually extremely broad. In private industry, the goal may be to manufacture a product that will make a profit for the company. Universities usually state their goals in terms of providing teaching, research, and service to society. Hospitals may state their goals in terms of provision of adequate care and treatment of patients.

Organizational goals can be divided into two categories: those that are primarily task achievement or output goals and those that are primarily system maintenance or throughput goals. Figure 8-3 provides examples of the two categories of organizational goals for health care agencies and universities.

Developing Organizational and Unit Goals and Objectives

Magula (1982, p. 24) defines goals as "descriptions of aspirations which represent fruition of the ideals established by values." Because goals are, by nature, value-laden as well as broad, they must be restructured into more tangible statements, the objectives. Organizational goals are usually articulated by the official controlling body; for example, the board of directors. Organizational objectives may be developed by the executive officers with input from others within the organization so as to give the specificity needed for goal achievement. Organizational objectives deal with time, place, quantity, and quality of change in persons or things. Units within an organization may also have objectives of their own. These, however, are subsidiary to the overall objectives and must be consistent with them. They are established to complement the

	Task Achievement Goals	System Maintenance Goals
Health Care Agencies	Provision of adequate care to clients	Recruitment and retention of adequate personnel; maintenance of a positive public image
Universities	Graduation of established students (teaching); reports of new knowledge through publications (research); provision of consultation to community agencies (service).	Effective faculty governance unit; provision of and support for research; provision of recognition for community service.

FIGURE 8-3. EXAMPLES OF GOALS OF HEALTH CARE AGENCIES AND UNIVERSITIES.

organizational objectives and give direction to the specific unit. Achievement of unit objectives contribute to the achievement of organizational goals (Rakich, Longest, & O'Donovan, 1977). Table 8-1 provides an example of the hierarchy of objectives within a health care agency.

Organizational objectives for both health care agencies and schools of nursing are usually set within the context of a written statement of philosophy and purpose. The philosophy states the significant beliefs that influence the goals of the organization or unit while the purpose defines its reason for existence. Other types of statements that influence the development of objectives are policies that define responsibilities and prescribe general actions in specific situations and procedures that describe specific actions to be taken in reaching objectives. Understanding of these documents precede any attempt to develop new objectives for an organization or unit.

Development of objectives that provide adequate direction to the activities of the organization or unit may initially be an extremely time-consuming activity. Objectives should be realistic yet challenging, explicit yet flexible, brief yet comprehensive. They should include the following information:

1. The activity to be done or change desired
2. The persons responsible for completion of the activity
3. The time frame in which the activity is to be finished
4. An acceptable outcome, in measurable terms if possible

Before adoption as objectives to be achieved by the organization or unit, they should be reviewed in reference to their contribution to overall goals, their relationship to acceptable standards, their realism and feasibility in terms of resources and time, and their priority of importance (Douglass & Bevis, 1979).

While organizational and unit objectives may be articulated initially by the executive or manager responsible, participative goal setting should be encouraged. It is perhaps easier for a head nurse or supervisor to write the objectives for the unit, but without the participation of the staff the objectives will rarely become unit objectives. They tend to remain the objectives the head nurse or supervisor has developed and little commitment exists to see that they are achieved. The time involved in meeting with all personnel who will be involved in the activities designated by the objectives will be balanced by the benefits derived from involved personnel. Persons involved in the

TABLE 8-1. EXAMPLE OF HIERARCHY OF OBJECTIVES

Organizational Goal	Organizational Objective	Unit Objective (Nursing Service)	Subunit Objective (Medical Unit)
Provision of adequate care to clients	Provision of direct care to all patients 24 hours/day	Develop program for providing quality nursing care to all patients: 1. Establish written policies and procedures 2. Establish system for development, implementation, and evaluation of a written care plan for each patient 3. Staff each unit with sufficient qualified personnel	Provide quality nursing care to patients with specific medical diagnoses: 1. Implement written policies and procedures based on standards of practice 2. Develop, implement, and evaluate a written care plan for each patient 3. Identify number of professional vs. non-professional hours of care needed for each patient and request appropriate personnel 4. Assign professional and nonprofessional personnel in accordance with patient needs

development of organizational and unit objectives have the opportunity to modify the organization to meet personal goals as well as to gain an understanding of their individual role within the organization.

The clarity of goal statements and the degree to which they are relevant to the employees determine to a large degree the extent to which goals and objectives will be achieved. McGregor (1960) discusses the integration of individual and organizational goals as the extent to which individuals and groups perceive their own goals as being satisfied by the achievement of organizational goals. For this integration to occur, both individual and organizational goals and objectives must be communicated through the management hierarchy. For example, the head nurse who knows that one objective of the hospital is to increase cost effectiveness can work with a staff nurse interested in research to collect necessary data for testing less costly staffing patterns that do not erode quality of care.

Management by Objectives
Management by objectives (MBO) is both a philosophy and a method of management. Introduced by Drucker in the 1950s (Drucker, 1954), the concept has been popularized and further refined by several other authors, notably Odiorne (1965) and Humble (1967). Management by objectives is defined as:

> a process whereby the superior and the subordinate managers of an enterprise jointly identify its common goals, define each individual's major areas of responsibility in terms of the results expected of him, and use these measures as guides for operating the unit and assessing the contribution of each of its members. (Odiorne, 1965, pp. 55–56)

The purpose of MBO is to minimize efficiency problems in reaching task-achievement goals by integrating organizational and individual goals and building intergroup team-work at all levels of management. System maintenance goals are also reached through utilization of information input and negative feedback.

Six steps are involved in the method of MBO (Odiorne, 1965):

1. Goals and objectives for the organization or unit are jointly developed by the manager of the unit and his or her superior.
2. Objectives for each individual within the unit are developed jointly between the individual and the manager of the unit.
3. All participants undertake the achievement of the planned objectives.
4. Interim reviews of performance occur.
5. Near the end of the specified time period, the actual performance of individuals is measured against their goals. Achievements and areas of lack of achievement are discussed by the individual and his or her superior.
6. The cycle is repeated for the next time cycle.

Figure 8-4 illustrates the process in detail.

It must be kept in mind that management by objectives is more than a method; it is also a philosophy of management. Implicit in MBO are the beliefs that all individuals within the organization are willing and able to participate; that individual goals will support and enhance the achievement of organizational goals; and that recognition of and input into organizational goals and objectives will encourage both greater task accomplishment and higher morale at the production level.

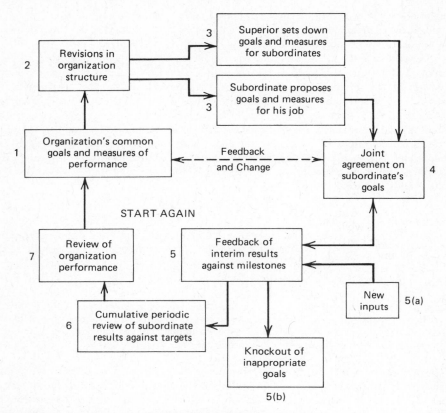

FIGURE 8-4. THE CYCLE OF MANAGEMENT BY OBJECTIVES.
Adapted from Odiorne G. *Management by objectives: A system of managerial leadership.* Copyright © 1965 by Pitman Learning, Inc., Belmont, Calif. Used with permission.

There are many case studies in recent literature detailing the successes and failures of MBO as a method of management (Bell, 1980; Frank & Haugh, 1981; Golightly, 1979; Jackson, 1981; Levinson & LaMonica, 1980). The successes seem to underscore the acceptance of the philosophical stance of MBO and to emphasize the need to establish realistic time frames for the implementation of the method. Such a time frame includes time for attitudinal changes of both superiors and subordinates and an internalization of the philosophy by all personnel involved. In cases where MBO has had limited success or seemed to fail, the major difficulties have included attempts to deal with too many objectives, failure to invest the necessary time for interpersonal goal setting, focus on future goals with concurrent neglect of necessary daily activities, and misunderstanding of the need for flexibility within individual and subunit objectives.

Management by objectives may be an extremely useful method by which to accomplish the functions of goal setting and achievement. However, it is not a panacea to be implemented without a great deal of thought, planning, and experience on the part of the total administrative structure of an organization. While some aspects, such as discussing organization and unit goals with personnel and encouraging subordinates to develop individual goals for a specific time period, may be implemented by a first-level or midlevel manager in isolation, the success of both the method and the philosophy of MBO rests on the support of all individuals within the organization.

Values Clarification and Ethical Considerations

Organizations are formed to accomplish goals that cannot be accomplished by single individuals. Therefore, the goals of organizations must in some way relate to the values of the society in which they exist. Furthermore, such organizations and their administrators are expected to develop and pursue identified goals in an ethical manner.

Webster's Third New International Dictionary (1971) defines values and ethics as follows:

Value—relative worth, utility or importance; status in a scale of preferences; something intrinsically desirable.

Ethics—discipline dealing with standards of good and bad or right and wrong; principles of conduct; standards of professional characteristics or ideals.

As indicated by the definition, values exist as a hierarchy and represent those things desired by an individual or group. Blum (1967) states that values provide a stimulus to goal setting as well as posing criteria by which the results may be judged. Even when some values are held in common, it is unlikely for any two persons or organizations to have the same hierarchy of values, thus, they will develop different goals and/or a different hierarchy of goals.

Values not only determine one's goals but also the methods of reaching those goals. Many times the methods devised for reaching some goals block or threaten other equally valued goals. For instance, the method of requiring all patients to attend preoperative teaching classes may aid in reaching a desired goal of patient education, but may conflict with the equally desirable goal of patient self-determination of care.

The nurse manager or supervisor must become aware of both his or her own hierarchy of values and those underlying the goals of the organization. Camus, the French journalist–philosopher, once said, "Ends do not justify means, but rather means justify means, and means have a way of becoming ends, so it is well to be scrupulous and uncompromising as to means" (cited in Clatterbuck & Proulx, 1981). In developing unit, subunit, and individual goals and objectives, nurses must identify the values implied in both the ends (goals) and the means (specific objectives) and resolve any conflict arising from either unclear values or differing hierarchies of values.

One approach for identifying values and diminishing conflict has been formalized as values clarification (Raths, Simon, and Merrill, 1966). This approach suggests that the strength of values may be analyzed through using seven criteria (Rath et al, 1966):

1. Is the object or action freely chosen?
2. Is the object or action chosen from alternatives?
3. Is it chosen after careful consideration of the consequences of each alternative?
4. Is the choice prized and cherished?
5. Is the choice publicly affirmed?
6. Does the individual act on the choice?
7. Does the individual repeat the choice through consistent and regular action(s)?

Clarification of underlying values provides a basis for the development of goals and objectives at all levels of the organization. It also provides the means to determine ethical standards of conduct in selecting methods of attaining objectives. It can be assumed that those choices one values are also those choices that one believes to be "right" or "good" based on a hierarchy of values.

Davis and Aroskar (1978) have outlined various historical and contemporary ethical theories as shown in the accompanying chart.

ETHICAL THEORIES AND CHARACTERISTICS

Theory	Right-Making Characteristics
1. Egoism	One should do what will promote his or her own greatest good
2. Deontology or formalism	One should consider other features of an act or rule than just its consequences
3. Utilitarianism	One should consider greatest possible balance of happiness over unhappiness for the greatest number—implies that good and evil can be balanced and measured in some way
4. Obligation: beneficence and justice	One should consider rules and actions from the basis of principles of beneficence and justice as equality
5. Ideal observer	One should consider actions and rules from a disinterested, dispassionate, omniscient, consistent point of view
6. Justice as fairness	One should consider rules and actions from point of view of least advantaged in society

Most nurses are familiar with ethical issues, such as euthanasia, abortion, informed consent, and use of technology, that occur in direct patient care settings. Nurse managers and supervisors, however, face other issues involving decisions of what is "right" and "good." Some of these arise during the process of goal setting and development of objectives. Others arise in the methods used to achieve the objectives. Let us use the goals and objectives as stated in Figure 8-3 as an example.

As stated, both the overall goal of providing quality care to patients and the unit and subunit objectives stating desirable (valued) outcomes in relation to staffing patterns seem reasonable and provide no dilemmas. However, daily staffing decisions often create the most conflict for the head nurse or supervisor who wishes to do the "right" thing. For instance, any of these ethical theories may be used in scheduling staff for holidays. While few nurses use egoism exclusively and schedule themselves off for every holiday, they may choose the holiday they value most. Attempting to achieve the greatest possible balance of happiness over unhappiness for the greatest number may be the basis for allowing the individual staff members to indicate first and second preferences and scheduling in such a way that as many people as possible get their first choice. Or, one can assume the role of an ideal observer and from a disinterested, dispassionate, omniscient point of view draw names out of a hat as a means of random selection. If, in addition, the nurse manager has a competing objective relating to cost containment and needs to use as few people as possible, preferably those at lower salaries, or if the patient census is extremely high and providing care requires that the same number of staff be scheduled regardless of a holiday, the "right" decision becomes extremely difficult.

Organizations and units frequently develop competing goals and objectives without exploring the ethical dilemma being created. While most health care agencies have an overall goal of quality patient care, they may also express a variety of objectives dealing with cost containment, staff development, and research. These all seem to be valued activities. Yet a hierarchy of values should be established to provide guidance. If, when the objectives are developed, it is clearly established that some will take precedent over others, a standard is established by which implementation decisions can be made. In addition, the underlying ethical theory needs to be explicit in the goal-setting process. For example, using a utilitarian approach to provide goals related to patient care, research, and staff development is an attempt to provide the greatest possible balance of happiness for the greatest number. Objectives must then be formulated that will balance patient care needs, research interests, and in-service education programs in such a way that more patients and staff are happy than unhappy. The dilemma arises when it is unclear whether it is more important for patients or staff to be satisfied.

Attempts at setting goals, developing objectives, and devising methods to achieve objectives must not only include skill and ability in defining what needs to be accomplished, but must also include a conscious understanding of the values and ethical considerations implied by the goals and objectives.

Planning

The function of planning has long been identified as a key element in the management process. What has not been as well identified is the need for adequate time and conceptual skill to implement planning as a specific activity. Planning may be defined as predetermining a carefully detailed course of action that will enable the organization, unit, or individual to achieve specific objectives or goals. Planning requires the ability to think, to analyze data, to envision alternatives, and to make decisions. The difficulty in most organizations lies in the fact that planning is a conceptual activity, and little value may be placed on the nonvisible activity required. Thus, while nursing care plans, for example, are required, little time is allocated in the daily routine to the thinking needed to design the plan of care. A nurse who is sitting at the desk or in an office "thinking" is frequently perceived as not being productive, that is, not getting the tasks done. The first-level and midlevel manager must learn to value the planning function and encourage subordinates to plan by allowing, or even requiring, time for this vital activity.

Time Frame for Planning

Many organizations are beginning to adopt a strategic planning program. In general, such a program requires all administrative personnel to develop a plan of action to meet the stated objectives of the unit or subunit and then to review these plans as a group to design an overall plan for the organization. This activity may take place on an annual basis, usually to be completed just prior to the start of the fiscal year. Thus, an *annual* planning cycle is established.

Other planning cycles may be shorter or longer. For example, plans to assure adequate staffing may be done on a biweekly or monthly basis. Plans for the purchase of major equipment may be developed every 3 or 6 months as needs and financial resources change. Some plans, such as the rotation of personnel for academic leaves, may be developed for several years at a time.

As a general rule, planning at the executive level will involve longer time frames that are seldom less than a year in scope. Plans at the managerial level, such as a division or department, will usually have some activities that can be accomplished in less than a year, as well as some long-range aspects. Supervisory plans, such as a single patient care unit or individual course, will more likely be dealing with day-to-day activities and have a relatively short time frame for completion.

Steps of Planning

Planning is essentially a decision-making process. Therefore, the steps of planning should be familiar since they parallel those of the nursing process. They include assessment of the system or subsystem, including goals and objectives; assessment of present strengths and weaknesses; establishment of planning premises; determining alternative courses of action; determining priorities; and selection of a course of action.

Assessment of the system.   It should be expected that an initial assessment of the system was made prior to the establishment of the goals and objectives and that the goals and objectives reflect areas of suggested changes. However, it is helpful at this stage to review the total system to focus on the current status as the baseline data against which goal achievement will be measured. Another review of goals and objectives is also useful in clarifying exactly what the end result should be and when it should be accomplished.

Assessment of present strengths and weaknesses.   A realistic appraisal of the system should include not only those factors that enhance the expectation that objectives will be met, but those factors that are likely to interfere. For example, an objective dealing with the recruitment of adequate nursing staff must not only consider the number of new nurse graduates in the area but the potential number of nurses retiring or leaving for other reasons. Information needed to assess the system and/or subsystem adequately includes: the number and capabilities of the personnel who will be involved, equipment and supplies available, location of activities required to meet objectives, and perceived time and cost constraints.

Establishment of planning premises.   Planning premises are the assumptions and forecasts that influence present activities. These deal with facts such as numbers of students or patients, policies such as minimum level of education for certain positions, and projections such as projected number of applicants. The nurse manager must assess the future in developing planning premises and use present facts and policies to predict what is likely to happen. Assumptions relating to continued levels of funding, sources of personnel, patterns of personnel assignment, cost of supplies and equipment, and continued need for the service provided should be stated as explicitly as possible. Since forecasting is likely to be an inexact science in the best of circumstances, the written assumptions upon which the projections are made provide information for changing projections as the plan is implemented.

Determining alternative courses of action.   Rarely is there only one way to achieve a goal. The principle of equifinality (von Bertalanffy, 1968) states that a system can reach the same end by a variety of means. Adequate planning requires that all possible alternative courses of action be explored. At this point, the nurse manager should involve as many people who will be participating in the implementation of the plan as possible. Many alternatives may not be feasible from the perception of the person doing the work, while an alternative presented by a staff nurse would not occur to the nurse manager. All alternatives should include information about relevance to organizational and unit objectives, anticipated cost-effectiveness ratio, acceptability to public, acceptability to staff, time frame, and extra dividend factors, if any (Arndt & Huckabay, 1980).

Determining priorities.   Since sufficient resources to accomplish all of the desirable objectives rarely exist, priorities within the organization or unit should be established.

Using the information provided with alternatives, the nurse manager can determine the priority to be given to each one. Factors such as expected impact of the alternative, relative cost, feasibility, acceptability, and desirability should be weighed. Those alternatives that receive the highest priority ratings can then be reviewed for final selection.

Selecting a course of action. Since several alternatives that seem of close to equal priority usually remain, a decision must be made and a cohesive plan completed. Making decisions is seen by many to be the primary job of the manager.

Good planning and good plans provide a framework within which the goals and objectives of the organization can be met. Longest (1976) identifies four generally accepted characteristics of a good plan:

1. The plan is based on clearly defined objectives, stated in quantitative terms, if possible.
2. The plan clearly spells out not only what is to be done, but how, by whom, and when.
3. The plan is a consistent part of the hierarchy of compatible and mutually supportive plans within the organization.
4. The plan is flexible and broad enough to contain provisions for alternatives if planning premises change.

PERT: A Planning Tool

Program Evaluation and Review Technique (PERT) is a planning tool developed in the 1950s as a method used by the U.S. Navy to plan and control the Polaris Missile program. PERT can be considered a road map of a particular project in which all major events have been identified and the relationships among events clearly indicated. The focus in a PERT network is on events that are defined as a specific completed accomplishment that occurs at a recognizable point in time. Events do not require time or resources. The interrelationships among events are indicated by arrows that represent activities. An activity is the work required to complete a specific event and require time and resources. After a PERT network has been completed, it is not difficult to determine the sequence of activities that will determine the earliest possible completion date. This sequence of events is called the *critical path*.

Figure 8-5 illustrates a PERT network for the completion of a self-study report for an accreditation visit in a school of nursing. Events are represented by boxes while activities are represented by arrows. Some events depend on the completion of a single prior event; other events are dependent on interrelated activities and events.

A PERT network can be used effectively in planning programs or projects with activities that are conducive to time estimates, that have definite start and end points, and that involve several activities taking place at the same time.

For the network to be usable, the activity time must be computed. While it is not always possible to project exactly how long an activity will take, a fairly accurate time estimate between events can be determined by estimating the most optimistic time, the most pessimistic time, and the most likely time. The most optimistic time is the estimated time if everything goes perfectly with no problems. There should be only a 1% chance that this would happen. The most pessimistic time is the estimated time if everything goes wrong. Again, there would be only a 1% chance that this would happen. The most likely time is the amount of time that the activity would most often require, under normal circumstances, if repeated again and again. Referring to Figure 8-5,

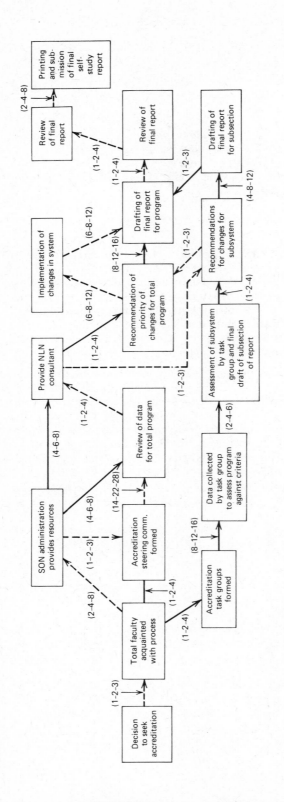

FIGURE 8-5. PERT NETWORK FOR ACCREDITATION SELF-STUDY REPORT.

——— critical

( ) weeks   Indicates in order of listing
             most optimistic, most likely,
             and most pessimistic completion
             times.

we can see that the time estimates between the first two events have been made as follows: most optimistic—1 week; most likely—2 weeks; most pessimistic—3 weeks.

The next step in using a PERT network is to determine the path through the network that takes the longest period of time to complete. This is called the *critical path*. In Figure 8-5, the critical path is shown by the dashed line. Since the critical path takes the longest time and determines project completion, events not lying along the critical path may be completed before they are needed. The time differential between scheduled completion of nonessential events and when they are needed is called *slack time*. When excessive slack time exists in a project, evaluation of what resources could be transferred to activities along the critical path in order to reduce total completion time should occur.

PERT illustrates the interrelatedness of planning and control and the basic role of decision making and can be used as a tool in many nurse management responsibilities.

Organizing

Organizing is the managerial function that identifies the roles and relationships necessary to implement the plans developed to achieve the objectives. Activities involved in this function include grouping tasks, delineating authority and responsibility, and establishing cooperative relationships among workers and subunits. These activities are carried out in a manner that meets both individual and organizational goals. The pattern of the relationships established is the formal organizational structure.

Effective organization structure is one that enhances organization performance. Magula (1982, p. 44) identifies six criteria for an effective structure:

1. Clearly identified lines of authority and accountability
2. Activities differentiated in such a way that they can be performed efficiently and effectively
3. Effective and efficient coordination and integration of the various activities in order to achieve organizational goals
4. Efficient communication system that provides the information needed by decision makers accurately, efficiently, and rapidly
5. Recognition of the informal structure with allowances for individualized behavior
6. Appropriate complexity and decentralization to allow the organization to respond to the environment

Organizations can be structured in many ways, depending on the goals, size, and complexity of the system or subsystem. There seems to be no "best" form of structure for all organizations. However, three basic models of structure can be identified. These can be designated as *functional, team,* and *matrix*.

Functional Structure
Organization by function can be observed in systems and subsystems that are organized by departments or on the basis of specialized knowledge and skills. Functional structure is based on the classic principles of organization developed in the early twentieth century. While some authors list from 10 to 30 classic principles (Fayol, 1949; Mooney & Riley, 1931; Urwick, 1943), this section will deal briefly with only the five that seem most commonly used.

Division of work.   The first principle of functional organization offers specialization of labor, or division of work, as the method by which more and better work can be produced with the same effort. Implementation of this principle results in depart-mentalization at the organizational level and specialization of activity at the subunit level. Thus, within hospitals, at the organizational level there are departments such as nursing, food service, and purchasing, and at the patient care level, personnel are assigned as treatment nurses, medicine nurses, or IV nurses.

Unity of command.   The classic principle of unity of command is derived from the bureaucratic concept of hierarchy and suggests that each participant in the system or subsystem should be responsible to, and receive orders from, only one supervisor. This principle is usually violated in both health care and educational settings where orders may be received from the immediate nursing supervisor, a member of another subsys-tem, such as a physician or another department chair, and from the person receiving the service, such as a patient or a student.

Equal authority and responsibility.   This basic premise ensures that if one is given re-sponsibility for the effective functioning of a system or subsystem, the authority to discharge that responsibility is also assigned. This legitimization of authority at a central source ensures that "the superior" has the right to command someone else and that the subordinate person has the duty to obey the command (Pfiffner & Sherwood, 1960, p. 75).

Limited span of control.   The principle of span of control in classic organization theory suggests that there should be a limited number of subordinates reporting to one superior. Factors such as level within the organization, type of work being performed, and abilities and availability of competent supervisors must also be taken into consider-ation. One should be aware that the number of relationships among a superior and each possible combination of subordinates increases dramatically with each addition to the number. For example, with five subordinates, the number of possible relationships among the superior and some combination of subordinates is 100. If the number of subordinates increases to 10, the number of possible relationships increases to 5210 (Longest, 1976). It can be seen from this example that attempting to deal with a large number of subordinates may decrease the effectiveness of the manager.

Delegation of routine matters.   Classic organization theory suggests that decisions should be made at the lowest level within the organization consistent with good decisions. The function of delegation will be discussed in a later section. The issue of centralization and decentralization, however, encompasses more than the function of delegation. It is a part of a philosophy of management. The selection of what decisions are to be held and what decisions are to be shifted to a lower level of the organization require careful study. The accompanying chart shows a comparison of the advantages of centralization and decentralization.

Most health care agencies and universities operate to some extent within a functional structure pattern. This design has a great advantage in that each person in the organiza-tion understands his or her own task and provides a high degree of stability. The accompanying chart compares the strengths and weaknesses of this design. Functional design works well in the situation for which it was designed—relatively small- to middle-sized organizations with few variables in the number of products or services, different skills required of the workers, and slow changes in technical innovations (Magula, 1982).

ADVANTAGES OF CENTRALIZATION AND DECENTRALIZATION

Centralization

1. Uniformity of policy and action
2. Lessens risks of errors by subordinates who lack either information or skill
3. Utilizes the skills of central and specialized experts
4. Enables closer control of operations

Decentralization

1. Speed and lack of confusion in decision making
2. Decrease in conflict between top management and departments
3. Informality and democracy in management
4. Development of a larger reservoir of promotable managerial manpower
5. High visibility of weak management through results of semi-independent departments
6. Thorough information and consideration of central management decisions

SOURCES: Flippo, 1970 (centralization), Drucker, 1946 (decentralization).

STRENGTHS AND WEAKNESSES OF A FUNCTIONAL ORGANIZATIONAL STRUCTURE

Strengths

1. Each individual clearly understands his or her own task

2. Functional structure when operating at best is highly economical

3. Makes least number of psychological demands in terms of work knowledge

4. High emphasis on standards of performance within the subsystem

5. Good communication if system is relatively small

6. Emphasis on acquiring and retaining high level of knowledge and skill in specialty subsystem

Weaknesses

1. Difficulty in understanding the total task of system and the relationship of individual tasks

2. Functional structure when operating at worst requires excessive managerial time and committee structure to decrease misunderstanding and increase communications among subsystems

3. May lead to extreme competition among subsystems since there is little knowledge or commitment to the task as a whole

4. Subordination of welfare of other subsystems and system as a whole to that of subsystem

5. Increasing size creates increased attention to subsystem and weakens communication

6. Poor preparation and development opportunity for management or broader scope of responsibility

Team Structure

Team structure has been proposed as an alternate to the classic functional design. This type of organizational structure should not be confused with team nursing which is often a modification of the functional approach. Organizational structure into teams has also been called project or program design. This approach to organizing pulls together a variety of specialists from varying fields to focus on a specific task. An example of this approach is the development of a "treatment team" within a psychiatric unit. The team may be composed of a psychiatrist, psychiatric nurse, social worker, occupational therapist, and other specialists. While the nurse or the psychiatrist may be officially designated as the team leader, each member takes personal responsibility for the success of the team effort. Thus, the leadership roles may be taken by any team member. The occupational therapist, for instance, may decide to countermand the doctor's order for therapy if the patient's condition seems to require such action. Leadership in a team structure places itself according to the logic of the work and there are no superiors or subordinates.

Successful team structure requires a continuing mission in which the specific tasks may change frequently. It also requires clear and sharply defined objectives, task-derived and focused authority, clarity of roles within the team with mutual understanding of each other's job, common understanding of the common task and individual acceptance of responsibility for the output and performance of the entire team, not just the individual task (Magula, 1982). The accompanying chart identifies some of the strengths and limitations of team design (Magula, 1982, pp. 63–64).

STRENGTHS AND WEAKNESSES OF A TEAM ORGANIZATIONAL STRUCTURE

Strengths

1. Common understanding of the work of the whole
2. Highly adaptable
3. Shared responsibility and authority
4. High involvement of all individuals
5. High degree of freedom for subsystem

Weaknesses

1. Potential lack of clarity about specific tasks
2. Poor stability
3. Potential lack of clarity in decision making and communication
4. Excessive time spent in maintaining internal relationships and exploring activities to other subsystems
5. High degree of self-discipline required to function as team member
6. Size must be limited for effective functioning

Team or program structure may be highly effective in systems where rapid changes are taking place, where there are many variables involved in the number of specialized skills required by workers, and where there are many variables in the types of products or services.

THE NURSING MANAGEMENT AND SUPERVISION PROCESSES   **107**

Matrix Structure

Matrix structure is a recent development that attempts to overcome the weaknesses of both functional and team designs while enhancing their strengths. A matrix structure imposes the team structure over an existing functional structure. Thus, individuals may be assigned to both a department or specialty subsystem and a project or team subsystem. Figure 8-6 illustrates a matrix structure within a school of nursing.

Like other forms of organization, a matrix structure has both strengths and weaknesses, as shown in the accompanying chart. Matrix structure, however, may provide the keys to making functional structure work in complex organizations such as a health care agency or educational institution.

STRENGTHS AND WEAKNESSES OF A MATRIX ORGANIZATIONAL STRUCTURE

Strengths

1. Focus on specific projects and yet retain specialization
2. Increased opportunity for innovation
3. Flexibility to move in and out of projects
4. Specialized knowledge is available to areas on equal basis

5. Management consistency can be maintained between team/program subsystems through functional subsystem

Weaknesses

1. Needs sophisticated management skills
2. Ambiguous structure
3. Individual is responsible to two superiors
4. More costly in time required for communication within both functional structure and program structure

---

As pointed out at the beginning of this section, there is no definitive way an organization should be designed for the most effective functioning. The concept of equifinality applies to the function of organizing as well as to other aspects of management. Cooperative relationships between and among subsystems can be designed in a variety of ways to meet the overall system goals. The nurse manager should be able to draw upon all three methods of organizing as inputs to the system.

Organizing at First and Middle Management Levels in Service Agencies

While the organizational structure of the total system will influence the structure of all subsystems, it is frequently possible for a first-level or midlevel nurse manager to develop some autonomy in the internal organization of a subsystem. For instance, although most hospitals are functionally organized, a single patient care unit may be internally organized using a team or matrix structure.

Functional nursing, team nursing, and primary nursing are the three methods of internal organization of subsystems in patient care settings. These roughly correspond to functional, team, and matrix structures as discussed previously. Functional nursing

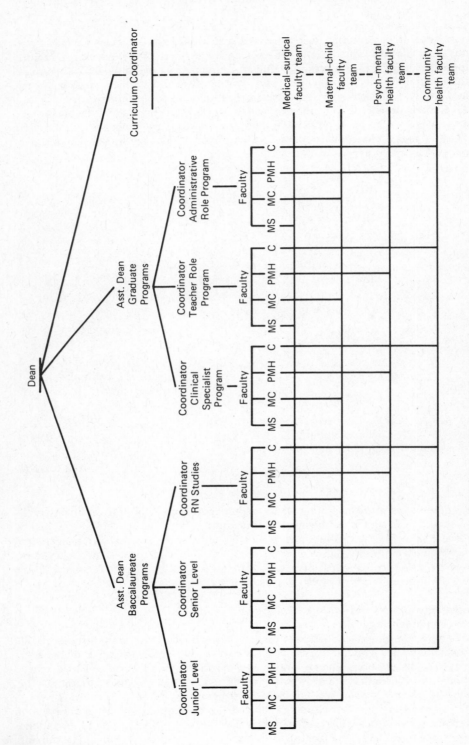

FIGURE 8-6. MATRIX STRUCTURE OF SCHOOL OF NURSING.

is based upon the classic principle of organization and the tasks of nursing care are assigned on the basis of the knowledge and skill of the nursing personnel. Each staff member is responsible only for those tasks assigned during a single shift. One weakness in this method has been that many professional tasks, such as development of care plans and patient teaching, are not included in the list of assigned tasks and are, therefore, not done. Another stated weakness has been the lack of continuity as personnel may be assigned to different tasks and/or patients each day. Both of these weaknesses can be corrected by the manager making the assignments.

Team nursing assumes that a variety of skilled care-givers within a specific subsystem (in a unit) will work together to ensure that all patient needs are met. A true team approach emphasizes the use of the capabilities of each member with all members being viewed as contributing equally to the planning, implementation, and evaluation of patient care. This creates difficulties when the majority of the team members are nursing assistants and licensed practical nurses. While these team members may offer valuable contributions regarding assessment data concerning the patients with whom they interact, they bring limited backgrounds in theoretical knowledge to the planning and evaluation aspects. Team nursing usually cannot be fully implemented in settings relying on large numbers of nonprofessional nursing staff.

Primary nursing offers a matrix approach to organizing care at the unit level. Registered nurses are assigned to a given unit and shift (functional organization) but are a part of a specific project team assigned to one or more patients. The composition of the team may be different for each patient. Thus, while Nurse A is primary nurse for three patients with Nurses B and C as associates, he or she may also be an associate nurse on a team with Nurses D and E. The primary nurse assumes the responsibility for planning and evaluating the care as well as implementation of the plan during the time he or she is working. Associate nurses assume the responsibility for the implementation during times the primary nurse is not available.

The choice of an appropriate method for organizing the unit requires careful assessment of several variables, such as the number and preparation of personnel, the variety of tasks and skill levels required, the philosophy of the personnel and the management skills of those persons who will be team leaders or primary nurses. The accompanying chart offers a few comparisons among the three organizational structures. Again, there are many ways of reaching the goal of good patient care. All three structures may be used with comparable results if effective leadership is provided.

Organizing at First and Middle Management Levels in Educational Settings

Most educational institutions remain highly specialized functional organizations. However, the concept of academic freedom has been used to establish varying degrees of autonomy for the subsystems or departments within the organization. In fact, many large universities have been described as a "collection of anarchists held together by a common parking lot"(Magula, 1982, p. 59). Effective use of this autonomy will allow the department chair or level coordinator to design the internal structure of the subsystem to meet the goals in the most appropriate manner. Most subsystems of educational institutions operate within a matrix structure. Some elements of functional organization, such as specialization, remain intact while aspects of team organization, such as integrated courses or curricula, are overlaid. As noted before, effective management within this type of structure requires a higher degree of conceptual and interpersonal skills because of the organizational complexities and ambiguities.

COMPARISON OF SOME ASPECTS OF FUNCTIONAL, TEAM AND PRIMARY ORGANIZATIONAL STRUCTURES

Aspect	Functional	Team	Primary
Personnel required	Sufficient numbers of varying skill levels to complete all tasks	Sufficient number of varying levels with all members able to contribute to delivery of total patient care	Sufficient number of professional staff to provide total care to primary patients and as well as associate patients
Assignments	Tasks assigned by manager to individual staff members on basis of job description	Task assignment agreed upon by team members on the basis of job description and experience	Individual patients (not tasks) assigned to individual nurse
Assessment, planning, evaluation	Related to specific patient; done by staff member assigned these tasks; continuity dependent on continuity in assignment	Related to specific patient; done by total team; continuity dependent on stability of team	Related to specific patient; done by primary nurse; maximum continuity
Implementation	Different staff members may do different tasks for each patient	Each team member does specific tasks for all team patients	Primary nurse does all tasks for assigned patients
Coordination and outcomes	Charge nurse is responsible for the coordination and outcomes of all tasks	All team members are responsible for coordination and outcomes of all tasks	Primary nurse is responsible for coordination and outcomes of all tasks
Communication between staff and patients	Difficult to identify a specific member with whom to communicate on continuing basis	Some confusion as to which team member should be given specific information	Clear identification of nurse with whom patient and family can communicate
Communication between subsystems	Communication addressed to charge nurse; may be some delay in obtaining information	Communication addressed to team leader; ideally all information is available to all team members	Communication addressed to primary nurse. May be some difficulty in locating specific nurse

Staffing

Staffing is the management function that assembles the people who will perform the work required to achieve the goals of the organization. The staffing function is complex and consists of the following steps:

1. Identification of the quantity and quality of the job to be done
2. Classification of workers needed to complete the job
3. Prediction of the number of workers needed in each classification
4. Recruitment of personnel to fill available positions
5. Selection of personnel from applicants
6. Optimum placement and utilization of personnel

While the nursing service director or dean at the executive level is responsible for the staffing program of the entire organization, first-level and middle-level managers must assume primary responsibility for the staffing of their specific subsystems. This requires thorough knowledge of the organization's goals, plans, and organizational structure.

Identification of Quantity and Quality of Job to Be Done

In order for staffing to be successful, there must be some understanding of the job to be done. In the past, this has been accomplished through a *job analysis*, a method by which information is obtained about the tasks involved in each job and the qualifications needed to perform them. On the basis of the job analysis, a job description is developed and personnel are employed to perform the designated tasks. The number of personnel needed is determined by the number of tasks to be done. This approach provides for sufficient staff in a functional structure, assuming all the tasks have been clearly identified. Unfortunately, in both health care agencies and educational institutions, many necessary tasks are of low visibility, that is, an observer is often unable to see the performance of the task or relate the value of the task to the job. Examples of low-visibility tasks are planning, reading of professional literature, brainstorming ideas for change, and talking with patients or students about subjects not immediately related to the illness or course. Consequently, low-visibility tasks may not be incorporated into job analyses or descriptions and may not become a part of the basis for staffing.

A more recent development in the health care system is the use of patient classification systems to define the quality and quantity of nursing care needed. Wolfe and Young (1965) devised a formula by which patient care needs could be categorized, direct and indirect patient care requirements could be determined, and nursing loads predicted. Although the original research is more than 15 years old, a recent extensive review of the literature on patient classification and assessment of the different types of classification systems in the United States has validated the earlier findings (Giovannetti, 1978). The accompanying chart presents Wolfe and Young's classification system.

Using this method of patient classification, it was determined that patients in category I required an average of 0.5 hours of direct patient care each day; category II patients required an average of 1 hour of direct patient care each day; and patients in category III required 2.5 hours of direct patient care. In addition, later studies have indicated that patients who are 65 years of age or older require from 10% to 22% more nursing time for direct care (Sauer, 1972; Thompson, Jacobs, Patchir, & Anderson, 1968).

In addition to direct care needs of patients, indirect care needs must also be calculat-

PATIENT CLASSIFICATION SYSTEM

CATEGORY I: SELF-CARE

Self-care patients fulfill any of the following combinations of criteria:
1. Ambulatory or can sit up in chair
   - Can feed self or may require help for cutting food
   - Can bathe in bathroom or at bedside with help for back and extremities
2. Ambulatory with assistance, can sit up in chair
   - Can bathe in bathroom or at bedside, but may need help with extremities
3. Same as number 1 or 2, but, in addition, fulfills *one* of the following:
   - Impaired vision
   - Requires occasional oxygen therapy
   - Requires IV feedings
4. Instructional needs that require no more than 15 minutes per 24 hours
5. Psychosocial needs that require no more than 15 minutes per 24 hours

CATEGORY II: PARTIAL OR INTERMEDIATE CARE

These patients fulfill the following combination of criteria:
1. Ambulatory with care
   - Can bathe self in bathroom or at bedside with assistance
   - Requires complete assistance with feedings (excludes IV feedings)
   - Has inadequate vision (optional; does not affect classification)
   - Requires oxygen therapy (optional)
2. Requires complete assistance to get up in chair and be bathed at bedside
   - Can feed self or may require help for cutting food or has IV feedings
   - Requires oxygen therapy (optional)
   - Inadequate vision (optional)
3. Same as number 2, but requires some assistance to get up in chair and be bathed at bedside
4. Requires some assistance to get up in chair
   - Can bathe self partially at bedside
   - Requires complete assistance with feeding
   - Inadequate vision and oxygen therapy (optional)
5. Requires bathing at bedside
   - Can feed self, but may require help for cutting food or have IV feeding
   - Inadequate vision, and oxygen therapy (optional)
6. Requires special (private) duty nurse or continuous nursing assistance to the extent that special duty nurse must be relieved for meals.
7. Instructional needs requiring approximately 15–30 minutes per 24 hours in addition to any of the above.
8. In addition to any of the above psychosocial needs require approximately 20–30 minutes per 24 hours.

CATEGORY III: INTENSIVE OR TOTAL CARE

These patients may fulfill the criteria of Categories I and II, but they also require the following:

- Suctioning therapy
- Isolation
- Care for incontinence
- Frequent change of bed linen because of wound drainage
- Constant observation and a private room because of marked emotional disturbance
- Instructional needs requiring more than 30 minutes per 24 hours

SOURCE: Patient classification system. Lucine M. Huckabay. *Patient classification: A basis for staffing.* New York: National League for Nursing, 1981, p. 9. Used with permission.

ed. Indirect patient care are those activities conducted for the patient's welfare and on his behalf which occur away from the bedside. The quantitative measures of indirect care should include the number of hours needed for:

1. Communication with persons other than the patient, such as physicians, social workers, family members, and other nurses
2. Preparation of medications and treatments
3. Documentation of nursing care and other paperwork
4. Escort services and other special errands
5. Housekeeping chores done by nursing staff
6. Physical environment, such as length of corridors, location of supplies and equipment, availability of supplies and equipment
7. Continuing education and travel
8. Development of policies and procedures
9. Administrative conferences
10. Nonproductive time, caused by factors such as fatigue, illness, and personal stress (Huckabay, 1981).

The concept of patient classification can also be used in educational settings where the direct and indirect student needs can be identified. The average amount of faculty time needed for each student in each course varies with the knowledge and skill level of the student as well as the complexity of the learning activity. In a classroom setting, one instructor can provide adequate instruction through a lecture to many students. Learning activities requiring active student participation, such as understanding group dynamics, require a smaller student–instructor ratio, and supervising students in giving patient care demands a different student–instructor ratio in each clinical setting.

The calculation of the number of nursing hours needed for direct and indirect patient care needs provides the quantity of the job. Quality is measured by the standards of nursing care expected within the agency. Standards of care and education are defined by the professional association (American Nurses' Association, 1973) but may also be defined by accreditation bodies, such as the Joint Commission on Accreditation of Hospitals and National League for Nursing, or governmental bodies, such as state or federal review boards. Each agency incorporates the broad standards into specific objectives, policies, and procedures. Thus, the quality of care is dictated by the philosophy and objectives of the system.

Classification of Workers Needed to Complete the Job

The decisions regarding how many workers are needed in each classification are dependent upon the objectives of the system and its organizational structure. A functional structure will usually require a larger mix of technical workers (those prepared for specific functions) than a team or matrix structure, which requires most personnel to be highly flexible and autonomous in performing a variety of functions.

Using the identified structures and information derived from the determination of job needs, the nurse manager decides which level of personnel should carry out each task. This requires a familiarity with the educational programs preparing the various levels of workers. The skill level, knowledge base, and attitudes of persons prepared as a nursing assistant, a licensed practical nurse, a registered nurse with an associate degree or a ·baccalaureate degree, or a clinical specialist are significantly different and cannot be used interchangeably. When various levels of personnel are substituted for each other, the quality component of the standards suffer and job performance is reduced to the level of the least-prepared worker. This can be called the "warm body" theory of staffing. An example is the assignment of a nursing assistant to replace a registered nurse who has called in ill. The theory can be stated as "any warm body is better than nobody." However, this method of staffing does not allow for the performance of those responsibilities that require the skills and knowledge specific to the registered nurse and states, in effect, that those aspects of the job are not important. Thus, if they are not important, why should they be included at any time by anyone? This interchangeable use of various categories of nursing personnel has promoted much of the confusion regarding educational requirements for providing various aspects of client care. The first-level and middle-level manager must carefully identify the levels of personnel needed to carry out the total scope of activities and accept no substitutes that compromise the quality and quantity of care.

Predicting the Number of Workers Needed in Each Classification

The prediction of the optimal number of workers in each classification can be successfully completed through the use of a systems approach. Inputs into the system for determining optimal staff composition include:

1. Organizational objectives
2. Nursing care standards
3. Nursing procedures and protocols
4. Patient census
5. Patient classification data
6. Patient care needs data
7. Organizational structure of staff
8. Legal and accreditation specifications (i.e., Medicare, Joint Commission on Accreditation of Hospitals)
9. Skill level and knowledge base expected in each classification

10. Amount and type of supervision required per person in each classification
11. Amount of nonproductive time (i.e., vacation, sick leave, holidays)

The process or throughput of the staffing system is the calculation of the optimal numbers and types of personnel to be recruited and assigned to each unit. A variety of formulas exist for this process and most can be adequately adopted to any given situation (see Arndt & Huckabay, 1980, pp. 242–243; Ramey, 1973).

Output for the staffing system consists of:

1. Recommended total number of personnel by classification for each unit
2. Recommended scheduling patterns that might include:
    a. Number and types of personnel for each day and shift on each unit
    b. Personnel on/off schedule for each unit for a specified period
    c. A list of all personnel assigned to a specific unit (Gillies, 1982)

It should be noted that scheduling is only one part of the output of the staffing system. The development of the schedule is not the primary purpose of staffing, although many managers spend more time on this single output activity than on adequate development of the inputs to the system.

Recruitment of Personnel to Fill Available Positions

Recruitment is the process of securing applicants for positions needed in addition to those already existing within the organization. While recruitment is usually carried out by a personnel department or nurses at the executive level, nurses in first-level and midlevel management positions should participate in developing the recruitment plan for their own subsystem.

The recruitment plan should be based on information from several areas:

1. Total number of personnel in each classification in the subsystem
2. Educational background of personnel in each classification (type of education, place of education)
3. Percentage of personnel in each 15 year age group in each classification (20–35; 36–50; 51–65)
4. Number of personnel in each classification enrolled in educational programs
5. Annual percentage turnover of personnel in each classification
6. Average length of employment for personnel in each classification
7. Average rate of absenteeism in each classification
8. Percentage of personnel living within the community who commute (Gillies, 1982)
9. Plans for changes and innovations in technology

This information can provide the basis for the recruitment of persons to meet specific needs. For example, if several nurses are new associate degree graduates in the 20–35 years of age bracket and turnover rates indicate that a high percentage of these persons leave within two years, recruitment efforts might be directed toward older nurses with a pattern of less mobility in order to provide stability. Conversely, if a large number of personnel are in the 51–65 age category with lengthy periods of employment, several younger persons may need to be recruited to provide for stimulation of change. A total recruitment plan is illustrated in the accompanying chart.

TOTAL RECRUITMENT PLAN

Activity	Person Responsible
1. Decision of specific requirement, number of personnel by classification and specific qualifications	First-level and midlevel manager
2. Develop source of qualified applicants	Personnel department or executive level
3. Conduct screening interviews	Personnel department or executive level
4. Interview and select from qualified applicants	First-level manager in consultation with supervisor

Selection of Personnel from Applicants

While frequently the selection of personnel to fill vacancies in both health care agencies and educational institutions has been restricted by the number of applicants, this should not mean that everyone who applies is automatically hired. It may be more beneficial to operate with a vacancy until a person who matches the job specifications is available. Selection criteria should be established before interviewing the first applicant and a standardized outline for obtaining desirable information should be developed. Areas of information to be obtained from the applicant should include: (a) personal information such as educational background, employment background (detail concerning specific types of assignments), membership in professional and community organizations, continuing education activities, professional strengths and limitations; and (b) career goals and job expectations. Changes in civil rights legislation has restricted some types of information previously sought in preemployment interviews. These areas include: marital status, plans or information about children, race, religion, national origin, and age (McLane, 1980).

Information given to the applicant should include: (a) review of organization, including philosophy, objectives, and structure; (b) job description and performance expectations; and (c) compensation and benefits program (Gillies, 1982). An additional area to consider in the selection of staff is the personal characteristics of the applicant. Although employment guidelines regarding discrimination are becoming very stringent, many job-related personal characteristics are valid bases for making employment decisions. However, they must be incorporated into selection criteria and applied to all prospective employees. Some examples of valid personal characteristics include grooming, skill in verbal and nonverbal communication, and ability to interact cooperatively with people of different ages, classes, races, and sex.

The selection process should include an opportunity for the prospective employee to meet and interact with the persons presently employed in the area or areas to which he or she will likely be assigned. Information from this activity can be used in the final selection and placement of employees.

Optimum Placement and Utilization of Personnel

The assignment of an employee to a specific job should be based on the match among information obtained in the selection process, the job requirements, personal preferences, and aptitudes of the employee and overall staffing needs of the organization. Reconciling the individual employee's goals and needs with those of the institution remains a major challenge for the nurse manager.

Gillies (1982) has identified eight steps to be taken by the nurse manager in placement and utilization of personnel or scheduling:

1. Determination of hours of maximum and minimum workload based on the analysis of work to be performed
2. Development of a pattern of on and off duty hours for available personnel that provides desired number and types of personnel for each hour of each day
3. Assignment of on- and off-duty time for each worker for a scheduling period in order to obtain the desired configuration
4. Review of completed schedule for errors
5. Submission of proposed schedule for administrative approval, if necessary
6. Distribution of schedule for notification to staff members of assigned time
7. Modification of schedule as needed to maintain desired staffing as workload changes
8. Review and analysis of schedules and policies on a regular basis to identify problems which require scheduling changes

Many variations from the traditional 3–8 hour shift/day schedule have been introduced during the past several years. Among these are scheduling by team (Froebe, 1974); the reconstructed work week, for instance 4–10 hour shifts (Bauer, 1971; Fraser, 1972); 2–12-hour shifts seven days on and seven days off (Ganong, Ganong, & Harrison, 1976); premium day scheduling (Fisher & Thomas, 1974); and flexitime.

Scheduling is the most recurring activity for a first-level manager within the staffing function. The basic pattern is developed from system and subsystem objectives and policies that dictate workload and numbers and classifications of personnel. The assignment of individual personnel to specific tasks and times must be accomplished through scheduling as an ongoing activity.

Budgeting

Budgeting as a management function has aspects of both planning and control. Because planning usually suggests expansion and change while control reflects a conservative stance, the development of a budget is a complex task. It requires a thorough understanding of the organization's objectives and planning priorities as well as the availability of resources. A budget may be defined as a preestablished standard of performance expressed in terms of controllable costs for a specific period of time. The primary purpose of budgeting is to ensure the most effective use of resources.

Types of Budgets

A variety of terms are used to describe different aspects or types of budgets. It is useful for the nurse manager to understand the usual connotations of the more common terms.

1. *Manpower budget*—the portion of the total institutional budget allocated for human resources; includes wages, salaries and fringe benefits for all regular employees and temporary or short-term contractual employees.
2. *Capital expenditure budget*—the portion of the total institutional budget allocated for

resources such as land, buildings, major equipment items, and major repairs of existing capital resources. Many institutions define a capital expenditure as any item costing over $200 and/or having a use expectancy of more than 5 years.

3. *Operational budget*—that portion of the institutional budget allocated for the purchase of supplies, minor equipment and repairs, and overhead costs, such as heating, electricity, and telephone.

4. *Open-ended budget*—financial plan with a single cost estimate for each department, program, or activity; does not provide alternatives if total funding is not available.

5. *Fixed-ceiling budget*—financial plan where an upper limit is established by executive level before individual unit plans are requested.

6. *Flexible budget*—several alternative financial plans representing different levels of activity and/or different financial expectations; executive level selects the level of activity that can be supported; plans can be changed as financial support changes.

7. *Performance budget*—based on functions and/or departments, such as direct nursing care, supervision, in-service, personnel, and x-ray.

8. *Program budget*—based on costs of a specific program, such as one-day surgery or continuing education; usually effective in identifying costs related to specific objectives.

9. *Incremental budgets*—based on historical expenditures; usually accepts the previous year's expenditures as the basis on which to increase or decrease allocations.

10. *Zero-base budget*—annual requests designed from zero; requires annual review of all programs and justification for all expenditures.

Role of First- and Middle-Level Managers in Budgeting
The responsibility for the development and monitoring of the total budget for nursing service or a school of nursing resides at the executive level. However, both the planning and controlling activities involved in budgeting can only be effective if the personnel using the resources are involved. Too often, head nurses and course coordinators carry out the daily activities of the organization as if there were an endless supply of personnel and material to meet their every wish. An awareness of the cost of supplies, equipment, and personnel is essential if first- and middle-level managers expect to be included in decisions concerning their areas.

Planning the budget.   The largest part of the budget of any health care agency or educational institution is allocated for personnel. The first-level manager should be responsible for translating the staffing policies and procedures of the institution into the specific number of nursing personnel or faculty needed for his or her subsystem. Each request for number and type of personnel necessary for the next fiscal period should be reviewed by the middle-level manager for compliance with policy and efficient utilization of personnel. Frequently, at the middle level of management, opportunities for the sharing of resources becomes apparent. For example, if the optimum staffing pattern indicates a need for 4.5 registered nurses and .5 orderlies on one unit and 6.5 registered nurses and .5 orderlies on another, the part-time requests may be converted into a single full-time position for people who will rotate between the two units. The middle-level manager is responsible for providing a comprehensive personnel request for his or her area.

The budget for equipment and supplies may be centralized through a special department, such as central supply, and projections based on inventory and data that is collected by that department. However, the head nurse or course coordinator is responsible for alerting the system if a change in the use of supplies and/or equipment is projected. For example, if an independent study activity is to be added to a required course, budget planning might need to include additional audiovisual equipment and software. Again, the role of the midlevel manager is to review the requests for equipment and supplies, offer alternatives, if necessary, and consolidate the requests into a single subsystem budget.

An effective budget plan will be a realistic indication of the resources needed to meet the objectives of the system and each subsystem. Difficulties arise when some subsystems inflate the budget request on the assumption that it will automatically be cut. When several subsystems ask for more than they need, the entire institutional budget becomes ineffective in determining what resources are actually needed. As a result, the executive level must either make decisions on fictitious data or carefully evaluate the budgets of each subsystem. In either case, it eventually becomes obvious that the projections are unrealistic and the reputations as effective managers of the persons involved are questioned.

Controlling the budget.   Resources are generally allocated on an extended period of not less than 1 year. It is important, therefore, that some control be exercised so that the resources planned for the end of the fiscal period are not used at the beginning. This calls for periodic review of expenditures and comparison with the planning estimates. Usually a monthly report of expenditures is developed by the accounting office for each subsystem. A detailed comparison will identify any variations. If more temporary personnel have been assigned to the unit or more equipment replaced than planned, the first-level manager will be asked for justification. Waste caused by loss, theft, misuse of equipment, or poor staff utilization reflects ineffective management. If, on the other hand, efficient use of resources has resulted in more being available than planned, this may provide an opportunity to implement an extra activity or service not originally seen as a high priority. However, careful allocation of funds throughout the year is required to avoid wasteful, end-of-the-year spending.

Motivating

Motivation implies behavior directed toward a goal. A clear distinction can be made between goals and motives. Goals are external to the individual and represent the value assumptions upon which decisions are based. Motives are the causes "that lead individuals to select some goals rather than others as the premises for their decisions" (Simon, 1964, p.3).

Most nurse managers are familiar with Maslow's hierarchy of needs, which views goals as needs in five categories: physiological, safety, social, esteem, and self-actualization. Needs theory suggests that as lower-level needs are met, they no longer exist as goals to motivate behavior and higher-level needs become the motivators (Maslow, 1970). The rewards chosen to motivate employees should be matched to their goals and needs. Previously, the effectiveness of a reward has been discussed in relation to the desirability of the goal, the connectedness of a reward to a behavior, and the amount of reward in relation to the effort expended (Katz & Kahn, 1978).

Hersey and Blanchard (1977) have suggested that motivation may be influenced by expectancy and availability. Expectancy is defined as the perceived probability of achieving a desired goal based on previous actual or vicarious experience. For example, if salary increases for all employees have occurred at regular intervals, an individual may reasonably expect to achieve a desired salary level (goal) at a specific time. Availability is determined by the perception of the accessibility of a goal. If instead of regular salary increases for all employees, only a very few individuals have received raises, the goal of a specific salary level may not be perceived to be available. Repeated failures to achieve a goal (low expectancy) or unavailability of a goal decreases the potential for that goal to influence behavior and thus be considered a motivator.

Before individuals or a group can be motivated a goal is necessary. Frequently what appears to be a lack of motivation is a misunderstanding about the goal. The effective nurse manager will make every effort to communicate the goals and objectives of the organization and the specific subsystem in a manner that provides direction for behavior. In addition, he or she will attempt to identify the individual goals of the employees. The integration of the needs and goals of individuals and groups with the interests and objectives of the organization will result in a higher degree of goal attainment for all.

Delegating

Delegating is the act of assigning to someone else a portion of the work that must be done. Delegation includes the assignment of the task, the allocation of authority, and the expectation of responsible and accountable completion of the work. A distinction must be made between *assignment* and *delegation*. When a task is *assigned*, it is to be carried out in a designated fashion and the person accepting the assignment has no authority to change the task or the manner of task completion. An example is the assignment of specific tasks of patient care to a nursing assistant. The nursing assistant has no authority to change the tasks assigned or to deviate from the policies and procedures controlling the tasks. If a decision is needed, he or she must return to the supervisor for instructions. The nursing assistant is, however, responsible for the completion of the tasks and accountable for the manner in which they were performed. *Delegation* of a task includes the authority to make the necessary decisions that arise in the completion of the task.

Effective delegation is a key element in the success of an organization. The totality of managerial tasks at any level usually requires more time and conceptual skill than is available to a single person. In addition, any activity that depends solely on one person is easily jeopardized if that person becomes unavailable, for instance when illness or resignation occurs. Thus, skillful delegation offers the opportunity to groom others to act as manager-surrogates and eventually assume managerial roles.

There are several steps to effective delegation:

1. Make sure everyone understands and is in agreement with the goals and objectives. If the objectives are not clear and/or there is disagreement concerning the value of the objectives, the likelihood of achieving the objectives is diminished.
2. Be specific about whether a task or a decision is being delegated. For example, the task of developing a care plan or a course outline based on accepted objectives is different from the decision about patient outcome goals or course objectives.
3. Be clear about the purpose for delegating the specific task or decision. Nothing should be delegated simply because it is unpleasant or boring. Tasks should be delegated on the basis of competence and interest as well as offering opportunity for growth.
4. Decide to whom the selected task or decision may be delegated. Some routine activities are included in job descriptions and are delegated to the individual holding that position. Decisions should be delegated to those persons who hold positions that have legitimate authority, such as a course coordinator or team leader, or to persons who are being groomed for managerial positions. When a

decision is delegated to a person not in position of legitimate authority, careful explanation to all involved is essential to avoid interpersonal conflicts.

5. Give the person to whom the task or decision is being delegated the authority to complete the activity. The individual accepting the delegated activity assumes the responsibility for its successful completion. He or she must, however, have the authority to use the resources required and to direct others in the performance of the activity. It is essential to be specific in the amount and kind of authority that is being delegated and this information should be communicated to everyone involved.

6. Set up controls for checking on the progress of the delegated activities. While a manager should not interfere with the authority of the person to whom an activity has been delegated, the ultimate responsibility for the achievement of the objectives remains with the manager. Therefore, it is essential to monitor the activity in a timely fashion. If the activity is not being completed, the quality of the performance is unacceptable, or the cost is becoming exorbitant, the person who delegated the activity must be able to correct the situation.

7. Be aware that the delegated activity will probably not be done exactly as the delegator would have done it. The ability to accept the concept of equifinality, that is, that different methods can still achieve the same goal, is essential to effective delegation.

8. Set the time frame for completion of the activity in cooperation with the person who will be responsible. This will provide logical checkpoints as well as ensuring timely completion.

9. Provide the person to whom an activity has been delegated for the first time with suggestions, coaching, and time to discuss the activity. A frequent comment from managers is "it's easier and quicker to do it myself." While this may be true, it stifles potential growth of others and leads to an unhealthy dependence on a single person.

10. Evaluate the performance upon completion of the activity. Providing feedback on both the positive and negative aspects of the person's performance is essential to the growth toward accepting additional responsibility. It is equally important to give public recognition and commendation to those people who have successfully achieved the completion of a delegated activity.

Delegation is perhaps one of the most difficult functions of management. If it is done well, others within the organization receive the public recognition of activities successfully completed and become less dependent upon the manager. Thus, delegation requires that the manager be a secure, mature individual who can feel rewarded by the growth and achievement of others.

Directing

Directing can be defined as the issuing of orders, assignments, and instructions that allow a subordinate to understand what is expected (Longest, 1976). The managerial function of directing is perhaps the most dependent upon leadership abilities of all the functions. The ability to give orders and instructions without antagonizing others is directly related to the manager's attitudes and assessment of the task and the persons who will be carrying out the orders. If the task is complex and/or the subordinate unfamiliar with it, the direction may require a high task form of communication, that is, a "telling" leadership style. On the other hand, if the staff is highly competent and the task relatively routine, the activity may be delegated rather than assigned, that is, directed.

When directions are given, it is essential that several characteristics of good direction be understood:

1. Directions must be clear, concise, consistent, and complete. Enough information should be included that the people receiving them know exactly what must be done, when it is to be done, and how it is to be done.

2. Directions should be based on an obvious rationale or the rationale should be explained. The worker who knows why the work must be done and done in a specific fashion is more likely to accept and follow through on the direction.

3. Directions must be understandable. Ambiguous words, poor sentence structure, overuse of pronouns, and use of abbreviations, technical terms, and jargon may lead to misunderstanding. The manager giving directions must make every effort to assure the directions are understood.

4. The tone and wording of the direction is important. Some directions are permissive in nature, such as "You may take a coffee break when you're finished with this task." Other directions are mandatory, "You must chart on each patient before leaving." Tone of voice also conveys the importance or urgency of a directive as well as the attitude of the manager.

5. Avoid giving too many directions at one time. Confusion results from having too many different tasks assigned at the same time, and priorities may not be clear. If it is essential to give several directions at once, for example, patient care assignments at the beginning of a shift, they should be written for ready reference as the work progresses.

6. The acceptance of a directive is influenced by the distance between the person issuing the order and the person who is assigned to carry it out. Orders and directives are most effective when given directly to the intended person rather than through others.

7. An order or directive implies a status difference that can lead to resentment. Depersonalizing the order or involving subordinates in identifying task assignments will help to decrease the friction created by status-conscious workers.

8. Always check to make sure the directions have been followed. While this is the essence of the function of controlling, it is also necessary to ensure that future direction will be effective.

Controlling and Evaluating

The function of *controlling* can be defined as the use of normal authority to assure the achievement of the stated objectives by the methods and procedures identified in planning (Tannenbaum, 1968). Control involves three steps: (1) establishing standards, (2) measuring performance and evaluating it against the standards, and (3) making corrections if deviations from the standards are found. Thus, evaluating is one aspect of the control function.

Establishing Standards
Standards are the criteria against which the performance is measured. Standards may be either quantitative or qualitative and should be developed in relation to the goals and

objectives of the organization. Most health care agencies and schools of nursing use standards developed by professional organizations and accrediting agencies as the basis for developing internal standards. In addition, recent concern about the quality of health care has resulted in the development of external standards or federal regulations, such as the Professional Standards Review Organization (PSRO); professional organizations quality assurance programs, such as the Performance Evaluation Procedure (PEP) of the Joint Commission on Accreditation of Hospitals; the quality assurance programs of the American Hospital Association; and the American Nurses' Association (Gillies, 1982).

Measuring Performance and Evaluating It Against Standards

Measuring performance consists of activities that provide information about the work of individuals and groups. This information may be collected in the form of records, reports, or direct observation. Usually records, such as patient charts, student files, and budget summaries, provide information about total quantitative outputs from the system. Direct observation provides qualitative information about the performance of individuals in meeting the objectives of the system or subsystem. Information should be obtained from consumers, such as students or patients; peers; interdisciplinary colleagues; and supervisors.

Information about task performance is compared with the established standards to identify areas of deviation. This evaluation activity is essential to the function of controlling. When evaluation is sporadic or ineffective, a loss of accountability for maintaining the standards frequently occurs.

Consistent performance appraisal may serve several purposes:

1. To provide back-up data for management decisions concerning salary standards, merit increases, selection of qualified individuals for hiring, promotion, or transfer, and demotion or termination of unsatisfactory employees
2. To serve as a check on hiring and recruiting practices and as validation of employment tests
3. To motivate employees by providing feedback about their work
4. To discover the aspirations of employees and to reconcile them with the goals of the organization
5. To provide employees with recognition for accomplishments
6. To improve communication between supervisor and employee, and to reach an understanding on the objectives of the job
7. To help supervisors observe their subordinates more closely, to do a better coaching job, and to give supervisors a stronger part to play in personnel management and employee development
8. To establish standards of job performance
9. To improve organizational development by identifying training and development needs of employees and designing objectives for training programs based on those needs
10. To earmark candidates for supervisory and management development
11. To help the organization determine if it is meeting its goals

In planning the performance appraisal activity, the nurse manager or supervisor should specify which person will be responsible for evaluating each worker. Usually, the evaluator is the person's immediate supervisor. More recently, increased emphasis has been placed on evaluation by peers, either in addition to or as a replacement for supervisor evaluations. Accurate evaluation requires frequent, direct, and prolonged contact to provide an adequate sample of the worker's performance.

Several principles of evaluation should be observed in conducting a fair and accurate performance appraisal (Gillies, 1982; Haar & Hicks, 1979):

1. The philosophy, purpose, and objectives of the organization are clearly stated so that performance appraisal tools can be designed to reflect these.
2. The purposes of performance appraisal are identified, communicated, and understood.
3. Job descriptions are written in such a manner that standards of job performance can be identified for each job.
4. The appraisal tool used is suited to the purposes for which it will be utilized and is accompanied by clear instructions for its use.
5. Evaluators are trained in the use of the tool.
6. The performance appraisal procedure is delineated, communicated, and understood.
7. An adequate and representative sample of the worker's behavior must be observed in order to evaluate consistent performance level.
8. Documentation of the performance appraisal should indicate those areas of outstanding and satisfactory performance as well as those areas needing improvement.
9. Indication of priority should be given when there is need for improvement in several areas.
10. The performance-appraisal should be scheduled as a routine part of the job. The evaluation interview should allow for discussion and be at a convenient time for both persons.
11. Plans for policing the appraisal procedure and evaluating appraisal tools are developed and implemented.
12. Performance appraisal has the full support of top management.
13. Performance appraisal is considered to be fair and productive by all who participate in it.

There are also obstacles to effective performance appraisal (Haar & Hicks, 1979, p. 22):

1. Lack of support from top management.
2. Resistance on the part of evaluators because:
   a. Performance appraisal demands too much of supervisors in terms of time, paperwork, and periodic observation of subordinates' performance.
   b. Supervisors are reluctant to "play God" by judging others.
   c. Supervisors do not fully understand the purposes and procedures of performance appraisal.
   d. Supervisors lack skills in appraisal techniques.
   e. Performance appraisal is not perceived as being productive.
3. Evaluator biases and rating errors, which result in unreliable and invalid ratings.
4. Lack of clear, objective standards of performance.

5. Failure to communicate purposes and results of performance appraisal to employees.
6. Lack of a suitable appraisal tool.
7. Failure to police the appraisal procedure effectively.

A variety of forms have been used in performance evaluation. Effective evaluation tools are designed to reduce bias, increase objectivity, and ensure validity and reliability. The accompanying chart provides information about several common types of evaluation devices.

ADVANTAGES AND DISADVANTAGES OF PERFORMANCE APPRAISAL DEVICES

Type of Performance Appraisal Device	Description	Advantages	Disadvantages
Essay technique/ free response report	Paragraph(s) on quality of performance, strengths and weaknesses, potential, personal characteristics	May provide in-depth analysis; suitable for identifying development needs and problem areas	Time consuming, vary in length, may not cover all aspects of job performance, may lack objectivity
Graphic rating scale	Assignment of numerical value or letter grade to activities in job description; judgments range from superior to unsatisfactory	Consistency; reliability; easy to construct	Limited depth of information; activities chosen may be poorly chosen
Checklist	List of activities and/or characteristics; evaluator records presence or absence of each item	Expectations clearly identified; efficient; objective	Difficult to construct; no indication of frequency or quality
Field review method	Several raters for each employee: all raters meet to establish consensus	Group judgment; more valid and fair	Time consuming
Forced-choice rating	Choice among statements which "best" and "least" describe worker; weighted statements	Reduces bias as score is established independent of rater	Costly to develop; implies lack of trust in rater

Type of Performance Appraisal Device	Description	Advantages	Disadvantages
Critical incident technique	Collection of instances that demonstrate performance in ways that are critical to success or failure	Identifies performance rather than personality	Requires written records on daily or weekly basis; time consuming
Management by objectives	Performance measured against specific predetermined objectives that are agreed upon jointly	Encourages worker participation in setting objectives and standards; decreases complaints of unfair standards	Incongruency of employee and organization goals; employee resistance to involvement

Making Corrections

When deviations from the established criteria have occurred, it is essential to determine the cause before corrective action can be taken. Careful consideration of the planning assumptions, work directives, and available resources may disclose the reasons for the deviation as an alternative to poor job performance by an individual or group. Once a cause is established, appropriate corrective action can be taken. This may consist of modifying the standard, revising planning forecasts, securing additional resources, or disciplinary action toward subordinates. Careful follow-up of the corrective action is necessary to determine if the desired results have been achieved (Longest, 1976).

Arndt and Huckabay (1980) have identified three types of control. Preaction control is intended to prevent deviations by assuring adequate quantity and quality of resources to meet the objectives. Concurrent control monitors the daily task performance to ensure the pursuit of the objectives. Feedback control focuses on the end results, which are then used to guide further action.

Collective Bargaining

Collective bargaining is usually defined as negotiation between an employer and a person representing the group of employees concerning issues such as wages, hours, fringe benefits, and working conditions. Representation of a group of employees implies a union in most contexts. The use of collective bargaining by unions representing trades and blue-collar workers is an acceptable part of our industrial society. The use of unilateral and largely unquestioned collective action by members of the long-established professions, such as medicine and law, to accomplish the same goals of economic security and adequate leisure is also acceptable since it is viewed as appropriate reward for their commitment to serve the public. There is, however, a middle group of "emerging professionals," such as nurses, teachers, and social workers, and white-collar workers who neither control their own destiny as professionals nor have the privilege of demanding action through the unions. This group is rapidly attempting to gain equity through either (a) adopting the philosophy and methodology of the labor unions, (b) attempting to achieve professional and autonomous control of their disciplines, or (c) achieve some compromise form of collective action (Colangelo, 1980).

A 1980 survey by the *American Journal of Nursing* (1980) identified 22 unions said to be actively soliciting registered nurses. Among these are the Office and Professional Employees International Union (OPEIU); the Federation of Nurses and Health Professionals (FNPH) of the American Federation of Teachers (AFT); District 1199 of the National Union of Hospital and Health Care Employees, a division of the Retail, Wholesale and Department Store Union; American Federation of State, County and Municipal Employees (AFSCME); the Teamsters; the National Education Association (NEA); and United Professionals for Quality Health Care (UP). In addition, it was noted that in 1980 the American Nurses' Association represented "more registered nurses for collective bargaining purposes than all other labor organizations combined" (Nichols, 1980, p. 61).

A survey of the growing number of articles describing the development of collective bargaining units in health care agencies and educational institutions leads to the conclusion that the underlying reason that such a unit is formed is ineffective leadership and/or poor management. Nurses and faculty members alike find themselves in the dilemma of owing loyalty to both the consumer (i.e., patient or student) and the employing institution. When the goals of the institution appear to conflict with the professional standards of nursing or faculty performance, or when the administrative activities within the institution seem to preclude achievement of personal goals, employees begin to consider forms of collective action to force institutional change.

The decision to organize a collective bargaining unit should consider the following questions:

1. Have sufficient attempts been made to identify the problem areas and discuss alternatives for change with the institution's administration?
2. What institutional factors are resisting change? Will the creation of a collective bargaining unit reduce or increase the resistance?
3. Is there sufficient agreement among the employees on the issues to be negotiated through collective bargaining? Are they concerned about economic security, fringe benefits, patient care issues, or some combination?
4. To what extent are the employees willing to force negotiations? Will they strike—for economic issues, patient care issues, or not at all?
5. What organization should represent the employees? A local unit with no organizational affiliation? A professional organization such as the ANA or NEA? A labor union, such as the AFT or OPEIU?
6. What are the laws affecting collective bargaining in health care institutions? In educational institutions? How do these affect who may belong to the collective bargaining unit?

Collective bargaining is a complex issue requiring extensive study before decisions are made. First-level and middle-level managers are frequently in the key position to encourage or discourage the perception that such activity is necessary to bring about change within the system.

SUMMARY

Management and supervision processes are administrative in nature and involve the implementation of policies and procedures within the institution. Management is the process by which organizational goals and objectives are accomplished through the use of technical, interpersonal, and conceptual skills to carry out defined functions. Supervision is the process in which the subordinate is encouraged to participate in activities designed to meet organizational goals and to develop as an employee and a person.

Functions within management and supervision processes include: goal setting, planning, organizing, staffing, budgeting, delegating, directing, controlling, and evaluating. These functions have been discussed from a theoretical base with some examples of theory application.

REFERENCES

American Journal of Nursing. Unions intensify organizing efforts among nurses, AJN survey reports. *American Journal of Nursing*, 1980, *80*, 195.

American Nurses' Association. *Standards for nursing practice*. Kansas City, Mo.: American Nurses Association, 1973.

Arndt, C., & Huckabay, L. *Nursing administration: Theory for practice with a systems approach*. St. Louis: Mosby, 1980.

Bauer, J. Clinical staffing with a 10-hour day, 4-day work week. *Journal of Nursing Administration*, 1971, *1* (6), 12–14.

Bell, M. Management by objectives. *Journal of Nursing Administration*, 1980, *10* (5), 19–26.

Blum, H. *Notes on comprehensive health planning*. San Francisco: Western Regional Office, American Public Health Association, 1967.

Bowers, D., & Seashore, S. Predicting organizational effectiveness with a four-factor theory leadership. In G. A. Gibbs (Ed.), *Leadership*. Baltimore: Penguin Books, 1969.

Clatterbuck, S., & Proulx, J. *A framework for ethical action in nursing service administration*. New York: National League for Nursing, 1981.

Colangelo, M. The professional association and collective bargaining. *Nursing Supervisor*, 1980, 27–29.

Cook, D. *Program evaluation and review technique: Application in education*. Washington D.C.: DHEW, Office of Education, 1966.

Davis, A., & Aroskar, M. *Ethical dilemmas and nursing practice*. New York: Appleton-Century-Crofts, 1978.

Donovan, H. *Nursing service administration: Managing the enterprise*. St. Louis: Mosby, 1975.

Douglass, L., & Bevis, E. *Nursing leadership action* (3rd ed.). St. Louis: Mosby, 1979.

Drucker, P. *Concept of the Corporation*. New York: John Day, 1946.

Drucker, P. *The practice of management*. New York: Harper & Row, 1954.

Fayol, H. [*General and industrial management*.] (C. Storrs, Trans.). London: Pitman, 1949.

Fisher, D., & Thomas, E. A "premium day" approach to weekend nurse staffing. *Journal of Nursing Administration*, 1974, *4* (5), 59–60.

Flippo, E. *Management: A behavioral approach.* Boston: Allyn & Bacon, 1970.

Frank, L., & Haugh, M. Management by objectives: A program that works. *Medical Laboratory Observer*, 1981, *13*, 117–130.

Fraser, L. The reconstructed work week: One answer to the scheduling dilemma. *Journal of Nursing Administration*, 1972, 2 (5), 12–16.

Froebe, D. Scheduling by team or individually. *Journal of Nursing Administration*, 1974, 4 (3), 34–36.

Ganong, W., Ganong, J., & Harrison, E. The 12-hour shift: Better quality, lower cost. *Journal of Nursing Administration*, 1976, 6 (2), 17–29.

Gillies, D. *Nursing management: A systems approach*. Philadelphia: Saunders, 1982.

Giovannetti, P. *Patient classification systems in nursing: A description and analysis*. DHEW Pub. No. (HRA) 78-22, HRP - 0500501. Washington, D.C.: U.S. Government Printing Office, 1978.

Golightly, C. MBO and performance appraisal. *Journal of Nursing Administration*, 1979, 9 (9), 11–20.

Griffiths, D. *Administrative theory*. New York: Appleton-Century-Crofts, 1959.

Haar, L., & Hicks, J. Performance appraisal: Derivation of effective assessment tools. *Journal of Nursing Administration*, September 1979, 8, 20–29.

Hersey, P., & Blanchard, K. *Management of organizational behavior: utilizing human resources* (3rd ed.). Englewood Cliffs, N.J.: Prentice-Hall, 1977.

Huckabay, L. *Patient classification: A basis for staffing*. New York: National League for Nursing, 1981.

Humble, J. *Management by objectives*. London: Industrial Education and Research Foundation, 1967.

Jackson, J. Using management by objectives: Case studies of four attempts. *Personnel Administration*, 1981, 26, 78–81.

Katz, D., & Kahn, R. *The social psychology of organizations* (2nd ed.) New York: Wiley, 1978.

Katz, R. Skills of an effective administrator. *Harvard Business Review*, 1955, 33–42.

Levinson, H., & LaMonica, E. Management by whose objectives. *Journal of Nursing Administration*, 1980, 10 (9), 22–30.

Longest, B., Jr. *Management practices for the health professional*. Reston, Va.: Reston, 1976.

Magula, M. *Understanding organizations: A guide for the nurse executive*. Wakefield, Mass.: Nursing Resources, 1982.

Maslow, A. *Motivation and personality* (2nd ed.). New York: Harper & Row, 1970.

McGregor, D. *The human side of enterprise*. New York: McGraw-Hill, 1960.

McLane, H. *Women executives*. New York: Van Nostrand Reinhold, 1980.

Mooney, J., & Riley, A. *Onward, industry!* New York: Harper, 1931.

Nichols, B. An open letter to the nurses of America. *American Journal of Nursing*, 1980, 80, 6l.

Odiorne, G. *Management by objectives: A system of managerial leadership*. New York: Pitman, 1965.

Pfiffner, J., & Sherwood, F. *Administrative organization*. Englewood Cliffs, N.J.: Prentice-Hall, 1960.

Rakich, J., Longest, B., & O'Donovan, T. *Managing health care organizations*. Philadelphia: Saunders, 1977.

Ramey, I. Eleven steps to proper staffing. *Hospitals*, March 16, 1973, 47, 98–104.

Raths, L., Simon, & Merrill. *Values and teaching*. Columbus, Ohio: Charles E. Merrill, 1966.

Sauer, J., Jr. Cost containment and quality assurance. *Hospitals*, November 1, 1972, 46, 78–90.

Simon, H. On the concept of organizational goal. *Administration Science Quarterly*. 1964, 9, 1–22.

Tannenbaum, A. *Control in organizations*. New York: McGraw-Hill, 1968.

Tannenbaum, R., Weschler, I., & Massarik, F. *Leadership and organization*. New York: McGraw-Hill, 1961.

Thompson, J., Jacobs, S., Patchir, N., & Anderson, G. Age a factor in amount of nursing care given, AHA study shows. *Hospitals*, March 1, 1968, 42 , 33.

Urwick, L. *The elements of administration*. New York: Harper & Row, 1943.

von Bertalanffy, L. *General systems theory: Foundations, development, and application*. New York: Braziller, 1968.

Webster's third new international dictionary. Chicago: Merriam, 1971.

Wolfe, H., & Young, J. Staffing the nursing unit. *Nursing Research*, 1965, *14*, 229–304.

Yura, H., Ozimek, D., & Walsh, M. *Nursing leadership: Theory and process*. New York: Appleton-Century-Crofts, 1976.

BIBLIOGRAPHY

Abdellah, F., Beland, I., Martin, A., & Matheney, R. *New directions in patient-centered nursing: Guidelines for systems of service, education, and research*. New York: Macmillan, 1973.

American Nurses' Association. *Standards for organized nursing services*. New York: American Nurses' Association, 1965.

Argyris, C. The impact of budgets on people. In J. Litterer (Ed.). *Organizations: Structure and behavior*. New York: Wiley, 1969.

Argyris, C. *Personality and organization: The conflict between system and the individual*. New York: Harper & Row, 1957.

Barba, M., Bennett, B., & Shaw, W. The evaluation of patient care through use of the American Nurses' Association Standards of Nursing Practice. *Supervisor Nurse*, January 1978, 42–54.

Block, D. Evaluation of nursing care in terms of process and outcome: Issues in research quality assurance. *Nursing Research*, July–August 1975, *25*(4), 256–262.

Brook, R., & Avery, A. *Quality assurance mechanisms in the United States: From there to where?* Santa Monica, Calif.: Rand Corp., 1975.

Budgeting procedures for hospitals. Chicago: American Hospital Association, 1971.

Chagnon, M., Audette, L., Lebrun, L., & Tilquin, C. A patient classification system by level of nursing care requirements. *Nursing Research*, March–April 1978, 27(2), 107–112.

Cleland, D., & King, W. *Management: A systems approach*. New York: McGraw-Hill, 1972.

Corwin, R. The professional employee: A study of conflict in nursing roles. In M. Abrahamson. *The professional in the organization*. Chicago: Rand McNally, 1967.

Daubert, E. Patient classification system and outcome criteria. *Nursing Outlook*, July 1979, 450–454.

Dimmock, M. *A philosophy of administration*. New York: Harper & Row, 1958.

Drucker, P. *Management: Tasks, responsibilities, practices*. New York: Harper & Row, 1973.

Drucker, P. *Technology, management and society*. New York: Harper & Row, 1970.

Eusanio, P. Effective scheduling: The foundation for quality care. *Journal of Nursing Administration*, January 1978, *8*(1), 12–17.

Fiedler, F. *A theory of leadership effectiveness*. New York: McGraw-Hill, 1967.

Filley, A., & House, R. *Management process and organizational behavior*. Glenview, Ill.: Scott, Foresman, 1969.

Getzels, J. Administration as a social process. In A. Halpin, (Ed.). *Administrative theory in education*. Chicago: Midwest Administration Center, University of Chicago Press, 1958, pp. 150–165.

Georgette, J. Staffing by patient classification. *Nursing Clinics of North America*, June 1970, 329–339.

Griffiths, D. The nature and meaning of theory. In D. Griffiths, (Ed.). *Behavioral science and educational administration*. The 63rd Yearbook of National Society for the Study of Education. Chicago: University of Chicago Press, 1964, pp. 95–119.

Herzog, T. The National Labor Relations Act and the ANA: A dilemma of professionalism. *Journal of Nursing Administration*, 1976, *6*, 34–36.

Hicks, H. *The management of organizations: A systems and human resources approach* (2nd ed.). New York: McGraw-Hill, 1972.

Joint Commission on Accreditation of Hospitals. *Accreditation manual for hospitals*. Chicago: Joint Commission on Accreditation of Hospitals, 1976.

Joint Commission on Accreditation of Hospitals. *Accreditation manual for hospitals.* Chicago: Joint Commission on Accreditation of Hospitals, 1970.

Kast, F., & Rosenzweig, J. *Organization and management: A systems approach.* New York: McGraw-Hill, 1970.

Koontz, H., & O'Donnell, C. *Principles of management.* New York: McGraw-Hill, 1964.

Levey, S., & Loomba, N. *Health care administration: A managerial perspective.* Philadelphia: Lippincott, 1973.

Lischke, N. *Application of Ramey's "eleven steps to proper staffing" to predict a staffing methodology for a university hospital.* Master's of nursing thesis, University of California, School of Nursing, Los Angeles, 1975.

Mager, R. *Preparing objectives for programmed instruction.* Belmont, Calif.: Fearon Publishers, 1961.

Mayo, E. *The social problems of an industrial civilization.* Cambridge: Harvard University Press, 1945.

McGregor, D. *The human side of enterprise.* New York: McGraw-Hill, 1960.

Moore, M. Philosophy, purpose and objectives: Why do we need them? *Journal of Nursing Administration,* May–June 1971, *1*(3), 9–14.

National League for Nursing. *A self-evaluation guide for nursing services in hospitals and related institutions.* New York: National League for Nursing, 1967.

Newport, G. *The tools of management.* Reading, Mass.: Addison-Wesley, 1972.

Pointer, D. The 1974 Health Care Amendments to the National Labor Relations Act. *Labor Law Journal,* June 1975, 350–359.

Professional Workers and Collective Bargaining. Selected papers. Los Angeles: Institute of Industrial Relations, UCLA, 1977.

Ramey, I. Setting nursing standards and evaluating care. *Journal of Nursing Administration,* May–June 1973, *3*(3), 27–35.

Ramphal, M. Peer review. *American Journal of Nursing,* January, 1974, 74(1), 63–67.

Somers, J. Purpose and performance: A system analysis of nurse staffing. *Journal of Nursing Administration,* 1977, 7(2), 4–9.

Stevens, B. *Nursing theory: Analysis, application, evaluation.* New York: Little Brown, 1979, pp. 121, 209–210, 212.

Stieglitz, H. Concepts of organization planning. In H. Frank (Ed.). *Organizing structuring.* New York: McGraw-Hill, 1971.

Taft-Hartley amendments: Implications for the health care field. Chicago: American Hospital Association, 1976.

Taylor, F. *Scientific management.* New York: Harper & Row, 1947.

Toffler, A. *Future shock.* New York: Bantam, 1971.

Traxler, R. The administrator's dilemma—The need for conceptual skills. *Hospital Administration,* 1964, *9* (1), 6–15.

Werther, W. *Labor relations in the health professions.* Boston: Little, Brown, 1977.

Williams, M. Quantification of direct nursing care activities. *Journal of Nursing Administration,* 1977, 7, 15.

Zimmer, M. Quality assurance in the provision of hospital care: A model for evaluating care. *Hospitals,* March 1, 1974, *48*(5), 91–95; 131.

PART THREE
DIAGNOSTIC AND INTERVENTION STRATEGIES FOR NURSING LEADERS, MANAGERS, AND SUPERVISORS

CHAPTER 9
ORGANIZATION DEVELOPMENT AND SYSTEM DIAGNOSES

French and Bell (1978) offer a comprehensive definition of organization development that is appropriate to health care organizations:

> Organization development is a long-range effort to improve an organization's problem-solving and renewal processes, particularly through a more effective and collaborative management of organizational culture—with special emphasis on the culture of formal work teams—with the assistance of a change agent, or catalyst, and the use of the theory and technology of applied behavioral science, including action research. (p. 14)

OVERVIEW OF ORGANIZATION DEVELOPMENT

Organization development (OD) is a problem-solving approach that enables the organization to examine the way it goes about diagnosing and making decisions about the opportunities and challenges of its environment. OD differs from many other organizational interventions because it is concerned with complete work teams and not just the manager/supervisor or a management group. OD specialists use a general systems perspective in developing an intervention strategy that will accomplish the goals of task accomplishment and system maintenance. In this process, collaboration between managers/supervisors and subordinates and between subsystems and the larger organization is essential.

THE ORGANIZATION DEVELOPMENT (OD) PROCESS

The components of the OD process are: data collection; feedback, data analysis, and system diagnoses; action planning and system intervention; and maintaining, managing, and evaluating the process. Integral to the entire OD process is the basic intervention model of action research.

> The action research model consists of (1) a preliminary diagnosis, (2) data gathering from the client group, (3) data feedback to the client group, (4) data exploration by the client group, (5) action planning, and (6) action. (French & Bell, 1978, p. 17)

Data Collection

An internal problem is generally the stimulus for a system to engage in OD. With the assistance of an internal or external consultant or change agent, the members of an organization or subsystem gather data related to the general problem area of concern. Diagnostic activities are designed to determine the present status of a system in relation to the problem area of focus. Diagnostic activities are also utilized to determine the outcomes of the change strategies/actions implemented.

The diagnostic focus can either be on the diagnosis of organizational subsystems *or* organizational processes (French & Bell, 1978). The target for the focus on organizational subsystems can be the total organization, large subsystems, small subsystems, interface subsystems, dyads or triads, individuals, roles, or between organization systems constituting a suprasystem. The targets for the focus on organizational processes include: communication patterns, styles, and flows; goal setting; decision making; problem solving; action planning; conflict resolution and management; managing interface relations; and superior–subordinate relations.

Self-assessment is begun through the data-collection process. System members begin to increase their understanding of their organization's processes, norms, values, and structure. As Fisher (1980) notes, "the process of collecting and sharing data is itself an intervention into the client system" (p. 34).

The nature of the data and the data-collection methods must be carefully selected. The data collection methods must be appropriate for the problem area and the client system.

Where appropriate, suggested assessment strategies have been incorporated in the chapters of this section. In addition, several major data-collection strategies will be described below. For a more detailed discussion, research texts should be consulted.

The Questionnaire

The major types of questionnaires are fixed-response, open-ended, and combination. In the fixed-response type, a fixed number of choices are designed for each statement or question. The respondent chooses the most appropriate response from among these choices. The open-ended type requires respondents to elaborate on their opinions. The combination type includes both fixed and open-ended responses. The questionnaire can be administered in two ways: face-to-face or by mail. The advantages of the questionnaire (depending on type and method of administration) are possible anonymity, elimination of interviewer bias, and low cost.

The Interview

The interview serves as an excellent tool by which to obtain descriptive data about a social system. Since it allows for exploration, the interview is useful in obtaining information about unexplored topics.

There are two major types of interviews: structured and unstructured. In the unstructured interview, little structure is provided the interviewer, thus optimizing a spontaneous response from the respondent. Black and Champion (1976) identify a number of advantages and disadvantages of the unstructured interview. Among the advantages are: the interview can approximate natural conversation, those areas of the problem most important to the respondent are identified readily, and the ability to explore aspects of the problem in an unrestricted fashion is fostered. Among the disadvantages are: questionable comparability of data, time wasted collecting information that is of little use, and time consumed in coding the collected data.

The interview can be structured by structuring the setting, regulating the questions and responses, and limiting the problem by means of the focused interview. In the latter, focus is placed on the experience as perceived by the organizational members.

There are a number of advantages of an interview, such as: in-depth data can be collected, unanswered questions can be reduced, misinterpretations can be corrected, and response rates tend to be good.

Observation

Participant observation and nonparticipant observation are useful in collecting data about behavior as it actually happens. Observation permits a graphic description of the system problem under investigation as well as the exploration of situations about which little is known.

The investigator is an active participant in the system under investigation in the participant observation method of data collection. Participant observation preserves natural behavior in the system. The drawback of this method is difficulty in replication.

In nonparticipant observation, the investigator collects data about the system by observation while not being an actual participant in the behavior or problem area under investigation.

A number of advantages and disadvantages of observational methods are noted by Polit and Hungler (1978). Data that may be impossible to collect by any other method can be collected through observation. It provides for a great deal of variety and depth of information, and, it captures a record of behavior as it occurs in the organization. The major drawback is that observational data is vulnerable to distortion and bias. Data analysis and interpretation is complex and subject to personal prejudice and emotion.

The PAS Model

The Processually Articulated Structural (PAS) model, as described by Loomis (1967), can be a useful tool in total system or subsystem analysis. Data is collected about each of the structural–functional categories and master processes. The structural–functional categories are (a) knowing; (b) feeling; (c) achieving; (d) norming, standardizing, patterning; (e) dividing the functions; (f) ranking; (g) controlling; (h) sanctioning; and (i) facilitating. The master processes are: (j) communications, (k) boundary mainten-ance, (l) systemic linkage, (m) institutionalization, (n) socialization, and (o) social control.

The internal or external OD consultant collects data in response to these categories and processes by posing relevant questions. A determination is then made in each area whether any problems or dysfunctional behaviors are present. A system comprised of nurses in independent practice will serve as a hypothetical example. (a) What are the general beliefs held by these nurses? What is the general knowledge base relevant to organizational goal achievement? (b) What is the overall sentiment or morale of these nurses? Strategies used for tension management? Liking or respect for each other? How is sentiment communicated? (c) What are the goals of this group? Goal-achievement activities? Commitment to goals and activities? (d) What are the group norms? Stan-dards? What is the degree of conformity? (e) How are the subsystem's functions divided among status-roles? Actual reponsibilities inherent in each role? (f) How are these nurses evaluated? What determines promotion to new status roles? (g) How does decision making take place? In what kind of power-oriented behavior do these nurses engage? (h) On what basis and in what manner are rewards and penalties administered? Any scapegoating? (i) Do these nurses have effective facilities to meet organizational goals? (j) Describe communication processes. Any perceptual distortions? Lack of feedback? (k) Describe the processes of boundary maintenance, that is, how does the subsystem keep its boundaries intact? (l) Describe systemic linkage, that is, how are aspects of the system of nurses linked to other systems in the community? (m) Describe institutionalization, that is, what are the aspects of the system which are perceived as "rightful," "the way things should be done?" (n) Describe socialization. What processes are used, for example, to make a new nurse in this group knowledgeable about the norms, values, and subculture prevalent among these nurses in independent practice? (o) How is deviant behavior eliminated or made more compatible with group norms and culture?

Data collected via this model can be used to delineate clearly problems in any of these aspects of the subsystem. Subsystem diagnoses can then be formulated.

Feedback, Data Analysis and System Diagnoses

Once the data is collected, various approaches to analyzing the data exist. The consultant can analyze the raw data and present the results to managers in the system. The consultant and representatives of management can analyze the data jointly; or, data feedback can be given to the members of the target subsystem. In this latter approach, the members of a subsystem participate in the analysis.

In the process of data analysis, the present status of the system is described, particularly as it relates to the target of the diagnostic activities. "From a comparison of 'what is' with 'what should be' comes a discovery of the gap between actual and desired conditions" (French & Bell, 1978, p. 60). The actual problem(s) existing in the system are identified and system diagnoses are formulated.

The initially collected data and results of the analysis are then used as a basis for formulating the action plans. In OD, data collection and analysis continues beyond this initial phase. Once action plans are implemented, data is collected and analyzed to determine their effects.

Action Planning and System Intervention

Based upon the identified problem areas and diagnoses, alternative intervention strategies are generated, goals are set, an action plan is developed, and the intervention strategies in the action plan are implemented.

Schmuck and Miles (1971) present a schema for classifying OD interventions. Organization development interventions can be designed to bring about improvement in the diagnosed problems in goals/plans, communication, culture/climate, leadership/authority, problem solving, decision making, conflict/cooperation, role definition, and other areas. Organization development interventions can focus on the total organization, intergroup, team or group, dyad or triad, and role. The mode of OD intervention can include training, process consultation, confrontation, data feedback, problem solving, plan making, OD task force establishment, and technostructural activity.

Maintaining, Managing, and Evaluating the OD Process

Implementing the action plan will have an effect on the target subsystem as well as on the larger organization. Are the intervention strategies timely, appropriate, and producing the intended effects? Are system members involved in and committed to the OD process? What is the impact of the action plan on the total organization? Is the OD consultant serving as a role model? Is data available that indicates a need to revise the action plan? Data must be continuously collected to answer these and other relevant questions. Feedback loops should be built into the process in order to monitor and alter the action plan as necessary. Maintaining, managing, and evaluating contributes to the constructive outcome of the OD endeavor.

SUMMARY

An important aspect of OD is action research. The process of action research is very similar to the steps in problem solving or to the components of the nursing process. Action research entails systematic data collection about the target area, feedback of the data to system members, data analysis, formulation of diagnoses, setting goals, developing action plans, implementing action plans, and evaluating the results. By means of such a process, OD becomes a useful tool in improving a social system's adaptive, goal-setting, problem-solving, and renewal processes. Whether to utilize OD in a nursing organization can be successfully determined by a nurse manager knowledgeable about the potential of OD for constructive system change.

REFERENCES

Black, J., & Champion, D. *Methods and issues in social research*. New York: Wiley, 1976.

Fisher, D. A review of organizational development. *Journal of Nursing Administration*, October 1980, *10*, 31–36.

French, W., & Bell, C. *Organization development*. Englewood Cliffs, N.J.: Prentice-Hall, 1978.

Loomis, C. *Social systems: Essays on their persistence and change*. Princeton, N.J.: D. Van Nostrand Company, Inc., 1967.

Polit, D., & Hungler, B. *Nursing research: Principles and methods*. Philadelphia: Lippincott, 1978.

Schmuck, R., & Miles, M. *OD in schools*. La Jolla, Calif.: University Associates, 1971.

BIBLIOGRAPHY

Blalock, H. *An introduction to social research*. Englewood Cliffs, N.J.: Prentice-Hall, 1970.

Diers, D. *Research in nursing practice*. Philadelphia: Lippincott, 1979.

CHAPTER 10
THE CONCEPT AND PROCESS OF PLANNED CHANGE

Managing change is an important function of nurses in leadership, management, and supervisory positions. The need for planned change emanates from problems identified in the input, throughput, or output processes in an organization, that is, a discrepancy is identified between a given state of affairs and a more ideal or functional state. Change also emanates from an organization's need to keep pace with a changing environment. Existing goals are altered or new goals are developed in order to contribute to organizational maintenance and survival and/or to stimulate organizational growth. The nurse leader who manages change by means of a planned process contributes to the maintenance of a positive staff morale, reduces conflict or resistance to a constructive level, enhances work-team productivity, and enables the achievement of the planned change objectives.

Problems arise in unplanned or improperly planned change. Unplanned change often leads to a process of staff denial of the problem followed by a period of rage including acts of sabotage, high anxiety levels, and finally a low level of morale, almost bordering on a subclinical depression. Change, for the sake of change, and change that is "unrelated to extant problems or goals is pernicious because it robs us of time and effort which could be directed to improving nursing practice" (Stevens, 1977, p. 27). The introduction of change at a too rapid and too frequent rate also depletes energy and leads to organizational instability.

RELEVANT DEFINITIONS

Change refers to an alteration, to becoming something different, to a tendency toward growth, progress, or development. Stevens (1977) cautions that the single word change can be used in two different ways. It can mean the *content* of the change itself, that is, those alterations being implemented; or, it can refer to the *process* of implementing these alterations. The former is labeled the activity plan, or "those activities and events specifically designed to reach a stated goal or to solve a particular problem" (p. 27). The latter is called the strategic plan and is comprised "of those activities and events designed to prepare the environment for acceptance of the activity plan" (p. 27).

Planned change refers to a deliberate, conscious, well-thought out effort or process to either alter and improve the operations of a system or to achieve changed organizational goals through the utilization of a knowledgeable change agent. In planned change, knowledge is consciously utilized and applied as a means for altering organizational practices.

The *change agent* is a person who possesses knowledge of the change process, examines the current state of a client system, and initiates alterations to bring about the achievement of planned change objectives. The *client system* refers to the individual, group, or community being helped.

MAJOR MODELS OF CHANGE

Three major models of change are described by Chin (1976): *system model, developmental model,* and *model for changing.*

System Model

A basic assumption of the system model is that interdependency, integration, and organization exist among the subsystems of a system. Change is perceived as a consequence of incompatibilities and conflicts among the subsystems of an organization or between the system and its surrounding environment. This structural stress and strain that is internally created or externally induced becomes the source for the change. Change is thus perceived as a process of tension reduction. Goals are emergent, arising either from imposed sources or from the structure itself, and focus on adjustment (internal equilibration) or adaptability (reaction of environment). The change agent is viewed as being separate from the client system.

Developmental Model

The source of change in this model is assumed to be in the nature of the organism itself. That is, a system constantly changes and develops, growing and decaying over time. "The direction of change is toward some goal, the fulfillment of its destiny, granting that no major blockage gets in the way" (Chin, 1976, p. 101). The need for change arises when a gap occurs between the system and its goals. The focus of the change agent is to assist in diagnosing the problem and removing the blockages.

Model for Changing

The model for changing incorporates elements from both system and developmental models. Change arises out of a perceived need. Change is a matter of choice for the client system. Change is both planned and controlled. Organizational stability is examined in order to unfreeze the system and induce forces to change it. Change goals are deliberately developed through a collaborative process and focus on improving the system. The change agent participates in the planned change process.

Elements from this model for changing, along with normative reeducative strategies, will be synthesized in a normative reeducative model for changing.

MAJOR TYPES OF PLANNED CHANGE STRATEGIES

Three major strategies for planned change are described by Chin and Benne (1976): power–coercive, empirical–rational, and normative–reeducative.

Power–Coercive Strategies

The change agent, using power-coercive strategies, seeks to achieve change goals by utilizing economic, political, or other coercive strategies. Economic sanctions bring about change in those to whom they are applied. Budget allocations to a continuing education department can be withdrawn, forcing the department to seek ways to become self-sufficient or be faced with decline and eventual phase-out. On the other hand, a nurse manager can bring about desired growth in a subsystem by allocating abundant resources to stimulate that growth.

Political power is also used in power–coercive strategies to bring about planned change. The force of legitimacy through laws, judicial decisions, and administrative rulings is used to bring about new programs or policies or to alter some traditional practices.

Moral power can be used as a power–coercive strategy by arousing guilt and shame in others in order to bring about change. By this means, conflicts in values can be generated, existing patterns can be challenged, and change can be induced.

In summary, power–coercive strategies bring about change by means of economic, political, or moral coercive means. Changing laws, making judicial rulings, issuing administrative directives, applying economic sanctions, or utilizing moral power does not reeducate people in new behaviors. Normative–reeducative strategies are needed in combination with power–coercive strategies in order to bring about new behavior that includes new knowledge and skills, new attitudes, and new value orientations. Used by themselves, power–coercive strategies often lead to failure.

Empirical–Rational Strategies

Empirical–rational strategies are based on the assumption that man is rational and acts in his own self-interest if the specific situation is rationally justified. The change agent introduces change known to be desirable, effective, and in line with the self-interest of the client system. It follows then that the client system will likely adopt the change since the change has been justified and the benefits have been clearly identified.

Knowledge is perceived as the main source of power in empirical–rational strategies for planned change. Ignorance and superstition, on the other hand, are perceived as the foes of introducing planned change successfully. Thus, emphasis is placed on basic and applied research as a means for generating and expanding knowledge. Systems analysts and operations researchers are also seen as important in generating a data base. Education is advocated as a means of diffusing such knowledge, stimulating the use of reason, and enhancing knowledge-based actions that lead to change.

Importance is likewise placed on putting the most knowledgeable and appropriate person into a specific job in an organization. Empirical–rational change agents view this essential for rationally based change to occur.

Nurse leaders, managers, and supervisors utilizing empirical–rational strategies put much effort into recruitment and selection of the most appropriate person for any given position vacancy. Resources are placed into staff development and staff are encouraged to remain current. Research and the dissemination of research findings are also encouraged. The nurse manager, or designated change agent, attempts to bring about planned change by justifying desired change goals and enhancing the knowledge of staff, showing them how they can benefit from the change.

For example, in changing from team to primary nursing, the nurse manager or delegated change agent who uses empirical–rational strategies would justify the desired change, elucidate all the negative aspects of team nursing, and highlight the expected positive outcomes of primary nursing. An educational program would be implemented to teach the nursing staff the principles and benefits of primary nursing.

Empirical–rational strategies work best when there is a high degree of readiness in acceptance of the change goals in the client system. If, in our example, the nursing staff possesses a favorable impression of primary care nursing and a readiness to implement it, then empirical–rational strategies for implementing planned change will work well. If, on the other hand, readiness for primary care nursing is not prevalent among the nursing staff and resistance is high, then empirical–rational strategies do not work as well. Additional attention must be given to deal with both the forces accountable for the resistance and the *process* of implementing change; that is, a strategic plan must be formulated. Attention to the content of the change, along with simply providing the client system with both information and a rationale, is not an appropriate strategy for bringing about change in all situations and contexts.

Normative–Reeducative Strategies

The underlying assumption for the normative–reeducative strategies is that man is perceived to be in active transaction with his environment while in quest of need satisfaction. Changes in patterns of behavior result from a person's potential ability to reshape his experiences in relation to the situational demands of the environment with which he desires continuity. This process of a more adequate fitting of man's needs with his environmental demands and resources is known as *adaptation.*

Normative–reeducative change strategies seek to influence and modify behavior while strengthening self-understanding and control. An adequate knowledge base is considered a key element in bringing about change in behavior. However, the importance of the noncognitive and sociocultural aspects are also considered in bringing about behavioral change. That is, changes are sought in a group's informational bases of operation; in the cognitive and perceptual basis of viewing phenomena; in habits, values, and internalized meanings at the personal level; and in normative structures and institutionalized roles and relationships (Chin & Benne, 1976).

GUIDELINES FOR PLANNED CHANGE

Before we discuss our normative–reeducative model for changing, there are several guidelines to consider when engaging in planned change (Benne & Birnbaum, 1969; New & Couillard, 1981; Schmalenberg & Kramer, 1979; Stevens, 1975, 1977).

Guideline 1. Recognize Symptoms Indicating Need for Change

Strive to recognize symptoms indicating a need for change. A problem may be encountered within the system that points to a failure in the system and a consequent need for change. The coordinator of an undergraduate faculty may notice, for example, that little effort is made by faculty to seek feedback from each other. Dysfunctional interpretations and behaviors, including dysfunctional "game playing," are prevalent. The general atmosphere is one of mistrust and tension. Clearly a need for change to more functional communications exists.

A need for change can also arise in the system because of the changing nature of its environment. For example, the associate dean of an undergraduate nursing program notices an ever-increasing demand from diploma- and associate degree-prepared nurses for career mobility options to obtain their baccalaureate degrees. The nursing program as it exists does not make accommodations to meet the needs of these students. New goals must be set by the school of nursing if it wants to meet the needs of its environment.

Guideline 2. Assess the Nature of the Problem

The nature of the problem must be assessed in order to formulate an accurate diagnosis. Both the forces that tend to maintain the status quo (restraining forces) and the forces promoting movement and change (driving forces) must be assessed. This includes those restraining forces labeled resistance.

Guideline 3. Set Change Goals

Change goals must be set, alternatives for achieving these goals examined, and activity and strategic plans designed based upon the selected alternative. That is, goals should be stated to reflect the desired outcome at the end of the change process. Activities and events must be specified to reach the goals (activity plan). For example, the activity plan might include the planning and implementation of a RN–BSN track to meet the educational needs of RNs. Activities must be designed to prepare the physical, psychological, or organizational environment to accept the activity plan (strategic plan). In the example given, faculty might be exposed to various approaches to designing such a program through staff development and sessions in which their views can be expressed.

Guideline 4. Analyze Resistance to Change

Resistance to change must be analyzed and understood in order to intervene constructively. The sources of resistance to change are many: threatened self-interest, inaccurate perceptions, objective disagreement, psychological reactance, and low tolerance for change. Although resistance is recognized as predictable when implementing change, open hostility may be expressed toward the change agent when there is a perceived or actual threat to one's job or personal integrity.

It is important for the nurse manager to recognize typical stages of resistance. Stevens (1975) identifies the typical stages of resistance as follows:

1. Undifferentiated resistance from various sources.
2. Pro and con sides line up, developing their stands in reasoned arguments or slogans.
3. Direct conflicts take place between the two sides.
4. Those favoring the change come into power as the executive institutes the change.
5. Old adversaries begin the stages of acceptance.
6. Few adversaries are to be found; most people do not recall that they ever opposed the change. (pp. 58–59)

The competent head nurse or nursing coordinator is also alert to the staff resistance a new nurse graduate may face in the clinical setting. Schmalenberg and Kramer (1979) present a sensitizing description of the stages of resistance often faced by these graduates.

In Stage 1—nullification—the suggestion for change is invalidated. Because the nurse is new, his or her suggestions are considered invalid. Besides, the traditional way of doing things has maintained the system so there is no reason to "rock the boat." The message communicated to the new graduate is: "You don't really know what you're doing, but thanks anyhow!" Eventually, any enthusiasm for making new suggestions is worn down and the new graduate is left with the feeling that he or she is "banging my head against the wall."

In Stage 2—isolation—the new nurse graduate is separated from peers and subordinates. The purpose of this isolation is to minimize the effects of suggested changes on the organization. Methods used to isolate the new graduate include swamping the nurse with work, closing links in the communications network, restricting freedom of movement, unresponsiveness, and limiting resources. The goal of isolation is to convince the change agent that attempting to change the system is futile unless directed to do so by superiors. The frustrations and sense of powerlessness induced by this strategy of isolation may cause the nurse to overreact. The overreaction may be used against the would-be change agent to demonstrate how "unstable and emotional" she or he is.

Stage 3—defamation—includes measures to cut the change agent off from any supporters through derogatory remarks. The change agent is accused of incompetence, emotional instability, sexual problems, or questionable motives. A great deal of mistrust of the nurse is generated in the work group. The goal of defamation is to make the change agent passive and retreat from initiating any more change efforts. The method of achieving this is to destroy the person's reliability, reputation, and competence.

In Stage 4—expulsion—the final stage of resistance to change is reached. The nurse insisting on bringing about change is forced to resign from the job. The obvious goal is to eliminate the "offensive" person and ideas from the organization. The group can then comfortably snuggle back behind its security blanket and continue "to do things the way we've always done them." Unfortunately, the nursing profession loses good nurses and ideas in this manner.

Guideline 5. Change Relevant Aspects of the Total System

In order to change a subsystem, relevant aspects of the environment or other parts of the total system will be affected and must be changed accordingly. Since the component parts of a system are interrelated, change in one subsystem will affect other subsystems. The potential impact of the change must be assessed and selected change may be necessary in related subsystems.

Guideline 6. Start Change at Points of Stress or Strain

Change should be started at those points in the system where some stress or strain is occurring. Benne and Birnbaum (1969) point out, however, that "one should ordinarily avoid beginning change at the point of greatest stress" (p. 333).

Guideline 7. Consider Both Formal and Informal Organizations

The effectiveness of planned change is enhanced when both the formal and informal organization of an institution are considered in the change process. Organizational members affected by the change should be involved in diagnosing the problem and formulating change strategies for best results.

Guideline 8. Evaluate and Stabilize the Change

The planned change must be evaluated and stabilized. The system must be permitted to return to homeostasis at the new level of functioning. Care must be taken to use appropriate timing to introduce any further change.

Keeping these guidelines, along with the described change models, and strategies in mind, attention is now turned to a normative–reeducative model for changing.

A NORMATIVE–REEDUCATIVE MODEL FOR CHANGING

In the normative reeducative model for changing— based on Bennis, Benne, Chin, and Corey, 1976; Chin, 1976; Davis, 1973; Lippitt, Watson, and Westley, 1958; Mayer, 1975; Schein, 1972—change is conceptualized as taking place when an imbalance occurs between the sum of restraining forces that tend to maintain behavior in the organization at the status quo and the sum of driving forces that tend to move behavior away from the status quo. When the driving and restraining forces are not in balance, a change in behavior will occur; that is, the imbalance unfreezes the pattern of behavior, with the eventual aim of creating a new balance between driving and restraining forces. Informational basis of operation, perceptions, habits, values, institutionalized structures, roles, and relationships are influenced to accomplish the unfreezing, to create movement in the desired direction, and to achieve change goals. To create the imbalance, the change agent can reduce the restraining forces and/or increase the driving forces. The model includes three change phases and seven change stages.

Phase 1. Unfreezing

Stage 1
The client system discovers the need for assistance. The need for change may arise from problems encountered within the system or be stimulated by a changing environment. The change agent sometimes serves as a catalyst to help the client system recognize the need for change and for assistance.

Three mechanisms can be used by the change agent to begin the process of unfreezing (Schein, 1972):

1. Inducing disconfirmation of presently held values, behavior patterns, attitudes, or beliefs
2. Inducing guilt and anxiety by pointing out the discrepancy between the actual and the ideal state
3. Creating psychological safety in order to reduce restraining forces and resistance

Stage 2
The change agent establishes and defines the helping relationship. The change agent participates in:

1. Diagnosing the client system's needs and problems
2. Assessing the client system's motivation and ability to change
3. Selecting relevant objectives for the change, with input from the client system
4. Selecting the helping role
5. Establishing and maintaining a relationship with the client system
6. Recognizing and guiding change phases and stages
7. Evaluating planned change results

If the change agent is external to the system, selecting a point of entry into the system is critical. Consideration should be given to the degree of access the change agent has in various parts of the system. What linkages does the entry subsystem or person have to other parts of the organization? What leverage will the change agent be able to exert on the entry point to facilitate the change process?

The change agent must be aware of personal responsibilities (those that have been jointly defined) to the client system. Strategies must be used by the change agent to augment the driving forces while making the environment "safe" enough for the client system to move toward change.

Schmalenberg and Kramer (1979) suggest the use of a change agent team, comprised of a new nurse graduate along with an established practicing nurse who possesses knowledge and empathy of the system gained through experience. This team can harness some of the ideas for change generated by the new nurse graduate and formulate realistic ways to engage the system in the change process.

Stage 3

The change problem is analyzed and clarified. A diagnosis is formulated. Schein (1972) points out that "a useful diagnostic tool for identifying and analyzing forces acting on a system with respect to any given change target is force-field analysis" (p. 85). Two columns are made, one for the restraining forces and one for the driving forces. Analyze the system with respect to the projected change. What are the driving forces that tend to move the system toward the change goals? List these under the driving forces. What are the restraining forces which keep the system at the present status quo? List these under the restraining forces.

The A VICTORY MODEL (Davis, 1973; Mayer, 1975) is useful in comprehensively analyzing essential elements in the field force analysis that could impinge on the target change. The major components of the model are *a*bility, *v*alues, *i*nformation, *ci*rcumstances, *ti*ming, *o*bligation, *r*esistance, and *y*ield. By such a model, the driving and restraining forces in relation to each of these components can be identified:

1. Ability
   - The willingness and capability of the client system to commit resources to the proposed change
   - The present knowledge level of staff to implement the change
2. Values
   - Attitudes and beliefs of the nursing staff or faculty toward the planned change
   - The agency's or school's general support for change
   - Other relevant characteristics of line and staff nursing personnel or faculty in the organization
   - Interpersonal relationships; employer–employee relations
3. Information
   - Procedures and channels for documenting and recording information about the planned change
4. Circumstances
   - Job responsibilities and job expectations of staff
   - Relationship of the client system with its environment
5. Timing
   - Other organizational activities occurring during the time of the planned change
6. Obligation
   - Felt need by the client system to do something about the problem
7. Resistance
   - Expected or feared negative consequences of the planned change
8. Yield
   - Expected or anticipated positive consequences of the planned change

Stage 4

Change goals are clearly identified and established. Exploration then occurs to identify possible alternatives to achieve these change objectives. The search for new alternatives can either focus on seeking a model with which to identify or scanning the entire environment for relevant information. In the former approach, the client system seeks to pattern its behavior after a model system it has found to be relevant to its change goals. In the latter, as much information is sought from the environment as possible. The alternatives that best fit the client system are selected for implementation. In developing the total plan for change, attention is given to both the activity plan and the strategic plan.

Phase 2. Changing

Stage 5

The change is implemented in the client system. Intentions and plans are transformed into actual change efforts. Feedback about the implementation of the planned change is sought.

The change agent should consider many guidelines when implementing change (Cizmek & Holland, 1979; Levenstein, 1976; Stevens, 1975, 1977):

1. Seek input from staff to be affected by the change early in the planned change process.
2. Select alternatives that will attain the change objectives but will affect staff in the least negative fashion.
3. Describe the proposed change in the simplest, most understandable terms.
4. Specify clearly what is to be done, when, and by whom.
5. Attempt to obtain attitudinal acceptance toward the projected change.
6. Inform staff of the projected positive consequences of the change.
7. Discuss the planned change openly with staff.
8. Introduce the change gradually, if possible.
9. Use an adequate time frame to implement the change.
10. Diagnose and solve any problems as they arise in the planned change process.
11. Disseminate information about the positive consequences from pilot testing the planned change.
12. Develop criteria for evaluating the change. Specify staff's role in the evaluation.
13. Continuously evaluate the results of the change efforts and provide feedback to the client system.

Phase 3. Refreezing

Stage 6

The change is generalized and stabilized. The change is evaluated to determine its effectiveness. Well-planned and executed change will eventually become integrated into the system. A state of equilibrium must be encouraged. The change that has been implemented must be given a sufficiently long enough trial period before its impact is evaluated.

Staff must be given assurance early in the planned change process that they will be involved in evaluating the change after a sufficient trial period. It should also be agreed upon whether the staff's recommendations resulting from the evaluation will be considered or accepted by management. The evaluation should be conducted as planned.

Stage 7
The change agent ends the helping relationship. Strategies need to be used to lessen any stress of separation produced. If viewed appropriate, on the other hand, the change agent defines and establishes a different type of continuing relationship.

A Case Example

A normative–reeducative model for changing served as the basis for the initiation and implementation of problem-oriented nursing records (PONR) in a nursing service (see Fig. 10-1). The setting in which the project was implemented was a single clinical division within a large, federal psychiatric hospital. This division had an average daily census of 315 clients during the time the project was implemented. Clients were admitted with a variety of psychiatric problems. Various treatment modalities were used on the eight wards of the division. The nursing staff included 27 registered psychiatric nurses who functioned in a number of different nursing roles and 133 psychiatric nursing assistants. The clinical nurse specialist assigned to the division served as the change agent in the project.

Prior to the initiation of the project, nursing notes were written in narrative style and were kept in a separate section of the medical record. Documentation of nursing plans, for the most part, was kept in a separate card file and discarded upon discharge of the client. The narrative notes did not permit efficient access to information in the chart regarding the client's presenting nursing problems and the progress made in their resolution, nor did the narrative form of charting permit easy review for purposes of determining accountability and for auditing the quality of nursing care. Problem-oriented nursing records were seen as a means for correcting these deficiencies.

Prior to the initiation of PONR, the clinical nurse specialist had also assessed a need among the nursing staff for improving their understanding and care of psychiatric clients. Approaches were often based on tradition rather than on an organized scientific approach to the assessment and resolution of the client's mental health needs, that is, more emphasis needed to be placed on operationalizing the nursing process—assessing, planning, implementing, and evaluating. Another purpose for implementing PONR was the reduction of these deficiencies.

Problem-oriented nursing records is a system of record keeping based on the problem-oriented medical records (POMR) developed by Weed (1969). The system includes essentially four parts. First, using a systematic, standardized form, data are collected about a client. In the described setting, a *nursing history* form was developed. This form clearly defined the information that was to be collected about the client by the nursing staff.

The information collected in the nursing history, along with information from other health team members, was used in the development of the client's *problem list* for use by nursing staff (the second part of PONR). Problems identified from this data base were numbered and titled.

In the *progress notes* (the third part of PONR), each entry has a number and a problem label corresponding to one appearing in the Problem List. The SOAP format is used—that is, the charting documented the client's point of view (subjective), the nurse's

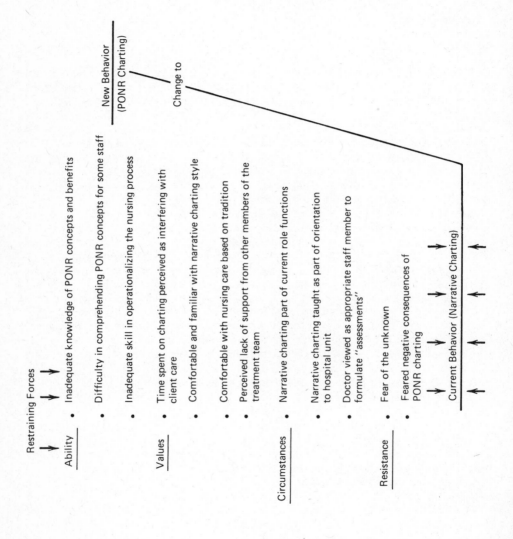

Restraining Forces

Ability
- Inadequate knowledge of PONR concepts and benefits
- Difficulty in comprehending PONR concepts for some staff
- Inadequate skill in operationalizing the nursing process

Values
- Time spent on charting perceived as interfering with client care
- Comfortable and familiar with narrative charting style
- Comfortable with nursing care based on tradition
- Perceived lack of support from other members of the treatment team

Circumstances
- Narrative charting part of current role functions
- Narrative charting taught as part of orientation to hospital unit
- Doctor viewed as appropriate staff member to formulate "assessments"

Resistance
- Fear of the unknown
- Feared negative consequences of PONR charting

New Behavior (PONR Charting)

Change to

Current Behavior (Narrative Charting)

150

Driving Forces

Ability

Values
- Desire to learn
- Optimal nursing care perceived as important and desired
- Prior positive interpersonal relations with nurse specialist and PONR project assistant
- Administrative support and sanction

Information
- Availability of learning packets and sessions on PONR concepts
- Change agent viewed as role model
- Availability of conferences with project staff
- Opportunity for formal and informal learning from nurse specialist and others

Circumstances

Obligation
- Desire to expand role of nurse
- Advocacy role of pilot unit staff to implement the change

Yield
- Hearing about actual PONR benefits from pilot unit staff
- Enthusiasm of pilot unit staff

FIGURE 10-1. SUMMARY OF MAJOR DRIVING AND RESTRAINING FORCES IN CHANGE PROCESS TO PONR.

observation about the client (*objective*), the nurse's conclusion about the data (*assessment*), and the short- and long-term goals and proposed nursing interventions (*plan*).

Administratively, the nurse specialist reported to the division chief nurse who supported the PONR project and delegated all responsibilities for the initiation, development, and implementation of the project to the specialist. The specialist sought input from nursing staff in developing the change objectives and in determining the most effective alternatives for implementing the change. Weekly meetings with the chief nurse afforded the opportunity to discuss these change alternatives and strategies. The chief nurse provided administrative sanction and authority when necessary since the specialist was employed in a staff position, in contrast to being a specialist employed in a line position.

The specialist had already worked with the nursing staff in a number of projects for a 10-month period. This was advantageous in implementing the PONR project since a good working relationship with the nursing staff had evolved. It had given the specialist enough time to assess the competencies of the nurses, as well as their readiness for learning and for change. In addition, being knowledgeable about the staff and the system permitted a comprehensive assessment of the driving and restraining forces relative to the intended change.

With input from staff, the assessment data was utilized in formulating change objectives and in generating some alternative strategies for the implementation of the change. Plans for implementation were formulated. These plans included the selection of a psychiatric staff nurse to assist in the project. This nurse was a baccalaureate graduate who had a number of years of staff and head nurse experience. This staff nurse was selected on the basis of her clinical competency, as well as for her ability to work collaboratively with other team members. Administrative approval was granted for this nurse to be partially released from her staff nurse duties in order for her to assist the specialist in the project. The specialist involved her in the development of plans for the project, as well as in its implementation, which included much teaching and supervision of the nursing staff. The plan also included the development of an extensive teaching packet, and the specification of a time schedule with specific assignment of responsibilities.

The implementation of the planned change included the pilot testing of the PONR project on one of the eight wards in the division. This unit was selected because the staff there expressed an interest in the project and demonstrated readiness for its implementation. The ward was also selected because the head nurse had good rapport and established linkages with the other head nurses in the division and could be counted on to serve as an advocate for a successful pilot project. In addition, the staff nurse assisting the specialist in the project was employed on that ward. Thus, her daily contact with staff afforded her with multiple opportunities to clarify the change objectives, to point out advantages of the planned change, to reinforce the teaching, and to determine immediately any problems which should be brought to the attention of the specialist.

The methods of instructing the staff for the conversion of charting to PONR were tested and revised on the pilot unit. Simultaneously, both a special meeting for all registered psychiatric nurses and a division in-service meeting for all nursing personnel were held in order to expose the staff to the purposes, advantages, and parts of the PONR. Emphasis was placed on the implications this project had for providing quality client care. Ample opportunities were provided staff for airing concerns, problems, and feelings about the planned change.

Upon analysis of the results of the pilot project, it was decided to introduce PONR on one ward at a time, allowing one month to train staff and to convert all records to the new system. Initially, a planning session was held with the head nurse and other key nursing staff members on the ward to discuss the adaptation of PONR to their particular ward. Each staff member, via small groups, was assisted in gaining a clear understanding of the system in a 1-hour training session. This also provided staff with the opportunity to discuss some of their reservations and concerns. The staff was then assisted and actively involved in developing problem lists and nursing treatment plans for each client. The staff was given the opportunity to report successes and problems via individual conferences, written reports, and group meetings. The project staff then conducted periodic chart audits to determine the degree of stabilization of the change on the wards where PONR had been implemented.

The change to PONR was well accepted by the nursing staff. PONR was first introduced on the pilot unit which created good momentum for the project. The pilot ward staff served as informal advocates by telling staff on other wards about the benefits of the project. The wards were selected for project implementation in order of their readiness for the change. By the time the project was to be introduced on the unit on which there had appeared to be the most resistance, the project had a good start in the rest of the division. In addition, the idea for the change had been around long enough that the resistance that remained was worked through with the staff without too much difficulty.

The major problem encountered during the implementation was the extra amount of time required to teach some of the psychiatric nursing assistants the basic concepts of PONR. In a few instances, the head nurse assisted the project staff in reviewing the concepts with the nursing assistant until they were understood. On some wards, the change objectives required a longer period of time than a month. It was necessary for project staff to continue their relationship with these staff members in a supportive role by holding periodic meetings during which questions could be answered and feedback given. On other wards, the project staff was able to resume their prior roles. That is, the specialist continued functioning in other ongoing projects, while the staff nurse severed the change relationship with the ward staff.

At the completion of the moving and refreezing phases, the major purposes and goals for the PONR project were accomplished. All charting followed the PONR format. Nursing care plans were documented and became part of the clinical record. Efficient access to information in the chart regarding the client's presenting nursing problems and the progress in their resolution were feasible. Determining accountability and auditing the quality of nursing care was made possible. Much more thought was given to the understanding of each individual client's needs and to the development of an individualized nursing plan to meet those needs. Charting began to reflect a more scientific approach to the understanding of the behaviors of the clients. The nursing process was operationalized as was reflected in the charting and in the nursing care conferences that were initiated and held on a regular basis.

In addition to the nursing care conferences, the PONR project stimulated other changes for improving client care. Staff, in thoroughly reading records, interviewing clients, and talking with other staff members, uncovered many learning needs. Some of these learning needs were handled via on-the-spot teaching by project staff. Others, however, served as the basis for in-service programs conducted initially by the specialist and eventually by the division ward instructor.

Other evidence of change stabilization and generalization was noted. In time, the problem lists developed by nursing staff began to be used in interdisciplinary planning meetings. As more interest was expressed by other disciplines in the PONR system, the responsibility for developing a teaching packet on POMR and conducting teaching sessions on an interdisciplinary basis were delegated to the division ward instructor. The PONR project had ramifications beyond the boundaries of the division in which it was implemented. Within the hospital, the specialist became cochair of a task force which functioned to study the feasibility of and to recommend methods for implementing POMR throughout the entire hospital. In addition, several publications and professional presentations evolved from the project.

SUMMARY

Planned change refers to a deliberate, conscious, well thought out effort or process to alter or improve the operations of a system or to achieve changed organizational goals by using a knowledgeable change agent. Three major models of change are discussed: the system model, the developmental model, and the model for changing. In addition, three major types of planned change strategies are explored: power–coercive strategies, empirical–rational strategies, and normative–reeducative strategies. Seven guidelines to consider in planned change are then presented. The chapter concludes with an in-depth exploration of a normative–reeducative model for changing and a case example built on this model.

REFERENCES

Benne, K., & Birnbaum, M. Principles of changing. In W. Bennis, K. Benne, & R. Chin (Eds.), *The planning of change*. New York: Holt, Rinehart, & Winston, 1969.

Bennis, W., Benne, K., Chin, R., & Corey, K. (Eds.). *The planning of change*. New York: Holt, Rinehart, & Winston, 1976.

Chin, R. The utility of system models and developmental models for practitioners. In W. Bennis, K. Benne, R. Chin, & K. Corey (Eds.), *The planning of change*. New York: Holt, Rinehart & Winston, 1976.

Chin, R., & Benne, K. General strategies for effecting changes in human systems. In W. Bennis, K. Benne, R. Chin, & K. Corey (Eds.), *The planning of change*. New York: Holt, Rinehart, & Winston, 1976.

Cizmek, C., & Holland, J. Coping with change during curriculum revision. *Nurse Educator*, 1979, 4, 30–35.

Davis, H. Planning for creative change in mental health services: A manual on research utilization (DHEW Publication No. (HSM) 73-9147). Washington, D.C.: U.S. Government Printing Office, 1973.

Levenstein, A. Effective change requires change agent. *Hospitals*, 1976, 50(24), 71–74.

Lippitt, R., Watson, J., & Westley, B. *The dynamics of planned change: A comparative study of principles and techniques*. New York: Harcourt Brace Jovanovich, 1958.

Mayer, S. Are *you* ready to accept program evaluation? *Program Evaluation Resource Center Newsletter*, 1975, 6(1), 1–5.

New, J., & Couillard, N. Guidelines for introducing change. *The Journal of Nursing Administration*, 1981, 11(3), 17–21.

Schein, E. *Professional education: Some new directions*. New York: McGraw-Hill, 1972.

Schmalenberg, C., & Kramer, M. *Coping with reality shock*. Wakefield: Nursing Resources, 1979.

Stevens, B. *The nurse as executive*. Wakefield: Contemporary Publishing, 1975.

Stevens, B. Management of continuity and change in nursing. *Journal of Nursing Administration*, 1977, *7*(4), 26–31.

Weed, L. *Medical records, medical education, and patient care*. Cleveland: Case Western Reserve University Press, 1969.

BIBLIOGRAPHY

Davis, H., & Salasin, S. The utilization of evaluation. In M. Guttentag & E. Struening (Eds.), *Handbook of evaluation research*. Los Angeles: Sage Publications, 1974.

Deal, J. The timing of change. *Supervisor Nurse*, 1977, *8*, 73–79.

Dean, L. The change from functional to primary nursing. *Nursing Clinics of North American*, 1979, *14*(2), 357–364.

Glenn, R., & Richards, D. Assessing the potential of change in institutions. *Psychiatric Quarterly*, 1977, *49*(4), 322–330.

Littlefield, N. The psychiatric nurse as a change agent. *Nursing Clinics of North America*, 1979, *14*(2), 373–382.

Marriner, A. Behavioral aspects of planned change: Reorganization. *Supervisor Nurse*, 1977, *8*, 36–37; 40.

Marriner, A. Planned change as a leadership strategy. *Nursing Leadership*, 1979, *2*(2), 9–14.

Miller, M. Task force—Genesis of a change. *Nursing Clinics of North America*, 1979, *14*(2), 347–356.

Mizer, H., & Barraro, A. Change—For nursing service and education. *Nursing Clinics of North America*, 1979, *14*(2), 337–346.

Olson, E. Strategies and techniques for the nurse change agent. *Nursing Clinics of North America*, 1979, *14*(2), 323–336.

Partridge, R. Education for entry into professional nursing practice: The planning of change. *Journal of Nursing Education*, 1981, *20*(4), 40–46.

Spradley, B. Managing change creatively. *The Journal of Nursing Administration*, 1980, *10*(5), 32–37.

Stevens, B. *Management and leadership in nursing*. New York: McGraw-Hill, 1978.

Welch, L. Planned change in nursing: The theory. *Nursing Clinics of North America*, 1979, *14*(2), 307–321.

CHAPTER 11
COMMUNICATION: PRINCIPLES AND SKILLS

Communication, as previously described, is an interactive process involving at least one other party and potentially impacting upon other members of the subsystem. The communication process is a major tool through which the nurse leader, manager, or supervisor directs the efforts of work group members toward goal achievement.

COMPONENTS OF THE COMMUNICATION PROCESS

The major components of the communication process are the sender, the message/mode, and the receiver.

The *sender* has certain goals in mind for the communication. These can include instructing, persuading, ordering, inquiring, informing, and so forth. The speaker encodes or puts the intended message to the receiver into analogic forms (gestures, facial expressions, voice inflection, body posture, etc.) and digital forms (words, written memos, etc.).

The *message* may be directed by the sender to one other person, to a small group, or to a large group. The communication *mode* may be face-to-face through conversation, meetings, or public speeches. The communication may be mediated through written memos and other correspondence, films, tapes, and other audiovisual media, or through mass media such as radio, television, newspapers, and brochures.

The *receiver* decodes the message—perceiving it and interpreting its meaning. Based on this perception, the original receiver responds, thus becoming the sender.

A number of variables can affect the communication process and become barriers to successful communication (McFarland & Wasli, 1982, p. 918):

a. Culture, customs, education, social background, physical and mental status, intellectual ability, and past experiences of the participants.
b. Channel, language, and words used to transmit message.
c. Context in which communication occurs.
d. Perceptions, feelings, thoughts, and motivations of receiver and sender prior to communication.
e. Nature of the relationship between sender and receiver.
f. Intentions or goals of sender.
g. Self-concept or self-perception of sender and receiver.
h. Anxiety or stress level of sender or receiver.

i. Sensory organ impairment or physical disorder interfering with mechanical ability to produce sound.

j. Discrepancies between the sender's and receiver's punctuation of the communication sequence of events—i.e., the particular aspects of the communication on which each focuses.

The interpretation of the communication by the receiver can be quite different from what was intended by the sender. This can be due to the sender's contradictory forms of analogic and digital communication. For example, Mr. Dawson, head nurse, says to Ms. Minetta, staff nurse, "You have certainly accomplished a great deal of work today." However, Mr. Dawson's voice is strained, he is scowling, and his hands are clenched. Preston (1979) points out that in such contradictions, the nonverbal message is usually the stronger one.

The interpretation of the communication by the receiver can also be quite different from what was intended by the sender because of the receiver's own frame of reference, perceptions, mental status, past experiences, motivations, feelings, or thoughts, that is, the sender's analogic and digital forms of communication are congruent and the message is otherwise clear. In such instances, the "noise" originates from the receiver and erroneous interpretations are made of the sender's communication.

COMMUNICATION WITHIN ORGANIZATIONS

Formal channels of communication coincide with the formal organization and formal lines of authority. As Stevens (1978) points out

> This type of channel is used by nurse-managers regardless of leadership style. Managers view this channel as the vehicle to disseminate orders and directives to unit members. (p. 166)

Formal channels of communication are also referred to as downward communication. The mode of communication can vary from face-to-face, to written memoranda, policy statements, or other written directives.

As nursing staff or faculty interact in the process of conducting the activities of the formal organization, personal and social relationships develop along with informal groups and informal communication networks, that is, the grapevine and rumors. These informal groups and communication channels can meet the nurse employee's needs for social interaction, self-esteem, constructive advice, or information about the organization.

The grapevine can serve as a speedy means of spreading information among employees and can be relatively accurate on noncontroversial topics. But, the grapevine can become quite dysfunctional as each person in the chain of information linkage edits, censors, alters, or adds to the original message. This is especially true for controversial topics. All the variables previously identified as affecting communication come into play here.

Information is sometimes also altered purposefully by persons in the informal, or formal system for that matter, for personal satisfaction or gain. When information is no longer accurate or factual, it becomes rumor (Schuldt, 1978). Rumor provides members in the organization with an outlet for psychological tension and helps to make sense out of a complex and poorly understood environment.

As Schuldt (1978) so aptly puts it

> If information were communicated accurately and promptly through formal channels there would be less need for the informal network to provide its members with news. In actual

practice, formal organizations often circulate news slowly, transmit it poorly, or even with-hold it. In these situations, the grapevine takes over and provides speedy communication for its members. (p. 22)

ASSESSING COMMUNICATIONS IN ORGANIZATIONS

It is important to diagnose problems in communication prior to taking corrective actions in an organization. As has been pointed out in the discussion of leadership, an analysis of communication includes the questions: Who communicates with whom? How often? For how long? In what mode? And, for what purpose?

Other questions to ask: What are the general outcomes of communication in the organization? Are there frequent misunderstandings? Conflicts? Disrupted relation-ships? Is there noncompliance with formal directives? What general principles of communication are neglected?

For example, in one group of nurse faculty, it was noted that conversation and nonverbal behaviors were perceived and interpreted without seeking clarification as to the receiver's accuracy through such strategies as seeking feedback. Receivers in the communication process instead acted as if they were fully justified in their perceptions. This dysfunctional communication pattern led to numerous misunderstandings, scape-goating, a general lack of trust among group members, as well as other dysfunctional behaviors.

There are in existence a number of commerically prepared tools to assess interper-sonal orientations and general communication styles, including the LIFO (Atkins, 1978, pp. 8; 21–24) method:

1. *Supporting/Giving.* The person believes that if personal worth is proven by hard work and pursuit of excellence, that good things in life will materialize.
Goals. To prove worth and be helpful.
Outer Actions. Is principled, cooperative, dedicated, and pursues excellence.
The effective supervisor for this person gives recognition, allows mutual goal setting, is accessible, tries to share, is dependable, and acknowledges trust.

2. *Conserving/Holding.* The person believes that if thinking occurs before acting and the most is gotten from what is possessed, that good things in life will materialize.
Goals. To go slow and be sure.
Outer Actions. Is systematic, analytical, maintaining, and tenacious.
The effective supervisor for this person is organized, shows purpose, is detail oriented, systematic, objective, fair, and consistent.

3. *Controlling/Taking.* The person believes that if competence is demonstrated and opportun-ities are seized, that good things in life will materialize.
Goals. To be competent and get results.
Outer Actions. Is persistent, initiating, urgent, and directing.
The effective supervisor for this person is confident, provides autonomy, rewards results, sets firm boundaries, appreciates initiative, and spars on an equal basis.

4. *Adapting/Dealing.* The person believs that if others are pleased and their needs are met first, that good things in life will materialize.
Goals. To be popular and fit in.
Outer Actions is harmonious, tactful, flexible, and aware.
The effective supervisor for this person expresses intent and preference, is friendly and informal, gives helpful feedback, provides lay of the land, shows flexibility, and displays sense of humor.

FOSTERING SUCCESSFUL COMMUNICATION

A few important principles useful in fostering successful communication are discussed in the following.

The Sender

Self-understanding and an appreciation for both digital and analogic forms of communication serve as foundations for effective nurse manager communications. Effort can then be directed toward anticipating how a given communication might be received by a nursing staff or faculty member given his or her orientation and background. Stevens (1978) suggests that anticipation and emphasis on receptivity should be stressed by nurse managers in their roles as senders of communications. Based on an understanding of the receiver, the communication and mode/channel can be revised from the approach initially intended. If a subject is quite complex or controversial, the nurse manager can provide orientation about the background and process leading to the specific issue at hand. This is especially important for issues affecting job responsibilities, working conditions, or other matters significantly impacting on the employee.

Message/Mode

The message sent must be clear, concise, understandable, and in the most appropriate mode, considering the goal of the communication and the intended receiver.

Benefits of either oral or written modes of communication should be considered. Nurse managers should use the written format when records or documentation are needed and for legal purposes. Written communication is generally more time-consuming and expensive to produce initially. However, clear, concise, and understandable written communication may be the most cost-effective mode in the long run.

Oral communication is quicker initially and can provide the nurse manager with immediate feedback for purposes of clarification. However, oral communication has its drawbacks. There is always the danger that not all persons needing the information received the communication. There is the danger, too, that the oral communication is not perceived the same by all nursing staff or faculty. Therefore, many nurse managers have found that communicating orally, seeking feedback, *and* providing a written follow-up is the most effective process.

It must be pointed out, too, that information must not be communicated to the group that should be communicated privately to an individual. On the other hand, the nurse manager must use care in communicating to only a few immediate staff members when all should be included.

The Receiver

The responsibility for effective communication is shared by all group members. Therefore, nursing staff and faculty need to listen to each other as well as to what is conveyed by their clinical supervisor or faculty coordinator. Likewise, the nurse manager has the responsibility for being an effective receiver of communication.

Effective listening is facilitated by (McFarland & Wasli, 1982; Stevens, 1975):

1. Listening to both facts and feelings
2. Listening actively

3. Avoiding judgmental attitude, prejudice, or stereotyping
4. Clarifying, that is, requesting feedback to make certain that the sender's communication is accurately understood
5. Avoiding selective attention, that is, hearing only the part of the message that is of interest
6. Avoiding selective perception, that is, selecting only the parts of the communication that conform to personal expectations
7. Assuming comprehension of the message sent before really listening to it in its entirety
8. Asking questions to clarify meaning
9. Giving sender full attention and not formulating a response in the meantime
10. Not focusing on and criticizing the speaker's appearance, habits, delivery, and so forth
11. Interpreting messages accurately

As a receiver, the nurse manager must be able to deal effectively with the informal organization's grapevine and rumor. As Schuldt (1978) points out, nurse supervisors must be able to assess, evaluate, and modify the existing culture of the informal organization if necessary. Information can be gained about the organization in this manner, but, extreme care must be taken to ascertain the validity of the content. The grapevine can also be used selectively as an adjunct to formal channels of communication to transmit information rapidly. Effort must be exerted promptly to correct any rumors or misinformation. A formal lateral system of information flow can be instituted as one means of reducing the need for the grapevine.

The nurse manager with a systems orientation will encourage the flow of communication *up* the hierarchical structure. This upward flow of communication can be used to seek feedback, to clarify communication, and to initiate the flow of new ideas from the nursing staff or faculty members.

> Encouraging the upward flow of ideas through the involvement process greatly assists unit members in feeling more a part of the total management process, and increases productivity and morale. (Stevens, 1978, p. 166)

Other Communication Techniques

A selected number of additional communication techniques are now described (McFarland & Wasli, 1982). These techniques can be used selectively by the nurse manager to facilitate effective communication, to ensure that the message sent is the message received, and to ensure accurate perception and interpretation of messages received.

Open-Ended Questions
These questions stimulate responses other than merely "yes" or "no." Such questions can be useful in obtaining additional information seeking clarification, or offering assistance, for example, primary care nursing coordinator to primary care nurse: "Your ideas about the teaching program needed by your patient are . . . ?"

Encouraging Verbalization
These include verbal and nonverbal messages to the sender to assist him or her to keep talking, for example, nursing faculty team leader to faculty member: "Go on," or "As you were saying," or "Hm-huh" and nodding head supportively.

Confrontation
With this technique, discrepancies are described between the verbalizations of the sender and other aspects of behavior, for example, clinical nurse specialist to staff nurse: "You have told me several times that you know how to formulate and utilize nursing diagnoses and yet I do not see their implementation in your care plans. Perhaps you can help me understand this."

Feedback
In this technique, some aspect of the sender's communication and its impact on the receiver is described, for example, charge nurse to nursing assistant: "You appear very upset about having to work on Saturday."

Focusing
In this technique, questions and other communication techniques are used to help the staff member stick to important subject matter in the conversation.

Restating
In this technique, a main thought is repeated using words very similar to those expressed by the staff member. Expansion of the subject matter is encouraged.

Clarifying
Feedback is requested in order to determine that the nursing team member's communications are accurately understood, for example, nurse practitioner to physician assistant: "By telling me . . . do you mean . . . ?"

Seeking Validation
Feedback is requested to check understanding and interpretation of the staff member's communications and perceptions.

Assertive Communication Skills

Nurse leaders who use assertive communication and behavioral skills set goals, act on those goals in a clear and consistent manner, and take responsibility for the consequences of those actions. Ideas are expressed firmly and positively with words that are congruent with nonverbal behaviors.

Assertive communication is direct, honest, and appropriate; its goal is to convey to others what you expect from others and what can be expected from you. (Clark, 1978, p. 12)

Assertive behavior also has these characteristics:

Sensitive to feelings, needs no threats, force used only when and where necessary, firm but gentle—unyielding where appropriate, based on human rights, negotiation a viable tactic, leads to good feelings, accepts workable outcomes. (Moskowitz, 1977, p. 17)

Aggressive communication and behavior patterns, on the other hand, try to control and manipulate others while disregarding their rights or feelings. Little responsibility is assumed for the consequences of actions. Other characteristics are:

insensitive to feelings; use of force and threats of force; attack oriented; either victory or defeat, no middle ground; leads to frustration, guilt, anger; demands preconceived outcomes. (Moskowitz, 1977, p. 17)

The third major type of communication/behavioral response is nonassertive/recessive behavior. In this pattern, rather than confronting an issue, the path of least resistance is taken. One method of doing this is to completely agree with the other person. "Smoothing things over" before really exploring the situation is another strategy used. Confrontation and conflict are avoided. Others are sought out to provide answers and behavior is reactive rather than goal-directed. Nurses using this pattern allow others to choose, decide, and speak for them. Thus, this nonassertive/recessive pattern is really a cover up for what is really wanted and does not help in obtaining personal goals. As a result, feelings of inadequacy, insecurity, depression, self-blame, self-punishment, and resentment develop. Characteristics can be summarized as follows: "insensitive to needs and desires; yields too often; sacrifices basic human rights; leads to frustration, guilt, bad feelings; accepts unwanted outcomes" (Moskowitz, 1977, p. 17).

Judgment must obviously be used in utilizing assertive communication skills. In general, however, assertive communication skills assist nurse managers in achieving their goals in a manner that respect the rights of other team members.

SUMMARY

The major components of the communication process described in this chapter were: sender, message/mode, and receiver. Variables affecting the communication process are identified.

Formal channels of communication coincide with the formal organization and formal lines of authority. As nursing staff or faculty interact in the process of conducting the activities of the formal organization, personal and social relationships develop together with informal groups and informal communication networks—the grapevine and rumor.

The assessment of communication in organizations is followed by a description of selected principles fostering successful communication.

In summary, considerable thought should be given by the nurse manager to the goals of the communication and to the best alternative mode to present the content to the receiver. Nurse managers should plan their communications.

REFERENCES

Atkins, S. *LIFO training discovery workbook*. Beverly Hills, Calif.: Human Resources Technology, 1978.

Clark, C. *Assertive skills for nurses*. Wakefield, Mass.: Contemporary Publishing, 1978.

McFarland, G., & Wasli, E. Psychiatric nursing. Part 2. In L. Brunner & D. Suddarth (Eds.), *The Lippincott manual of nursing practice*. Philadelphia: Lippincott, 1982.

Moskowitz, R. *Assertiveness for career and personal success*. New York: AMACOM, 1977.

Preston, P. Communication for managers. *American Health Care Association Journal*, 1979, *5*, 10–11, 14, 16.

Schuldt, S. Supervision and the informal organization. *Journal of Nursing Administration*, 1978, *8*(7), 21–25.

Stevens, B. *The nurse as executive*. Wakefield, Mass.: Contemporary Publishing, 1975.

Stevens, W. *Management and leadership in nursing*. New York: McGraw-Hill, 1978.

CHAPTER 12
THE PROBLEM-SOLVING PROCESS AND IDEA GENERATION

A common assumption—finding problems to solve is easy; dreaming up solutions to these problems is far more difficult—must be dispelled. To the skilled problem solver, the reverse is often true. With proper strategies, good solutions will come quickly and easily while problem choice, definition, and analysis will often be difficult.

THE PROBLEM-SOLVING PROCESS

The problem-solving process begins long before the first ideas for solution begin to come into one's mind. Practiced and skilled problem solvers may pass from stage to stage in the process without being aware of the manner of progress. Slighting or leaving out any of the critical links, however, will result in an inferior product or a serious impass.

Koberg and Bagnall (1974) identified the following steps in the creative process: problem birth, acceptance of the problem, problem analysis, problem definition, generating ideas for problem solution, selection of best ideas, implementation of ideas for problem solution, and evaluation of results.

Problem Birth

Problems are born in many ways. Problems will be brought to the attention of the nurse manager by subordinates and superiors. The nurse manager may observe that something on the patient care unit requires replacement, alteration, or repair so that performance may be improved. In many cases, the solution of one problem will uncover other problems that require attention.

Problem Acceptance

Many potential problems are generated each day, but equal attention cannot be given to all of them. By necessity, successful managers establish priorities, deciding to accept some problems for attention while ignoring others temporarily or permanently. Unsuccessful managers dive into problems indiscriminantly without assessing whether the problem is important, whether they have sufficient personal interest in solving the problem, or even whether they have the qualifications to continue to the end.

A few problems come in a form that require further refinement to produce creative solutions. Koberg and Bagnall (1974) gave a simple example of an initial problem in need of refinement. The distraction of buzzing flies may lead a person to spend his or her energies buying a fly swatter. Greater care in accepting this problem might lead to seeing the holes in the screen as the more relevant problem.

When a problem has been identified as warranting a manager's attention, the issue of personal acceptance emerges. To accept a problem means to assume responsibility for it. Before assuming such responsibility, the effective manager will be wise to ask, and honestly answer, several questions: What's in it for me? Does this fit into my personal priorities? Can I manage any resulting stress? Am I willing, if necessary, to make sacrifices in other areas to solve this problem? Commitments to projects without a cold-blooded look at the personal consequences for the manager as well as for the system often lead to half-hearted and unsuccessful problem-solving efforts.

Problem Analysis

Once a problem has been accepted as worthy of further attention, the process of problem analysis begins in earnest. Problem analysis involves two basic methods (Koberg & Bagnall, 1974): questioning and comparing. It requires seeking information through active curiosity and comparing the problem to other problems to determine the ways in which they are similar or different.

The same authors suggested that the problem solver ask the following "basic questions" to begin an analysis, even if she or he feels timid about the pursuit:

> Usually, the mere asking of a question calls for courage, however. It means throwing off fear and pride to determine what, why, where, when and who. The basic questions tend to be:
> Where can information be found?
> Who can help me solve this problem?
> What has already been tried to solve this problem?
> Are there books or references available?
> What are my resources and what is required?
> What is the total scope or world of this problem?
> What limits can I control and which are fixed?
> What is allowed and what is ruled out?
> Can the rules be changed?
> (Koberg & Bagnall, 1974, p. 48)

The discovery of the interrelationship of problems can be facilitated by a process termed *synectics* (Gordon, 1968, 1971). Synectics employs analogy, metaphor, and simile so that the problem solver may learn (make the strange familiar) and innovate (make the familiar strange). To accomplish learning and innovation, strategies are employed to get the problem solver both inside and outside of the problem. One assumption is that it is easier to solve someone else's problems than to solve one's own problems.

Gordon (1968, 1971) suggests that the problem solver adopt four attitudes toward the problem: (a) detachment and involvement (getting outside of and inside of the problem); (b) deferment (tolerating input until all decisions have been considered); (c) speculation (questioning, examining related superstitions, analyzing personal dreams); and (d) autonomy of object (focusing on the *process* of solution, not the *product* of the solution).

While maintaining these important attitudes toward the problem-solving enterprise, the manager using synectics employs three basic problem-solving methods: (a) direct analogy (finding out how the problem is like other problems); (b) personal analogy (role-playing elements of the problem in various human, animal, vegetable, mineral, and abstract contexts); and (c) compressed conflict (searching for subproblems within the main problem, looking for something to solve).

A key concept in synectics is "stretch." By looking at a problem from the outside, by developing *outsight* rather than *insight*, the manager stretches away from the original problem to problems that are analogous and interrelated to the original problem.

In typical use, synectics has three stages. In the first stage, existing viewpoints are stated and the mind is purged of preconceptions. In the second stage, the problem solver attempts to "stretch" away from the original problem into other areas using any or all of the three synectics mechanisms (direct analogy, personal analogy, and compressed conflict). During the third stage, the problem solver uses these new experiences in completing the analysis of the original problem. In these ways, novel and fresh views of the problem may be obtained.

An example may help the reader gain greater understanding of how synectics might be used. A nurse manager in a large general hospital observed that day nursing staff made decisions about patient care without advising or consulting with the evening or night nursing staff. Consequently, patient care was inconsistent throughout the 24-hour period and conflict had emerged among the three shifts.

To aid in analyzing the problem, the nurse manager might use synectics methods in the following ways. The nurse manager might note a direct analogy between the staff and the problem of "coordinating" the electrical charges to the spark plugs in an automobile engine. Without coordination, the spark plugs will not fire when the pistons are in the correct positions. The net result is an engine that will run poorly or not at all. By studying the way engineers have solved the spark plug problem, the nurse manager may discover new ways to analyze and solve the staff problem.

To gain a greater understanding of the dynamics occurring among the three staff groups, the nurse manager might employ the personal analogy method by role-playing each staff group as a different animal. The day staff might be role-played as a lion, the evening staff as a mule, and the night staff as a mole, if those are the animals that come to mind when he or she thinks of each staff group. A variation of this method would be to enlist the help of colleagues in role-playing these animals fighting, playing, and working together. These role-playing experiences may shed more light on the relationship of these three staffs.

Finally, the compressed conflict method could be employed by identifying the smaller subproblems contained within the larger problem: making sure medication is administered consistently throughout the three shifts, preventing the patients from identifying the evening staff as the "good guys" and the night staff as the "bad guys,"and so forth.

Outsights discovered through these methods could be brought back to the original staff problem to complete problem analysis. From the spark plug analogy might come the recognition of a need for a group to perform a *distributor* function (distributing information in the right frequency and order to the various staff groups). From the role-playing experiences might come an awareness of the various roles each staff group plays with each other, the relative power each group has with each other, and even an awareness of some of the unconscious processes involved in each staff group's behavior.

Problem Definition

A definition of the problem will frequently result from successful analysis. Simply stated, a definition is a refined objective (Koberg & Bagnall, 1974). It states the essence of the problem and marks a turning point in the problem-solving process from discovery to solution. It is often a "eureka" statement. Frequently, successful definition indicates that the problem solver is halfway to the solution. This is implied in the popular aphorism, "A job well begun is half done."

From the synectics exercise, the following definition of the problem might be distilled: representatives from all three staff groups need to be involved in making decisions and disseminating information about patient care. This statement serves as a goal statement in efforts to generate ideas. This definition, however, is not set in concrete and may be modified with further experience.

GENERATING IDEAS FOR PROBLEM SOLUTION

All too frequently, problem solving begins with dreaming up ideas to solve vaguely defined problems without considering the previous steps. By analogy, this process resembles an ocean voyage in a boat with no rudder and no planned destination. The process will be frustrating enough if one embarks on this voyage alone, but it will result in confusion, acrimony, and even mutiny if attempted with a group. Is it any wonder that groups are often so unproductive in solving problems?

On the other hand, the potential problem-solving capability of groups is considerable. Although groups may be involved in any step within the problem-solving process, there is considerable evidence (Hall, Mouton, & Blake, 1963; Osborn, 1979) that groups can be particularly useful in generating problem-solving ideas.

This statement cannot be made unequivocally, however, since the method of group problem solving is critical to its superiority in relation to individual problem solving (Bouchard, 1969; Osborn, 1979; Parnes & Meadow, 1959). Freely interacting groups have many characteristics that interfere with or inhibit creative thinking. Such groups tend to evaluate ideas prematurely. This restricts creativity, originality, and practicality of ideas generated and arouses individual defensiveness (Collaros & Anderson, 1969). Interacting group members tend to react to the opinions of others rather than to generate their own ideas (Van de Ven, 1974). By prematurely evaluating the ideas of others and arousing defensiveness in contributing members, much group energy is tied up in preserving intragroup harmony and is diverted from the task of generating ideas (Campbell, 1968). Another characteristic of freely interacting groups is a tendency to focus on a single train of thought for extended periods of time, thereby halting further search for alternative ideas (Van de Ven, 1974).

Norms for conformity of opinion often develop in unstructured problem-solving groups that constrain the felt freedom of members to be open with their ideas and thereby inhibit creativity in the group (Delbecq, Van de Ven, & Gustafson, 1975). These effects are emphasized in groups with members varying in degree of status. There is a tendency for low-status members to agree with the opinions of high-status members (Torrance, 1957). There may be implied threats of sanctions from more knowledgeable or powerful members that inhibit creativity (Hoffman, 1965). Members with dominant personalities frequently inhibit the creativity of more timid members (Chung & Ferris, 1971).

Freely interacting groups tend to resolve conflict by smoothing over differences among members to provide an appearance of harmony and goodwill among members (Van de Ven, 1974). When this method fails and differences do come up for open discussion, it has been observed that contending members become polarized on issues and criticism becomes personalized (Van de Ven, 1974).

Unfortunately, these conflict-resolution methods lead to inferior problem solving. Burke (1970) reports that direct confrontation of problems (rather than people) is consistently related to creative problem solving, while smoothing-over methods lead to inconsistent creativity (sometimes positive, sometimes negative). When some members remain silent while others confront each other on a personal basis, as frequently happens in polarized groups, creativity is consistently inhibited.

Another characteristic of freely interacting groups is a tendency to fail to gain closure on issues and to table decision making until later (Van de Ven, 1974).

Many of these drawbacks to group problem solving can be eliminated or reduced by selecting an appropriate working structure for the group. Three alternate methods— *brainstorming* (Osborn, 1979) *nominal group technique* (Delbecq & Van de Ven, 1971), and the *Delphi technique* (Dalkey, 1967)—will be discussed. Each has particular strengths as well as some drawbacks for use by the problem solver.

Brainstorming

Brainstorming is a simple and versatile method that was introduced by Osborn (1979). Osborn identified four principles of brainstorming that *must* be followed if the group is to avoid many of the pitfalls of group creativity described in the previous section.

1. List every idea. Quantity is desirable. Try to list the ideas *exactly* as stated. Do not try to paraphrase, consolidate, integrate, or differentiate a new idea from the other ideas.
2. Do not judge ideas as they are offered. There will be plenty of time later for criticism.
3. Encourage members to "tag on" or "spin off" ideas from previous ideas. Apparent repetition of ideas is acceptable. There may be subtle but important differences in ideas that seem alike.
4. Do not discuss ideas as they are presented. The primary purpose of brainstorming is to *generate* ideas.

Lippitt and Schindler-Rainman (1977) suggested further refinements of the brainstorming technique. Before beginning a brainstorming session, participants are instructed to list on newsprint or blackboard, "all the ways to develop a workshop, revise a form, solve a scheduling conflict, or whatever. In other words, state the name of the problem to be solved." This establishes a psychological attitude or set that encourages quantity of ideas. With regard to the problem of premature evaluation of ideas, it is suggested that the brainstorm leader *immediately* cut off criticism or even ring a bell to alert the group to this problem. Lippitt and Schindler-Rainman caution that even nonverbal gestures ("relationship" messages) such as head noddings, smiles, or scowls can signal approval or criticism and inhibit group creativity. Brainstorming sessions often have periods of silence. It may be very tempting to stop a brainstorming session at the first long silence. Lippitt and Schindler-Rainman, however, encourage brainstorm leaders to tolerate these silences since many of the most creative ideas will frequently follow.

The structure of brainstorming sessions eliminates several of the serious drawbacks of freely interacting groups: premature evaluation is prohibited, focusing effects are avoided, all members are encouraged to contribute regardless of rank, status, or intellectual ability, and the lack of discussion at the start frees the group from worrying about harmony.

The necessity of adhering to *all* of the principles of brainstorming is reemphasized. In recent years, the term has come to mean the process of groups meeting to freewheel ideas with little or no additional structure. These groups have little advantage over freely interacting groups that have many, if not all, of their drawbacks. A case example follows.

A workshop designed to introduce organization development to the nursing education section of a large federal psychiatric agency was conducted. During the afternoon of the first day, members of the workshop were introduced to the problem of diagnosing the system and its processes from a general systems theory viewpoint through a lecture process. At this point, the workshop design called for breaking the membership into three or four small groups to work on concrete and relevant problems facing the nursing education section. The staff believed that these problems would best be identified by members themselves rather than imposed by fiat by the workshop staff. It was at this point that a group brainstorming session was *planned* into the program.

Approximately 20 minutes were allotted for this process. The group was instructed to think of "all the problems facing the nursing education subsystem at the agency that needed solving." By this method, 35 problems were identified quickly as worthy of the attention and effort of the workshop members.

With this data, the group established priorities for problems and collapsed problems into three primary problem areas: problems in the large nursing system (large subsystem), problems in the smaller nursing education system (small subsystem), and problems concerning the interface between these two systems (interface groups), which served as a basis for developing three task groups.

This example illustrates the flexibility of the brainstorming technique. In this case, the brainstorming technique was used to identify problems in need of solution. Later on in the same workshop, it was used to generate solutions to the identified problem of maintaining the organization development process after the workshop ended. This latter brainstorming session generated a number of novel and creative solutions.

Nominal Group Technique

The nominal group technique (NGT) was developed by Delbecq and Van de Ven (1971) as an improved version of Osborn's original brainstorming technique. It incorporated findings from social-psychological studies of decision conferences, management science studies of aggregating group judgments, and social work studies of problems involving participation in program planning (Delbecq, et al., 1975).

At the beginning of a NGT session, group members are instructed not to talk to one another as they write down ideas related to a predefined problem. At the end of 5–10 minutes, each member in turn shares an idea, which is displayed on newsprint or a blackboard for all in the group to see. This round-robin sharing continues until all the ideas are presented. As in brainstorming, no discussion is allowed to occur until all the ideas have been presented.

The next phase of NGT involves clarifying and discussing the merits of each idea. When the discussion is completed, the group privately gives priority to the ideas by rank-ordering them or rating them. A mathematical solution represents the group decision.

This method is presumed to encourage more balanced participation than the brainstorming technique since shy and nonassertive members are given their turn at offering ideas as often as anyone else. A method of group decision making is also built into the NGT. Similar decision-making methods, however, could easily be added to brainstorming sessions.

There are several drawbacks to NGT. Due to the time required to give everyone their turns during the round robin, groups larger than seven to ten members require excessive time to generate ideas. Some preparation is necessary for a NGT session, thus reducing its usefulness as a spontaneous idea-generating technique. As with brainstorming, all participants need to be in the same room together. The next idea-generating method, the Delphi technique (Dalkey, 1967, 1969) does not make this requirement and is an innovation in idea generation that allows members in separate locations to participate in the decision-making process.

The Delphi Technique

The Delphi technique (Dalkey, 1967, 1969) is really an approach to problem solving that has many variations. Developed by Dalkey at the Rand Corporation in 1950, it was first used to forecast technological developments (hence the name, relating to the "Delphic Oracle").

The process involves the systematic solicitation and collation of judgments from respondents on a particular topic by means of a series of questionnaires. Summarized information and opinions are obtained by each wave of questionnaires and fed back to the respondents along with further requests for more refined judgments.

Turoff (1970) suggests that there are at least three separate groups performing within distinct roles:

Decision maker(s)—the individual(s) expecting some sort of product from the exercise that is used for making final decisions.

A staff group—the group that designs the initial questionnaire, summarizes the returns, and redesigns the follow-up questionnaire.

A respondent group—the group whose judgments are being sought and who are asked to respond to the questionnaire.

Variations in the Delphi technique include whether the respondent is anonymous, whether open-ended or structured questions are used, how many series of questionnaires are employed, and what decision rules are employed to aggregate the judgments (Delbecq et al., 1975).

The following hypothetical problem will be used to exemplify use of the Delphi technique. Assume that nurses across the country wish to develop a nomenclature of acceptable nursing diagnoses. Leaders in the field of nursing who would be polled by mailed questionnaires for their ideas and opinions on this subject could be identified. When these questionnaires are returned, the staff group would commence to compile and summarize the acquired information.

A feedback report and second questionnaire would then be prepared and mailed back to the respondents. Having received the feedback reports, the respondents would evaluate earlier responses independently. Respondents would be instructed to place in order of priority the ideas included in the second questionnaire and to mail their responses back to the staff team. This process would continue until the staff team concluded that sufficient consensus had been obtained concerning a nomenclature of acceptable nursing diagnoses. The staff group would then submit a summarizing report to the decision maker(s).

The Delphi technique has many unique advantages over other idea-generation methods. It requires little time from respondents, it can involve large numbers of respondents, and it does not require physical proximity of respondents. With no verbal interaction, inhibiting group dynamics are not present.

On the other hand, respondents frequently report a sense of detachment from the problem-solving process and a lowered sense of accomplishment with the final product (Van de Ven, 1974). The lack of opportunity for verbal clarification in the questionnaire and feedback reports makes communication and interpretation difficulties common (Delbecq et al., 1975). Difficulties in resolving conflicts become apparent since solutions picked by pooling or adding votes prevent efforts to reach more integrative solutions (Delbecq et al., 1975). There is some evidence, as well, that NGT produces a higher-quality product than Delphi techniques (Gustafson, Shukla, Delbecq, & Walster, 1973). Open discussion of ideas and alternative solutions does seem to play an important role in producing high-quality solutions and participant satisfaction with derived solutions.

Selection of the Best Ideas

NGT and Delphi techniques have idea selection methods already built into the problem-solving process. Lippitt and Schindler-Rainman (1977) added an idea selection method to the variation of Osborn's brainstorming technique. When the group has finished the idea-generation phase, each participant is instructed to select their top priority ideas from among the larger list of ideas generated by the group. The participants, in turn, verbally disclose their choices to the newsprint and place check marks next to their choices. The group's selection of high priority, importance, or quality ideas is the simple sum of individual voting for each idea.

Another cluster of methods for idea selection that may be used by individuals as well as groups involves using simulations to "test" each potential solution in advance. Individuals or groups may role-play application of the solutions to identify critical stages, unexpected obstacles, personal reactions to the planned change, and so forth, Koberg and Bagnall (1974) termed this the "Indian scout" method and likened its use to the Indian scouts of the last century who traveled ahead to see what the main force would be that they would encounter when they arrived. Program Evaluation Review Technique (PERT) (Cook, 1966) uses this strategy to determine "the most critical path" in anticipating the feasibility of idea implementation.

Implementation of Ideas for Problem Solution

Several methods of implementing ideas to solve problems will be considered. One method is to develop time-task schedules (Koberg & Bagnall, 1974):

1. Decide how many and what kinds of tasks are involved in performing the selected idea requirements. Find the answer to the question, "What are all the steps which must be taken in order to complete this thing?"
2. Determine the exact amount of time you have for the overall project.
3. Assign in the most reasonable way you can, portions of the total time to each of the steps required.
4. Prepare a graphic display (a piece of paper will do) which shows the relationship of time to your tasks.
5. Allow the time-task schedule to guide you through the implementation phase. (p. 82)

Another method presented by Koberg and Bagnall is termed performance specification. In this method, ideas are broken down in the specific and intended behaviors implied by the idea. When the exact performance desired has been specified, it then becomes possible to translate the idea into real materials and actions. The method serves to stabilize the needed actions to implement an idea.

For example, if the problem involves implementing a new ward work schedule, the specifications for performance might include: (1.) Staffing must be adequate on all shifts, (2.) Shift changes must not occur during meals or periods of treatment, and (3.) The hospital will not incur overtime expenses for staff.

A last implementation method involves the process of delegation of responsibility for various parts of the projected solution (Koberg & Bagnall, 1974). Find members of the work team who have expertise in the various subareas of the solution that has been identified by performance specification and the time-task schedules. A consulting team will then have been developed.

Evaluating Results

Evaluation of the results of idea implementation requires matching results to the goals. This often takes the form of simple observations when the desired outcomes are visible or easily quantifiable. In management, however, many desired outcomes involve attitudes, opinions, or subjective judgments of one sort or another.

Evaluation in these cases involves many additional problems of measurement that the nurse manager is not typically qualified to solve. The problems of psychological scaling and measurement require specialists who are often not available to the nurse manager.

Simplified evaluation questionnaires may be constructed, however, using the following guidelines that will yield quite valuable information concerning the success of the solution efforts:

1. Be direct and do not ask general questions. Make the objectives into evaluation questions.
2. Avoid strange, unfamiliar, or highly symbolic language.
3. Avoid questions that beg answers that support personal opinion. The manager will be guilty of being a self-fulfilling prophet.
4. Give a reward to encourage completion of the questionnaire.
5. Employ a numerical scale to simplify scoring and interpretation. One widely employed scale is a 5-point Likert Scale (1932) with the following form:

   Rate the degree to which a specific goal was attained.
   Circle a number below to record your response

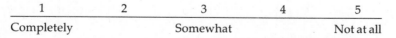

1	2	3	4	5
Completely		Somewhat		Not at all

(Adapted from Koberg & Bagnall, 1974.)

When the problem-solving sequence is completed for one problem, evaluation may suggest return to an earlier stage in the problem-solving process for reanalysis based upon the new data that has been collected. The manager may also become aware of new problems to tackle that become apparent in the evaluation phase. Rarely does evaluation leave the problem solver completely satisfied and content with the product of his or her efforts.

SUMMARY

Some readers may have noted the similarity between the problem-solving processes described in this chapter and the organization development model (French & Bell, 1978). Through organization development, specific methods designed to improve an organization's problem solving and renewal processes are employed. The problem-solving methods offered in this chapter may be applied generally to any problem in need of solution.

The problem-solving sequence that we have offered is an expanded form of OD's basic steps: data collection; feedback, data analysis, and system diagnoses; action planning and system intervention; and maintaining, managing, and evaluating the process. Koberg and Bagnall's problem analysis and problem definition steps correspond to the diagnosis step in OD. In a similar way, the generation of ideas for problem solution, the selection of the best ideas, and the implementation of ideas for problem-solution steps are contained within the new actions/intervention step in OD. In both approaches, evaluation of results leads to finer tuning of the problem-solving process. The problem birth and acceptance of the problem steps contained in the Koberg and Bagnall model would correspond to a system entry stage in the OD process. As the nurse manager becomes more skilled as a problem solver, she or he will also become more creative and effective as an organizational manager and system change agent.

REFERENCES

Bouchard, T. Personality, problem-solving procedure, and performance in small groups. *Journal of Applied Psychology*, 1969, 53(1, Part 2), 1–29.

Burke, R. Methods of resolving superior-subordinate conflict: The constructive use of subordinate differences and disagreements. *Organizational Behavior and Human Performance*, 1970, 5, 393–411.

Campbell, J. Individual versus group problem solving in the industrial sample. *Journal of Applied Psychology*, 1968, 52(3), 205–210.

Chung, K., & Ferris, M. An inquiry of the nominal group process. *Academy of Management Journal*, 1971, 14(4), 520–524.

Cook, D. *Program evaluation and review technique: Application in education.* Washington, D.C.: DHEW, Office of Education, 1966.

Collaros, P., & Anderson, L. The effect of perceived expertness upon creativity of members of brainstorming groups. *Journal of Applied Psychology*, 1969, 53(2), 159–163.

Dalkey, N. *Delphi.* Santa Monica, Calif.: Rand Corporation, 1967.

Dalkey, N. *The delphi technique: An experimental study of group opinion.* Santa Monica, Calif.: Rand Corporation, 1969.

Delbecq, A., & Van de Ven, A. A group process model for problem identification and program planning. *Journal of Applied Behavioral Sciences*, 1971, (July-August).

Delbecq, A., Van de Ven, A., & Gustafson, D. *Group techniques for program planning.* Glenview, Ill.: Scott, Foresman, 1975.

French, W., & Bell, C. *Organization development.* Englewood Cliffs, N.J.: Prentice Hall, 1978.

Gordon, W. J. *Synectics.* Riverside: Macmillan (Colliers), 1968.

Gordon, W. J. *The metaphorical way: Learning and knowing.* Cambridge: Porpoise Books, 1971.

Gustafson, D., Shukla, R., Delbecq, A., & Walster, G. A comparative study of differences in subjective likelihood estimates made by individuals, interacting groups, Delphi groups, and Nominal groups. *Organizational Behavior and Human Performance*, 1973, 9, 280–291.

Hall, E., Mouton, J., & Blake, R. Group problem-solving effectiveness under conditions of pooling versus interaction. *Journal of Social Psychology*, 1963, 59, 147–157.

Hoffman, L. Group problem solving. In Berkowitz, L. (Ed.) *Experimental social psychology, Part II.* Oshkosh: Academic Press, 1965.

Koberg, D., & Bagnall, J. *The universal traveler.* Los Altos, Calif.: William Kaufman, 1974.

Likert, R. A technique for the measurement of attitudes. *Archives of Psychology*, 1932, No. 140.

Lippitt, R., & Schindler-Rainman, E. Mimeographed proceedings from Laboratory in Designing Consultation and Training Activities. Bethel, Maine: NTL, 1977.

Osborn, A. *Applied imagination.* New York: Scribners (1979). (Originally published, 1957.)

Parnes, S., & Meadow, A. Effects of brainstorming instructions on creative problem solving by trained and untrained subjects. *Journal of Educational Psychology*, 1959, 50, 171–176.

Torrance, E. Group decision making and disagreement. *Social Forces*, 1957, 35, 314–318.

Turoff, M. The design of a policy Delphi. *Technological Forecasting and Social Change*, 1970, 2.

Van de Ven, A. *Group decision-making effectiveness.* Kent, Ohio: Kent State University Center for Business & Economic Research Press, 1974.

CHAPTER 13
DECISION MAKING

The methods and strategies described in Chapter 12 provide the necessary ingredients for an effective decision. If an appropriate decision-making strategy is not employed, however, the results of the problem-solving process will be poor.

In this chapter, the characteristics of an effective decision are compared with typical decision-making behavior. A model is then presented to allow the nurse manager/supervisor to make effective decisions. The emphasis is upon methods that use the resources of the health care system in an efficient manner to ensure that a *quality* decision that will be *accepted* by subordinates and superiors emerges.

IDEAL DECISION-MAKING PROCESSES

While it is difficult to judge whether a given decision is of high quality, Janis and Mann (1977) identify seven procedures that generally ensure high-quality decisions. Their review of the literature suggests that decisions satisfying the seven ideal procedural criteria given in the following have "a better chance than others of obtaining the decision maker's objectives and of being adhered to in the long run" (p. 11).

The decision maker, to the best of his or her ability and within his or her information-processing capabilities,

1. Thoroughly canvasses a wide range of alternative courses of action;
2. Surveys the full range of objectives to be fulfilled and the values implicated by the choice;
3. Carefully weighs whatever he knows about the costs and risks of negative consequences, as well as the positive consequences, that could flow from each alternative;
4. Intensively searches for new information relevant to further evaluation of the alternatives;
5. Correctly assimilates and takes account of any new information or expert judgment to which he is exposed, even when the information or judgment does not support the course of action he initially prefers;
6. Reexamines the positive and negative consequences of all known alternatives, including those originally regarded as unacceptable, before making a final choice;
7. Makes detailed provisions for implementing or executing the chosen course of action, with special attention to contingency plans that might be required if various known risks were to materialize (p. 11).

These are ideal criteria and very few decisions would be rated highly on all seven dimensions. Janis and Mann (1977) assume that decision quality is diminished with each criteria that is not successfully met. If all seven criteria are substantially met, however, the decision-maker's orientation is characterized by "vigilant information processing" (Janis & Mann, 1977, p. 12).

DECISION MAKING IN ACTUAL PRACTICE

The vigilant information processing described by Janis and Mann would be termed an "optimizing" strategy (Young, 1966). Optimizing strategies require the decision maker to compare the value of every viable alternative in terms of expected benefits and costs. A familiar procedure using the optimizing strategy is the construction of a list of every viable choice with the pros and cons associated with each choice.

A number of difficulties, however, are encountered when trying to make an optimum decision. In many cases, humans simply do not have "the wits to maximize" (Simon, 1976, p. xxviii). A complete compilation of all relevant information concerning alternative choices quickly overwhelms the mind's ability to process information (Miller, 1956). Simon (1976) notes that the decision-maker's attention "shifts from one value to another with consequent shifts in preference" (p. 83).

Decision makers seldom have the time required to engage in a complete search and analysis of all viable choices (Janis & Mann, 1977). Most managers are forced to make decisions in the midst of a crisis. This is hardly the best environment for dispassionate search and analysis of alternative choices.

It is also difficult to place a comparative value on alternative choices. One choice may be best in terms of monetary concerns but may be considered unethical. How does one compare monetary and value outcomes? Many managers/supervisors also have difficulty comparing short- and long-term benefits. Is it any wonder that people prefer to avoid decision making altogether given the complexity of achieving an optimum decision outcome (Janis & Mann, 1977)? The optimizing strategy is frequently viewed as "an excellent normative (or prescriptive) model—that is, a set of standards the decision maker should strive to attain when making vital decisions" (Janis & Mann, 1977, p. 25).

Satisficing

Simon (1976) has suggested that most managers and supervisors *satisfice*, rather than maximize. The decision maker chooses the first course of action that is "good enough" to meet a minimal set of requirements. This strategy seems to be compatible with the limited information-processing capabilities of people. Using this strategy, the decision maker constructs a list of minimum requirements for an acceptable choice and selects the first choice that meets these standards or, at most, the best choice of the first two or three acceptable choices.

Simon (1976) argues that decision makers are only capable of bounded or limited rationality and resort to gross simplifications with complex decisions. As a result, decision makers accept courses of action that are only slight improvements of the status quo.

While satisficing decisions are considerably less than optimal, they also tend to be conventional and conservative. The manager/supervisor may believe that a satisficing decision is "safe" and will not create waves with his superiors (Johnson, 1974). There are several variations of satisficing that are frequently used by managers and supervisors.

Moral Decision Making

In many situations, a small number of moral precepts are used as the major criteria in making decisions. Schwartz (1970) has referred to this process as moral decision making. Instead of considering the choice as minimally satisfactory, the choice is considered the best or only choice. Health care organizations have a number of traditional values regarding life and death that result in moral decision-making behavior. The existence of such moral precepts or values tends to reduce the number of viable alternative choices and simplifies the decision-making problem.

Elimination-By-Aspects

A quasi-satisficing strategy has been described by Tversky (1972) as the elimination-by-aspects approach. This approach uses a hierarchy of criteria in a sequential narrowing-down process. If a choice under analysis meets the most important criteria, it is evaluated by the next most important criteria for acceptability. The first option that meets all the criteria is selected. The process is quite similar to the familiar game of Twenty Questions.

The nesting of criteria allows the decision maker to use a simple satisficing procedure to consider a large number of alternative choices. The sequential process of the elimination-by-aspects avoids the problem of simultaneous comparison of many options required in optimizing procedures. The decision trees currently used in medical diagnosis represent a useful example of an elimination-by-aspect procedure.

Incrementalism

Although satisficing strategies frequently result in suboptimal decisions, the cumulative effect of such decisions allows for slow progress toward an optimal goal (Janis & Mann, 1977). Lindblom (1959) has referred to this process as "the science of muddling through." When problems arise, the successful "muddler" considers a very narrow range of alternatives that differ slightly from existing policy. The sin of "omission" is chosen over the sin of "confusion" (Lindblom, 1965, p. 146).

EFFECTIVE DECISION MAKING

An effective decision must be (a) of high quality, (b) accomplished without unjustifiably taxing the decision makers's and organization's resources, and (c) accepted by those who must approve and carry out a decision.

Mixed Scanning

The mixed scanning strategy proposed by Etzioni (1967) is a synthesis of the stringent optimizing and the muddling approach of satisficing. The mixed scanning procedure has the virtue of being well-structured, allowing the decision maker to work through a series of decisions in a step-by-step manner. The decision maker is also asked to estimate, prior to entering decision making, how much time, energy, and money he or she is willing to allocate for search and appraisal activities. An implementation phase that encourages the decision maker to consider how a decision will be carried out is also included.

Scanning, as used by Etzioni, refers to the search, collection, processing, evaluation, and weighing of information in the processing of making a choice (Janis & Mann, 1977).

A mixed scanning method could be used by decision-makers on strategic occasions in the following manner (Etzioni, 1967). In the first step all relevant alternatives raised by decision-makers are listed (including alternatives not normally considered feasible). Next, all alternatives that have a "crippling objection" are eliminated (alternatives for which means are not available, which violate the basic values of the decision-makers, or which violate the basic values or interests of those whose support is crucial to successfully implement a decision).

Remaining alternatives are scrutinized in successively greater detail until only one alternative remains. The implementation process, when possible, is broken into several sequential steps. The commitment to implement and necessary assets are divided into several serial steps thereby maintaining a strategic reserve. In this process, costly and less reversible decisions are implemented after decisions which are more reversible and less costly.

Etzioni (1967) also suggests that decision-makers review the implementation process after the first sub-set of work is completed. If the implementation process is successful, longer review periods are employed. This author strongly suggests that decision-makers "scan" at set intervals in full, over-all review, even if no problems appear. Decision-makers are also encouraged to formulate a rule for the allocation of assets and time among the various levels of scanning.

Implicit in the mixed scanning strategy is the notion that decision makers should use different decision-making strategies for differing kinds and levels of decisions. No single decision-making model or rule is appropriate for all decisions.

Procedures That Ensure the Acceptance of Decisions

Acceptance of and commitment to a decision are enhanced by informing and involving those above and below the manager/supervisor who will be affected by the decision and who will be expected to carry out the decision. Many procedures are available for gaining the involvement of superiors and subordinates: information dispersal, formal requests for input concerning up-coming decisions, advise and consent, formation of representative committees and task forces, and group decision-making procedures. Some of the procedures eventually place the decision back in the hands of one person (an autocratic decision) while others require the approval of many people for enactment (a consensual decision).

Decision Rules for Quality and Acceptance

Decision rules specify who will be involved in making a decision and how much power and influence each person participating in a decision will have. In autocratic decisions, one person has the formal power, although others may have influence and informal power, concerning the decision. In democratic decisions, such as simple or two-thirds majority decision rules, formal power is vested in the majority and the minority has no means of legitimately blocking decision enactment. In consensus decisions, on the other hand, each participant in a decision must approve the final choice and, in effect, has a personal veto over any choice unacceptable to her or him. Figure 13-1 presents decision rules on a continuum from autocratic to consensual.

No particular decision rule is appropriate for all types of decisions. Maier (1970) has presented a model that will help the nurse manager/supervisor choose the best decision rule for a specific situation. The first step in this process is to consider the requirements of a decision in terms of two dimensions: (a) the necessity of a high-quality decision and (b) the necessity for acceptance of a decision by those who must carry out the decision. A useful question to ask is whether a decision is likely to fail because it lacks quality or because it lacks acceptance.

| Autocratic | Oligarchic | Majority | Two-thirds | Three-fourths | Consensual |

FIGURE 13-1. CONTINUUM OF DECISION RULES.

Some decisions require neither quality nor acceptance. For example, it hardly matters whether a nursing aide filing patient charts in a rack does so alphabetically from A to Z or Z to A. The consequences of making a mistake are limited and there is little likelihood that the nursing aide will not carry out the decision. The supervisor or manager may save time by personally making a policy that charts must be filed by the end of the shift.

If the quality of a decision is crucial and acceptance is likely to be obtained easily, the decision can be made at the leadership level with input from subordinates and consultants. Decision by a few leaders is most appropriate when needed information and skills are held by a few individuals and lengthy discussion by the entire team would add little to the quality of a decision. For instance, nursing staff input will add little to the diagnosis being made by radiologists or other highly technical medical specialists.

On the other hand, considerable research indicates that groups make higher-quality decisions than individuals in situations where no one person has all the required knowledge and skill (Barnlund, 1959; Davis & Restle, 1963; Husband, 1940; Kanekar & Rosenbaum, 1972; Lane, Mathews, Chancy, Effmeyer, Reher, & Teddlie, 1982; Shaw, 1932; Taylor & Faust, 1952; Tuckman & Lorge, 1962). While more time is required in group decision making, the improvement in quality may be well worth the additional expenditure of resources.

When acceptance of a decision is clearly a top priority and the quality of that decision is not of high concern, a group decision-making procedure is best. For instance, in making a decision about shift assignments, any arrangement of nurses will be satisfactory as long as patient care is adequate and the assignments are appropriate and fair. Much more cooperation will be achieved if nursing staff are actively involved in this decision.

When both high quality and high acceptance are required of a decision, active involvement of the nursing leader and her or his subordinates is crucial. Since so much is at stake in this type of decision, however, the nursing leader may insist upon having the "final say" in such a decision. The nurse manager/supervisor may ask for input and make the final decision. If the final decision is not consistent with advice from staff, the leader may be seen as autocratic and unwilling to use constructive input. Acceptance of such a decision is therefore reduced.

Another option in this case is to use a consensual decision rule in which both the leader and staff have veto power over options they believe to be unacceptable. This process, though time-consuming, results in a high-quality decision that will be supported by the staff. Figure 13-2 presents the appropriate decision rules for given requirements for quality and acceptance using Maier's model (1970).

GROUP DECISION MAKING

Involving an entire group or team in the problem-solving and decision-making process accomplishes two objectives. First, the knowledge, expertise, and resources of an entire group are mobilized to accomplish a task. When no one person has all the necessary knowledge, skills, and resources to solve a problem, the resulting group decision is normally of higher quality than would be obtained if *any* one of the group made the decision alone (Watson, 1928). Secondly, by involving the group in the decision-making process, individual group members feel some ownership and commitment to the

Acceptance

	Low	High
Low **Quality**	Rule: autocratic— leader decides Time required: little	Rule: democratic—simple majority Time required: moderate
High	Rule: oligarchic— leader decides with input from experts and consultants Time required: moderate	Rule: consensual, two-thirds or three-fourths Time required: extensive

FIGURE 13-2. APPROPRIATE DECISION RULES FOR GIVEN REQUIREMENTS FOR QUALITY AND ACCEPTANCE.

decision. This bolsters motivation to implement the decision and minimizes attempts to ignore or sabotage the decision.

The increase in decision quality and acceptance, however, must be balanced against the additional time required. In many cases the demand for quality and acceptance is not sufficient to warrant a group decision-making procedure (Husband, 1940; Marquart, 1955; Taylor & Faust, 1952).

Majority Decision-Rules Versus Consensus

Consensus decisions are reached only when all members of a decision-making group find a particular solution acceptable. Each member must be willing to support the decision and no "minority" opinion must exist. The process of proposing and modifying solutions until acceptable to everyone is very time-consuming. Japanese management has used consensus-building procedures to ensure high-quality decisions and long-term profitability (Ouchi, 1981).

Majority decision rules requiring 50%, 67%, or 75% approval by group members are often employed as compromise group decision-making procedures that partially achieve the goals of quality and acceptance and save considerable time and energy. There are several major drawbacks, however, to majority decision rules. Ultimately, group leaders seldom support a decision when they are part of the losing minority. In addition, group members desiring approval from the leader will support the leader's position even if they do not believe that it is the best option. These processes make a mockery of majority decision rules.

The existence of minority opinions plants the seeds for coalitions to form that attempt to block, delay, or sabotage decisions that they do not support. The loyalty of these "minority" members is often suspected by the majority, damaging group cohesiveness.

As the importance or gravity of a decision increases, so does the percentage of group members required to approve the decision. For example, ordinary bills in the U.S. Congress require a simple majority, overriding a presidential veto requires a two-thirds majority, a constitutional amendment requires three-fourths of the state legislatures for approval, and a criminal conviction requires the agreement of all jury members. This principle is useful in management practice. The nurse manager/supervisor may employ individual or simple majority decision rules for everyday decisions that will have limited impact on team performance. For important decisions, however, the approval of the manager/supervisor and a substantial majority, if not a total consensus, may be most appropriate.

Hare (1980, p. 142) has presented procedures that improve quality and shorten the time necessary to reach a consensus.

Do's:

1. Secure agreement to follow rules for consensus, i.e., look for a solution that incorporates all points of view or is best for the group at this time.
2. Give your own opinions on an issue. Approach the task on the basis of logic. Seek out differences of opinion to obtain more facts, especially from low-status members.
3. Address remarks to the group as a whole. Show concern for each individual opinion.
4. Although the main function of the group *coordinator* is to help the group formulate a consensus and the main function of the group *recorder* is to record each decision as it is reached, all members should help formulate statements about solutions to which all can agree. Even if there appears to be initial agreement, explore the basis of the agreement to make sure there is agreement at the fundamental level.
5. If consensus is reached, make it clear that each group member is responsible to apply the principle in new situations.

Don'ts:

1. Don't use a win/lose solution or use a majority rule, averaging or trading rule as conflict reduction devices.
2. Don't argue for your opinions.
3. Don't use confrontation and criticism. Try to build onto the ideas of others.
4. Don't change your mind *only* to reach agreement.
5. Don't press for a solution because the time for the meeting is over. If consensus is not reached, postpone the decision until another meeting and do more homework on the problem

SUMMARY

Decision makers rarely have the time, energy, mental capacity, knowledge, and skills to make optimizing decisions. More frequently, decision makers employ a satisficing strategy that results in a decision that is "just good enough" to satisfy minimal requirements. Mixed scanning procedures may be used to focus energy on really important decisions while using energy-saving satisficing strategies for less important decisions.

Effective decision making requires flexibility in the use of decision rules. In some cases, individual decision making is satisfactory, saving a great deal of time and energy. When quality and acceptance are required of a decision, group decision-making strategies are more appropriate. Simple majority decision rules may be used for decisions requiring quality and acceptance but have serious drawbacks. Consensus decision rules result in the greatest acceptance and highest quality but are time-consuming.

REFERENCES

Barnlund, D. A comparative study of individual, majority, and group judgment. *Journal of Abnormal and Social Psychology*, 1959, *58*, 55–60.

Davis, J., & Restle, F. The analysis of problems and prediction of group problem solving. *Journal of Abnormal and Social Psychology*, 1963, *66*, 103–116.

Etzioni, A. Mixed scanning: A third approach to decision making. *Public Administration Review*, 1967, *27*, 385–392.

Hare, R. P. Consensus versus majority vote: A laboratory experiment. *Small Group Behavior*, 1980, *11* (2), 131–143.

Husband, R. Cooperative versus solitary problem solution. *Journal of Social Psychology*, 1940, *11*, 405–409.

Janis, I., & Mann, L. *Decision making: A psychological analysis of conflict, choice and commitment*. New York: Free Press, 1977.

Johnson, R. Conflict avoidance through acceptable decisions. *Human Relations*, 1974, *27*, 71–82.

Kanekar, S., & Rosenbaum, M. Group performance on a multiple-solution task as a function of available time. *Psychonomic Science*, 1972, *27*, 331–332.

Lane, I., Mathews, P., Chancy, C., Effmeyer, R., Reher, R., & Teddlie, C. Making the goals of acceptance and quality explicit: Effects on group decision. *Small Group Behavior*, 1982, *13*(4), 542–554.

Lindblom, C. The science of muddling through. *Public Administration Review*, 1959, *19*, 79–99.

Lindblom, C. *The intelligence of democracy*. New York: Free Press, 1965.

Maier, N. *Problem solving and creativity in individuals and groups*. Belmont, Calif.: Brooks/Cole, 1970.

Marquart, D. Group problem solving. *Journal of Social Psychology*, 1955, *41*, 103–113.

Miller, G. The magical number seven, plus or minus two. *Psychological Review*, 1956, *63*, 81–97.

Ouchi, W. *Theory Z: How American business can meet the Japanese challenge*. New York: Avon, 1981.

Schwartz, S. Moral decision making and behavior. In J. Macauley & L. Berkowitz (Eds.), *Altruism and helping behavior*. New York: Academic Press, 1970.

Shaw, M. A comparison of individuals and small groups in the rational solution of complex problems. *American Journal of Psychology*, 1932, *44*, 491–504.

Simon, H. *Administrative behavior: A study of decision-making processes in administrative organization* (3rd ed.). New York: Macmillan, Free Press, 1976.

Taylor, D., & Faust, W. Twenty questions: Efficiency of problem solving as a function of the size of the group. *Journal of Experimental Psychology*, 1952, *44*, 360–363.

Tuckman, J., & Lorge, I. Individual ability as a determinant of group superiority. *Human Relations*, 1962, *15*, 45–51.

Tversky, A. Elimination by aspects: A theory of choice. *Psychological Review*, 1972, *79*, 281–299.

Watson, G. Do groups think more effectively than individuals? *Journal of Abnormal and Social Psychology*, 1928, *23*, 328–336.

Young, S. *Management: A systems analysis*. Glenview, Ill.: Scott, Foresman, 1966.

CHAPTER 14
JOB SATISFACTION
AND THE NURSE EMPLOYEE

An understanding of job satisfaction and how to motivate staff is important to the nurse manager. With this knowledge, the supervisor is in a better position to assist nursing staff or faculty in their initial adjustment to the job as well as with continued satisfaction in the role. Given this knowledge, the nurse manager is able to manipulate and influence factors found to be related to job satisfaction. The result—increased job satisfaction—has been related to productivity (Herzberg, Mausner, Peterson, & Capwell, 1957; Herzberg, Mausner, & Snyderman, 1967; Ivancevich & Donnelly, 1968; Vroom, 1967) and tenure, while job dissatisfaction has been related to job absenteeism and turnover (Diamond & Fox, 1958; Hulin, 1966, 1968; Morse, 1953; Ronan, 1970; Ross & Zander, 1957; Saleh, Lee, & Prien, 1965; Taylor & Weiss, 1969). And lest it be forgotten, the cost of replacing a nurse lost due to job dissatisfaction is high.

THEORIES OF JOB SATISFACTION

Three major orientations to theoretical formulations and research in job satisfaction are identified: aspects involving the job, aspects involving the individual, and the interaction of individual and job aspects (Vessey, 1973).

Job aspects are emphasized by such job theorists and researchers as Hoppock (1935, 1967), Smith, Kendall, and Hulin (1969), and Vroom (1967). Hoppock's theory postulates that a person's job satisfaction is dependent upon the degree to which that job meets the individual's needs. In Smith, Kendall, and Hulin's theory, job satisfaction is described as the affective responses to facets of the job situation. These affective responses are associated with the perceived difference between what is expected as a fair return and what, in fact, is experienced on the job. The employee utilizes a personal frame of reference to make the evaluation of a "fair return," including alternatives available to the person, internal standards, and comparisons with other people. Valence, instrumentality, expectancy, and force are central concepts in Vroom's theory. Employees have preferences among outcomes. Valences, which can encompass a wide range of positive and negative values, are the affective orientations toward these outcomes. Job satisfaction is described as the valence of the job or work role to the person performing it.

Individual aspects are emphasized by such job theorists as Super (1953, 1957, 1969), Super and Bohn (1970), Super, Starishevsky, Matlin, and Jordaan (1963), and Korman

(1966, 1970). The works of Super and associates view the process of vocational development essentially as one of developing and implementing one's self-concept. The phases through which the employee moves in the process of forming this self-concept are those of exploration, self-differentiation, identification, role-playing, and reality testing. The self-concept is translated into occupational terms through identification, experience, and awareness. As the young employee enters the work world, the self-concept is implemented. The young employee finds out whether the job permits the kind of role desired and whether that role is compatible with the individual's self-concept. This entails the process of testing the self-concept against reality. Consequently, job satisfaction and life satisfaction depend upon the extent to which the individual finds adequate outlets for abilities, interests, personality traits, and values. Korman uses the term self-cognition to describe an individual's self-awareness. Self-esteem is described as a moderating variable in job selection. Persons with a high level of self-esteem possess perceived needs that have been satisfied in the past and seek out roles in which these needs can be met in the future. The person with low self-esteem is not similarly motivated, becoming more accepting of situations that do not satisfy personal needs. Persons will involve themselves in those roles that maximize their sense of cognitive balance.

Herzberg (1971); Herzberg, Mausner, Peterson, & Capwell (1957); Herzberg, Mausner, & Snyderman (1967); Lofquist and Dawis (1969); and Holland (1959, 1966) are interaction theorists stressing the interaction of the individual and job aspects. The theory of Herzberg and associates proposes that factors associated with job satisfaction (called satisfiers or motivators) are qualitatively different from factors related to job dissatisfaction (called dissatisfiers or hygienes). The satisfiers—achievement, recognition, work itself, responsibility, advancement, and growth—are job *content* factors and satisfy the employee's need for self actualization. The dissatisfiers—company policy and administration; supervision; interpersonal relations with superiors, subordinates, or co-workers; working conditions; salary; personal life; and job security—are job *context* factors and satisfy the employee's need to avoid unpleasantness. They are preventive in that they remove conditions impeding satisfaction. Job satisfaction and dissatisfaction are viewed as two unipolar traits. That is, job satisfaction is a general positive feeling toward one's work controlled primarily by the satisfiers. If the satisfiers are removed, indifference, but not dissatisfaction, will result. The factors responsible for dissatisfactions, the dissatisfiers, are perceived separately from those associated with job satisfaction. Job dissatisfaction will occur only when the negative aspects of the dissatisfiers are present, while the positive aspects of the dissatisfiers are an essential but not sufficient condition for job satisfaction.

Holland proposes that a person's job behavior can be explained by the interaction of the environment and individual's personality pattern. A developmental hierarchy of personality variables, describing six personality orientations and six occupational environments, with labels complementing these personality orientations, are contained in the theory. These six personality-environmental orientations are realistic, investigative, conventional, social, artistic, and enterprising. Individuals seek out work environments that permit them to exercise their skills and abilities, express their attitudes and values, and assume agreeable roles. The person's choice of jobs is explained in terms of a desired fit between a personality pattern and the environment that best meets that pattern.

With this general overview of theories of job satisfaction, the theory that will serve as the framework for the remainder of the chapter will be discussed.

The Theory of Work Adjustment

Another major interaction theory, the theory of work adjustment (Dawis, Lofquist, & Weiss, 1968; Lofquist & Dawis, 1969) is a relevant framework for exploring job satisfaction and motivation of nursing staff and faculty.

The employee's personality is described in terms of *needs* and *abilities* (see Figure 14-1). *Ability requirements* and the *reinforcer systems* are the two major sets of variables defining the work environment. Each person seeks to achieve and to maintain *correspondence* with the environment. Correspondence means the suitability of the individual to the work environment as well as vice versa, *between both abilities and ability requirements* and *between needs and the reinforcer system of the job*. The outcome of a fit between the employee and the job is tenure. Instability in this fit or correspondence leads to termination of the job.

Job satisfaction and *satisfactoriness* are concepts denoting the outcome of this process by which the employee interacts and comes to terms with the work environment. Job satisfaction is an internal indicator of this correspondence, the employee's evaluation of how well the work environment meets personal needs. Satisfactoriness is an external indicator of correspondence that is an evaluation of the worker's fulfillment of the requirements of the work environment.

According to Dawis et al. (1968, pp. 9, 11) there are several key propositions in the work adjustment theory:

1. An individual's work adjustment at any point in time is indicated by his or her concurrent levels of satisfactoriness and satisfaction.
2. Satisfactoriness is a function of the correspondence between an individual's abilities and the ability requirements of the work environment, provided that the individual's needs correspond with the reinforcer system of the work environment.
3. Satisfaction is a function of the correspondence between the reinforcer system of the work environment and the individual's needs, provided that the individual's abilities correspond with the ability requirements of the work environment.
4. Satisfaction moderates the functional relationship between satisfactoriness and ability-requirement correspondence.
5. Satisfactoriness moderates the functional relationship between satisfaction and need-reinforcer correspondence.
6. The probability of an individual being forced out of the work environment is inversely related to her or his satisfactoriness.
7. The probability of an individual voluntarily leaving the work environment is inversely related to her or his satisfaction.
8. Tenure is a joint function of satisfactoriness and satisfaction.
9. Work personality–work environment correspondence increases as a function of tenure.

The instruments used to operationalize and measure the concepts are (a) the Minnesota Satisfaction Questionnaire, which measures an individual's job satisfaction; (b) the Minnesota Job Description Questionnaire, which measures the kinds of reinforcers available in a job; (c) the Minnesota Importance Questionnaire, which measures an individual's vocationally related needs; and (d) the Minnesota Satisfactoriness Scales, which measure how satisfactorily people perform on their jobs (see Fig. 14-2).

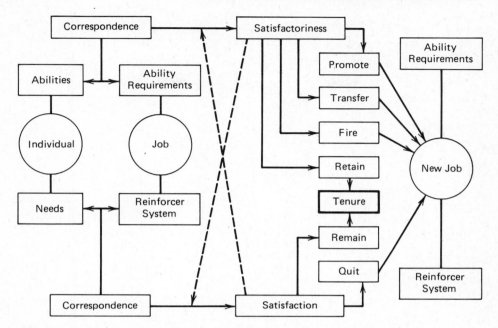

FIGURE 14-1. THE THEORY OF WORK ADJUSTMENT IN THEORETICAL TERMS.

From Dawis, R. V., Lofquist, L. H., & Weiss, D. J. A theory of work adjustment. *Minnesota Studies in Vocational Rehabilitation*, 1968, 23(47), 1–15. Reproduced by permission of Vocational Psychology Research, University of Minnesota. Copyright 1968.

The 20 job aspects measured by the Minnesota Satisfaction Questionnaire are ability utilization, achievement, activity, advancement, authority, company policies and practices, compensation, co-workers, creativity, independence, moral values, recognition, responsibility, security, social service, social status, supervision-human relations, supervision-technical, variety, and working conditions (Weiss, Dawis, England, & Lofquist, 1967).

The Minnesota Job Description Questionnaire contains 20 scales that parallel those in the Minnesota Satisfaction Questionnaire as well as in the Minnesota Importance Questionnaire (Borgen, Weiss, Tinsley, Dawis, & Lofquist, 1968a). The Occupational Reinforcer Patterns that can be developed using this Minnesota Job Description Questionnaire indicate the relative strength of the 20 needs measured by the Minnesota Importance Questionnaire for the profession being measured (Borgen, Weiss, Tinsley, & Lofquist, 1968a, 1968b; Rosen, Weiss, Hendel, Dawis, & Lofquist, 1972). Autonomy completes the 21 scales of the instrument.

The Minnesota Importance Questionnaire measures a person's vocationally related needs or the importance to the person of the work reinforcers (Gay, Weiss, Hendel, Dawis, & Lofquist, 1971).

JOB SATISFACTION AMONG NURSES: RESEARCH FINDINGS

What are the aspects of the job with which clinical nurse specialists, supervisors, and staff nurses are most or least satisfied? The theory of work adjustment already described

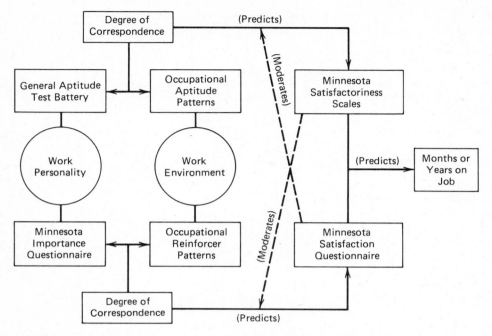

FIGURE 14-2. THE THEORY OF WORK ADJUSTMENT IN OPERATIONAL TERMS.

From Dawis, R. V., Lofquist, L. H., & Weiss, D. J. A theory of work adjustment. *Minnesota Studies in Vocational Rehabilitation*, 1968, *23*(47), 1–15. Reproduced by permission of Vocational Psychology Research, University of Minnesota. Copyright 1968.

served as the theoretical framework for a research study designed to answer this and related questions about job satisfaction among nurses (McFarland, 1977).

The job aspects with which the clinical nurse specialists were found to be most satisfied were (in descending order of satisfaction): creativity, activity, social service, moral values, variety, responsibility, and achievement. The clinical nurse specialists found the least satisfaction in hospital policies and practices, advancement, working conditions, social status, compensation, recognition, and supervision-technical (McFarland, 1977). In contrast, full-time nurses in general duty staff nurse positions reported the most satisfaction with social service, moral values, co-workers, achievement, activity, security, and responsibility, and the least satisfaction with compensation, advancement, hospital policies and practices, creativity, recognition, social status, and supervision-technical (Weiss et al., 1967) (see Fig. 14-3).

The supervisory nurses, on the other hand, were found to be most satisfied with social service, moral values, co-workers, responsibility, activity, achievement, and ability utilization, and the least satisfaction with compensation, hospital policies and practices, advancement, recognition, supervision-human relations, supervision-technical, and independence (Weiss et al., 1967) (see Fig. 14-4).

The research study by McFarland (1977) also focused on the difference between the Occupational Reinforcer Pattern for clinical nurse specialists and general duty staff nurses. Significant differences were found in ability utilization, authority, co-workers, creativity, recognition, responsibility, security, social service, and autonomy (see Fig. 14-5). The clinical nurse specialists were found to use their individual abilities (ability

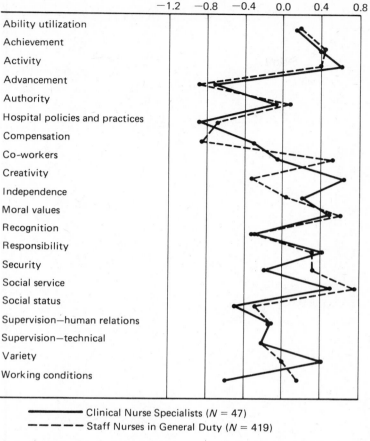

FIGURE 14-3. A GRAPHIC COMPARISON OF THE SATISFACTION WITH 20 ASPECTS OF THE JOB EXPRESSED IN TRANSFORMED MEAN SCALE SCORES BETWEEN CLINICAL NURSE SPECIALISTS AND FULL-TIME STAFF NURSES IN GENERAL DUTY.

From McFarland, G. *An investigation of selected factors as related to job satisfaction . . . .* Doctoral dissertation, Catholic University of America, 1977. (University Microfilms No. 77-19, 973)

utilization), try out their own ideas (creativity), receive recognition for the work they do (recognition), make decisions on their own (responsibility), and plan their work with little supervision (autonomy) significantly more so than the registered nurse in a general duty position. Staff nurses, however, tell other workers what to do (authority), have co-workers with whom it is easy to make friends (co-workers), have steady employment (security), and have work in which they do things for other people (social service) more so than clinical nurse specialists.

IMPLICATIONS FOR THE NURSE MANAGER AND SUPERVISOR

What relevance does the previous discussion of theory and research have for the midlevel nurse manager, supervisor, or leader? First, the correspondence existing

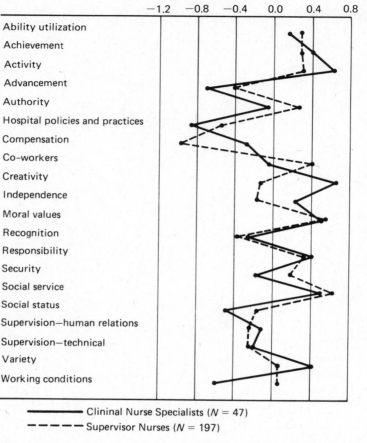

Clininal Nurse Specialists ($N = 47$)
------ Supervisor Nurses ($N = 197$)

FIGURE 14-4. A GRAPHIC COMPARISON OF THE SATISFACTION WITH 20 ASPECTS OF THE JOB EXPRESSED IN TRANSFORMED MEAN SCALE SCORES BETWEEN CLINICAL NURSE SPECIALISTS AND SUPERVISOR NURSES.

From McFarland, G. *An investigation of selected factors as related to job satisfaction* . . . . Doctoral dissertation, Catholic University of America, 1977. (University Microfilms No. 77-19, 973)

between the job *content* requirements—the skills and abilities required by a given job—and the nurse employee in that job must be evaluated. Does the employee possess the abilities and skills that are needed to meet the performance standards set for his or her job? Knowledge of the position description, the performance standards, and the evaluation of the actual performance of the nurse employee in that position helps make this determination.

What are the findings? Are there areas of performance in which improvement is needed? If so, explore the problem area with the nurse employee. Set mutually agreeable performance goals and develop a "contract" or action plan with the employee, along with a realistic time frame, to improve performance in the identified problem area.

As a public health nurse supervisor, for example, the identified performance problem area for one of the public health nurses is the quantity of work output. After further exploration with the nurse, it is found that inability to set priorities in caseload manage-

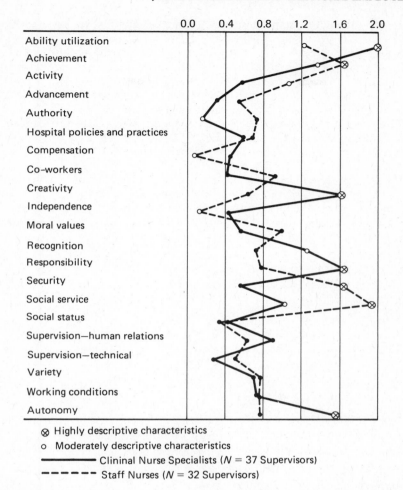

⊗ Highly descriptive characteristics

o Moderately descriptive characteristics

────── Clininal Nurse Specialists (N = 37 Supervisors)

─ ─ ─ ─ ─ Staff Nurses (N = 32 Supervisors)

FIGURE 14-5. OCCUPATIONAL REINFORCER PATTERN FOR CLINICAL NURSE SPECIALISTS AND STAFF NURSES IN GENERAL DUTY.

From McFarland, G. *An investigation of selected factors as related to job satisfaction* . . . . Doctoral dissertation, Catholic University of America, 1977. (University Microfilms No. 77-19, 973)

ment and the inability to utilize other time management principles are contributing factors to the poor performance. The overall goal that is developed is to increase the quantity of work output by the next formal performance review. More specific subgoals are jointly determined. The mutually developed action plan is as follows: The public health nurse will (a) set caseload management priorities each morning, (b) attend a time management workshop, and (c) utilize additional time-management principles. The nurse supervisor will meet biweekly with the nurse to review progress, provide constructive feedback, and offer support and encouragement when needed.

Second, correspondence between the job *context* requirements (occupational reinforcer pattern), that is, the reinforcers or set of need-satisfying characteristics of the work environment for a given job, and the *needs*—the preferences for specific job-related reinforcers—for the nurse in that job should be evaluated. Does the job offer the nurse performing it those need-satisfying characteristics that are important to the nurse?

Two sets of data will be important in making this determination. Research data on occupational reinforcer patterns for positions such as staff nurse or head nurse is very useful. It provides information about the need-satisfying characteristic of the work environment for that job. If research data is not already available, data can be obtained by (a) conducting formal research to determine the Occupational Reinforcer Pattern of a given job utilizing the Minnesota Job Description Questionnaire (MJDQ), (b) collecting data informally by having all supervisors of a given job in the agency complete this questionnaire, or (c) informally appraising the job using the reinforcers in the MJDQ as a guide.

In the latter approach, for example, the need-satisfying characteristics of a given job are specified. Although the data will not be of the same quality as from formal research, this personal assessment of the job can nevertheless give a better understanding of that job. Using the reinforcers in the MJDQ as a guide (Borgen et al., 1968a), determine for example, whether and to what extent the nurses in the staff nurse jobs supervised:

1. Make use of their individual abilities (ability utilization)
2. Get a feeling of accomplishment (achievement)
3. Are busy all the time (activity)
4. Have opportunities for advancement (advancement)
5. Tell other workers what to do (authority)
6. Have a hospital that administers its policies fairly (hospital policies and procedures)
7. Are paid well in comparison with other workers (compensation)
8. Have co-workers who are easy to make friends with (co-workers)
9. Try out their own ideas (creativity)
10. Do their work alone (independence)
11. Do work without feeling that it is morally wrong (moral values)
12. Receive recognition for the work they do (recognition)
13. Make decisions on their own (responsibility)
14. Have steady employment (security)
15. Have work where they do things for other people (social service)
16. Have the position of "somebody" in the community (social status)
17. Have supervisors who back up their employees (with top management) (supervision-human relations)
18. Have supervisors who train their employees well (supervision-technical)
19. Have something different to do every day (variety)
20. Have good working conditions (working conditions)
21. Plan their work with little supervision (autonomy)

Next, the needs (preferences for each of these specific job-related reinforcers) for each of the staff nurses who are supervised must be determined. This can again be done formally by having the staff nurse complete the Minnesota Importance Questionnaire (MIQ). Informally, assess the staff nurse's needs by means of observation or interview, using the MIQ as a guide. The need dimensions, stated in terms of a preference for a given occupational reinforcer must be considered. They are: ability utilization, achievement, activity, advancement, authority, company policies and practices, compensation, co-workers, creativity, independence, moral values, recognition, responsibility, security, social service, social status, supervision-human relations, supervision-technical, variety, and working conditions (Gay et al., 1971).

Determine, for example, how important it is to Staff Nurse A to make use of individual abilities in a job (ability utilization). How important is it to Staff Nurse A to get a feeling of accomplishment in the job (achievement)? How important is keeping busy all the time on the job (activity)? How important are opportunities for advancement in the job (advancement)? How important are each of the other reinforcers?

Another approach in determining the correspondence between the job context requirements and the preferences for specific job-related reinforcers is to administer the Minnesota Satisfaction Questionnaire to the staff nurse. This measures the employees satisfaction with 20 job aspects: ability utilization, achievement, activity, advancement, authority, hospital policies and procedures, compensation, co-workers, creativity, independence, moral values, recognition, responsibility, security, social service, social status, supervision-human relations, supervision-technical, variety, and working conditions.

Once the problem area(s) are identified for a specific employee an action plan can be designed. For example, Mr. O'Brien, staff nurse, has a very high need for creativity, trying out original ideas on the job. The reinforcer—creativity—is not a highly or moderately descriptive characteristic of the staff nurse position in the agency. As a short-term approach, Mr. O'Brien can be given special job assignments in which he can use his creativity. Mr. O'Brien's potential and motivation for advancement can be explored. Perhaps preparation for a clinical nurse specialist role would offer him the opportunity for creativity he desires. As a long-term goal, the staff nurse position can be explored with administrative staff in the organization. Perhaps the position description needs to be changed.

In another example, it has been identified that Dr. Domer, a nurse faculty member on your team, has a high need for ability utilization. A large curriculum revision project is scheduled to be undertaken in the future. It is decided to hold a conference with Dr. Domer to determine what aspects of the project would be challenging to her and permit maximum utilization of abilities.

SUMMARY

The theory of work adjustment can serve as a framework to determine what each member of the nursing staff or faculty considers important in the job (needs), what the job as currently structured offers in the way of job reinforcers, and what problem area(s) exist for any given employee. Action plans can then be designed with the employee. The result of this process should be a more job-satisfied nurse staff or faculty member. As described earlier, a process should also be used to remedy any identified problems between the employee's skills and the performance requirements actually demanded by the job. The theory of work adjustment predicts that then the employee is likely to be satisfied in the job, function competently, and remain in the job for a longer period of time.

REFERENCES

Borgen, F., Weiss, D., Tinsley, H., Dawis, R., & Lofquist, L. The measurement of Occupational Reinforcer Patterns. *Minnesota Studies in Vocational Rehabilitation*, 1968, 25(49), 1–89. (a)

Borgen, F., Weiss, D., Tinsley, H., Dawis, R., & Lofquist, L. Occupational Reinforcer Patterns (first volume). *Minnesota Studies in Vocational Rehabilitation*, 1968, 24, 1–263. (b)

Dawis, R., Lofquist, L., & Weiss, D. A theory of work adjustment (a revision). *Minnesota Studies in Vocational Rehabilitation*, 1968, 23(47), 1–15

Diamond, L., & Fox, D. Turnover among hospital staff nurses. *Nursing Outlook*, 1958, 6(7), 388–391.

Gay, E., Weiss, D., Hendel, D., Dawis, R., & Lofquist, L. Manual for the Minnesota Importance Questionnaire. *Minnesota Studies in Vocational Rehabilitation*, 1971, 28(54), 1–83.

Herzberg, F. *Work and the nature of man.* Cleveland: World, 1971.

Herzberg, F., Mausner, B., Peterson, R., & Capwell, D. *Job attitudes: Review of research and opinion.* Pittsburgh: Psychological Service of Pittsburgh, 1957.

Herzberg, F., Mausner, B., & Snyderman, B. *The motivation to work.* New York: Wiley, 1967.

Holland, J. A theory of vocational choice. *Journal of Counseling Psychology*, 1959, 6(1), 35–45.

Holland, J. *The psychology of vocational choice.* Waltham, Mass.: Blaisdell, 1966.

Hoppock, R. *Job satisfaction.* New York: Harper & Row, 1935

Hoppock, R. *Occupational information.* New York: McGraw-Hill, 1967.

Hulin, C. Job satisfaction and turnover in a female clerical population. *Journal of Applied Psychology*, 1966, 50(4), 280–285.

Hulin, C. Effects of changes in job satisfaction on employee turnover. *Journal of Applied Psychology*, 1968, 52(2), 122–126.

Ivancevich, J., & Donnelly, J. Job satisfaction research: A manageable guide for practitioners. *Personnel Journal*, 1968, 47(3), 172–177.

Korman, A. Self-esteem variable in vocational choice. *Journal of Applied Psychology*, 1966, 50(6), 379–486.

Korman, A. Toward an hypothesis of work behavior. *Journal of Applied Psychology*, 1970, 54(11), 31–41.

Lofquist, L., & Dawis, R. *Adjustment to work, a psychological view of man's problems in a work-oriented society.* New York: Appleton-Century-Crofts, 1969.

McFarland, G. An investigation of selected factors as related to job satisfaction; and selected concepts—needs, occupational reinforcer pattern, job satisfaction, satisfactoriness—in clinical nurse specialists (Doctoral dissertation, Catholic University of America, 1977). (University Microfilms No. 77-19, 973).

Morse, N. *Satisfactions in the white-collar job.* Ann Arbor: University of Michigan, 1953.

Ronan, W. Individual and situational variables relating to job satisfaction. *Journal of Applied Psychology Monograph*, 1970, 54 (1, Pt. 2), 1–31.

Rosen, S., Weiss, D., Hendel, D., Dawis, R., & Lofquist, L. Occupational Reinforcer Patterns (second volume). *Minnesota Studies in Vocational Rehabilitation*, 1972, 29, 1–313.

Ross, I., & Zander, A. Need satisfactions and employee turnover. *Personnel Psychology*, 1957, 10(3), 327–338.

Saleh, S., Lee, R., & Prien, E. Why nurses leave their jobs—An analysis of female turnover. *Personnel Administration*, 1965, 28(1), 25–28.

Smith, P., Kendall, L., & Hulin, C. *The measurement of satisfaction in work and retirement*, Chicago: Rand-McNally, 1969.

Super, D. A theory of vocational development. *The American Psychologist*, 1953, 8(5), 185–190.

Super, D. *The psychology of careers.* New York: Harper & Row, 1957.

Super, D. Vocational development theory: Persons, positions, and processes. *The Counseling Psychologist*, 1969, 1(1), 2–9.

Super, D., & Bohn, M. *Occupational psychology.* Belmont, Calif.: Wadsworth, 1970.

Super, D., Starishevsky, R. Matlin, N., & Jordaan, J. *Career development: Self-concept theory.* New York: College Entrance Examination Board, 1963.

Taylor, K., & Weiss, D. Prediction of individual job turnover from measured job satisfaction. *Proceedings of the 77th Annual Meeting of the American Psychological Association*, 1969 (pt. 2), 587–588.

Vessey, T. A longitudinal study of the prediction of job satisfaction as a function of the correspondence between needs and the perception of job reinforces in an occupation (Doctoral dissertation, University of Minnesota, 1973). (University Microfilms No.: 73-25,667).

Vroom, V. *Work and motivation*. New York: Wiley, 1967.

Weiss, D., Dawis, R., England, G., & Lofquist, L. Manual for the Minnesota Satisfaction Questionnaire. *Minnesota Studies in Vocational Rehabilitation*, 1967, 22(45), 1–120.

BIBLIOGRAPHY

Appelbaum, S. Attitudes and values: Concerns of middle managers. *Training and Development Journal*, 1978, 32, 52–58.

Baird, L. Managing dissatisfaction. *Personnel*, 1981, 58, 12–21.

Brown, M. The relationship of values and job satisfaction: Do birds of a feather work well together? *Personnel*, 1980, 57, 66–73.

Burton, D., & Burton, D. Job expectations of senior nursing students. *The Journal of Nursing Administration*, 1982, 12(3), 11–17.

Council, J., & Plachy, R. Performance appraisal is not enough. *The Journal of Nursing Administration*, 1980, 10(10), 20–26.

Davidson, D. Employee participation can mean increased employee satisfaction. *Supervisory Management*, 1979, 24, 33–36.

Discontent is growing among middle managers. *Training and Development Journal*, 1981, 35, 8–9.

Duxbury, M., & Armstrong, G. Calculating nurse turnover indices. *The Journal of Nursing Administration*, 1982, 12(3), 18–24.

Ginzberg, E., Patray, J., Ostow, M., & Brann, E. Nurse discontent: The search for realistic solutions. *The Journal of Nursing Administration*, 1982, 12(11), 7–11.

Gordon, G. Developing a motivating environment. *The Journal of Nursing Administration*, 1982 12(12), 11–16.

Gordon, G. Motivating staff: A look at assumptions. *The Journal of Nursing Administration*, 1982 12(11), 27–28.

Grant, P. A model for employee motivation and satisfaction. *Personnel*, 1979, 56, 51–57.

Haar, L., & Hicks, J. Performance Appraisal: Derivation of effective assessment tools. *Journal of Nursing Administration*, 1976, 6(7), 20–29.

Hanson, R. Managing human resources. *The Journal of Nursing Administration*, 1982, 12(12), 17–23.

Hofmann, P. Accurate measurement of nursing turnover: The first step in its reduction. *The Journal of Nursing Administration*, 1981, 11(11–12), 37–39.

James, L., & Jones, A. Perceived job characteristics and job satisfaction: An examination of reciprocal causation. *Personnel Psychology*, 1980, 33, 97–135.

Keller, R., & Szilagyi, A. A longitudinal study of leader reward behavior, subordinate expectancies, and satisfaction. *Personnel Psychology*, 1978, 31, 119–129.

McNurlin, B. Managing staff retention and turnover. *EDP Analyzer*, 1977, 15(8), 1–13.

Pfeffer, J., & Lawler, J. Effects of job alternatives, extrinsic rewards, and behavioral commitment on attitude toward the organization: A field test of the insufficient justification paradigm. *Administrative Science Quarterly*, 1980, 25(1), 38–56.

Skinner, W. Big hat, no cattle: Managing human resources, Part 1. *The Journal of Nursing Administration*, 1982, 12(7–8), 27–29.

Skinner, W. Big hat, no cattle: managing human resources, Part 2. *The Journal of Nursing Administration*, 1982, 12(9), 32–35.

Vecchio, R. Individual differences as a moderator of the job quality–job satisfaction relationship: Evidence from a national sample. *Organizational Behavior and Human Performance*, 1980, 26(3), 305–325.

White, B. The criteria for job satisfaction: Is interesting work most important? *Monthly Labor Review*, 1977, 100, 30–35.

CHAPTER 15
METHODS OF SOCIALIZATION

Professional socialization is the process of becoming indoctrinated into the knowledge, skills, attitudes, and sense of identity characteristic of a particular occupational group (Moore, 1970). This process involves internalizing the group norms and values into one's own self-concept and behavior. It neither begins nor ends with the educational system of the profession.

For the purposes of this chapter, the following definitions will be used:

Socialization—"process by which persons acquire the knowledge, skills and attitudes which make them more or less able members of their society" (Brim, 1966, p. 3).

Resocialization—"the process wherein an individual, defined as inadequate according to the norms of a dominant institution, is subjected to a dynamic program of behavior intervention aimed at instilling and/or rejuvenating those values, attitudes and abilities which would allow him to function according to the norms of said institution" (Kennedy & Kerber, 1973, p. 39).

Profession—"an occupation whose members create and explicitly use systematically acquired knowledge in the solution of problems posed by clientele" (Moore, 1970, p. 71).

Role—"standardized patterns of behavior required of all persons playing a part in a given functional relationship, regardless of personal wishes on interpersonal obligations irrelevant to the functional relationship" (Katz & Kahn, 1978, p. 43).

THEORIES OF SOCIALIZATION

Socialization begins in infancy with nonverbal communication between parent and child. Mead (1964) believed that behavioral phenomena, such as fondling, play activity, and physical manipulation, are essential to understanding symbolic interactions and instill such feelings as affection, security, or fear. With the acquisition of language, a person becomes capable of planning, evaluating, and consciously conveying the meaning of symbolic interactions. Language provides the categories and systems by which the person perceives both physical and abstract reality. Through the response of persons on the family and other groups, the individual develops behavior which reflects the knowledge, skills, and attitudes expected by the group (Kennedy & Kerber, 1973).

The socialization that occurs in childhood is insufficient as preparation for all the roles expected in adult life. Thus, the skills and attitudes acquired earlier are used as a foundation for more demanding, and often conflicting roles, in later life. Adult socialization, in contrast to childhood socialization, is more concerned with overt behavior than motives; synthesis of knowledge rather than acquisition of new knowledge; realism rather than idealism; dealing with conflict among expectations rather than developing expectations; and role-specific expectations rather than general societal demands (Brim, 1966).

Socialization into a role requires acquiring specific knowledge of the status structure of the group or organization in which the role exists, and expected behaviors of persons assuming the role. This knowledge is learned in an interactional process in which role negotiation occurs. Role negotiation suggests that each participant influences the behavior of each other participant in significant ways, with the result that the behavior of each is altered to some degree. The ability to negotiate roles successfully can be fostered by nonauthoritarian leadership and is influenced by the distribution of power within the interactional system and the internalization of values and standards of conduct inhibiting the use of personal power (Hurley, 1978).

Outcomes of the socialization process include learning verbal or language skills; development of the capacity to take on the role of another; development of the self; and development of interpersonal competence and presentation of the self (Hurley, 1978).

SOCIALIZATION OF WOMEN

Nursing remains predominantly a woman's field of endeavor. The art of nursing involves comforting and supporting activities that are traditionally viewed as mothering. Therefore, the cultural roles into which girls are socialized have had a tremendous impact on acceptable roles and role behaviors in nursing.

The process of socialization from infancy develops the self-image of what it means to be masculine or feminine. Men are said to be active, aggressive, autonomous, competitive, analytic decisionmakers who initiate ideas, take risks, and lead others. Women are passive, peaceful, intuitive, nurturing, empathic responders who meet others' needs. Men are socialized for achievement, women for affiliation. Girls excel in verbal and social skills, boys excel in visual–spatial ability and mathematical skills (Yeaworth, 1978; Yura, Osimek, & Walsh, 1976). The socialization process has reinforced women in their nurturant, docile, and submissive roles and has inhibited self -assertion, achievement, and independence (Montager, 1974). Women have described themselves as "waiting to be chosen, discovered or invited to accept a position," as "waiting to be told what to do," and "feeling conflicted and confused about their own goals" (Hennig & Jardim, 1977, p. 178).

> They fear the unknown, do not accept criticism objectively, are afraid to take risks and feel they must become super-women in order to deal with both career and family. (Andruskiw, 1983)

Cultural norms inherent in the socialization process have provided psychological barriers that inhibit women in seeking careers and attaining leadership positions. Some of these cultural inhibitors are the beliefs that being successful in both a career and marriage is not possible and that marriage and homemaking are more important than a career (Arter, 1972; Elder, 1975; Epstein, 1975; White, 1975). Other beliefs that serve as barriers to a successful career are that administration is a masculine role; that women in professions are socially deviant; that successful performance by women is related to luck or effort, whereas successful performance by men is related to ability; and that men have higher job expectations and are more likely to achieve better performance (Dean &

Emsweller, 1974; Diggary, 1966; Frieze, 1978; Hennig & Jardim, 1977; Ramaley, 1978; Schlossberg, 1974; Tyler, 1958; Valle & Frieze, 1976).

Studies of students in schools of nursing and professional nurses consistently found a high need for succorance, submissiveness, order, and blame avoidance and a low need for risk taking (Mauksch, 1977). Further, both the educational setting for nursing education and the practice settings in most health care agencies reinforce dependency, obedience, and low self-esteem (Cohen, 1980). Williamson (1972) states that nursing faculty are

> responsible for socializing the student to the professional value system, but to be able to socialize one must first be socialized to the set of norms considered acceptable to that role. (p. 360)

Since most nursing managers/supervisors have been socialized into the culturally accepted norms of the roles of women, they tend to display behaviors of a mother surrogate rather than those of a consultant/coordinator in their professional interactions with students or staff. Thus, the necessary reinforcement of role models for autonomous, risk-taking, decision-making behavior is absent. Young men and women now entering nursing whose socialization process has encouraged a more galitarian perception of the roles of men and women may be discouraged or hampered in becoming nurses since the values espoused by nursing often conflict with the behavior of nurses.

PROFESSIONAL ROLES IN NURSING

Formal socialization for the role of a nurse begins in the first nursing education experiences although expectations and ideas of the role may have been developed much earlier.

Nursing education must, therefore, address the issue of what constitutes a profession as well as the appropriate knowledge, skills, and attitudes expected of its members. Flexner (1915) declared that a profession is intellectual, learned, practical, based on techniques, organized, and guided by altruism. These criteria have served as the basis for distinguishing between those occupations that deserve the status of a profession and other types of occupations.

Jacox (1978) identified three characteristics essential to the professional role as a nurse: (a) a strong commitment to act in the best interests of the patient; (b) a strong commitment to education—both lifelong learning as an individual and the development of a specialized body of knowledge through research; and (c) increased autonomy. Added to these attitudes is the wide variety of technical and cognitive skills and the rapidly expanding knowledge base required to function adequately in any specific setting. Providing the interactional environment for this socialization to occur is a challenge to the faculty of any educational institution.

Another facet of the discussion surrounding preparation for professional roles is the controversy of socialization versus resocialization. Socialization speaks to the acquisition of knowledge and attitude required in a new role. Resocialization implies a deficiency that must be corrected. Nurses in practice settings frequently speak of the need to resocialize new graduates into the values of the work setting. Kramer (1974) suggests that this discrepancy in role perception between education and service is a major factor in job dissatisfaction. Registered nurses returning to school for a baccalaureate degree or new faculty members may face the perception that they need to be resocialized, rather than socialized into a different role. Clarification between inadequate preparation for a role and additional preparation for a new role will result in decreased resistance to required behavior changes and a more positive attitude toward accepting new roles.

STRATEGIES FOR SOCIALIZATION

Before the nurse leader can successfully socialize a new employee into the appropriate role behaviors expected by the organization, a thorough assessment of the role expectations, the individual, and the leader must be done. While most organizations have job descriptions that define the tasks to be accomplished, many are not sufficiently detailed to provide information on the knowledge base and attitudes expected. Once these have been identified, the nurse leader has a standard against which to assess the individual.

Using situational leadership theory, the nurse leader assesses the new employee in relation to both job maturity and psychological maturity. A head nurse who is responsible for the socialization of a new staff nurse will want to look at previous employment, nursing knowledge, understanding of what is required of a staff nurse, problem-solving ability, and ability to assume responsibility. Psychological maturity components of willingness to take responsibility, achievement motivation, commitment, initiative, and independence must also be assessed.

The nurse leader must also be aware of his or her own role behaviors and attitudes. Group and Roberts (1974) suggest that the authoritarian model of early nursing derived from the military and church hierarchies is not conducive to developing autonomous professional practitioners. However, this model still persists in both education and service settings, and the majority of nurses have been socialized in a system in which regimentation, obedience, conformity, and appearance are emphasized (Raabe, 1978). The nurse leader who has accepted these values will have difficulty in implementing strategies that are aimed at socializing an independent change agent.

Planning for the Socialization of Personnel

Planning socialization strategies begins with the identification of expected outcomes. Several general goals should be kept in mind. Among these are: knowledge of the status structure of the organization, expected behaviors of the role, acquisition of the specialized language, development of the self-image, and development of interpersonal competence. Most of these goals are initially addressed in orientation programs for new employees, but a variety of ongoing activities can be developed to enhance the socialization process. Examples of specific activities for an orientation program can be seen in the accompanying chart. Ongoing activities include regularly scheduled individual and/or group conferences, informal chats over coffee (which should also be carefully planned), and assigning a mentor or "buddy" to provide role modeling.

Implementation of Socialization Interactions

The process of socializing a person into a new role is an interactive process. Styles (1982) has identified eight elements of a socializing relationship:

1. Identification with the person to be socialized; being convinced and convincing him or her that the relationship is significant, that individual success and failure, past and future are linked with each other.
2. Exemplification of the traits, values, processes and roles perceived to be deserving of development and transmission within nursing; among these are a strong sense of social significance, ultimacy of performance and collegiality.

3. Instruction, in person and through professional literature, when and where he or she wants to be better informed; the leader has special knowledge, experience or conviction; demonstration of eagerness to learn from each other.

4. Appraisal according to understanding of the standards of professional performance and perception of his or her capacities for professional achievement; informing him or her of this appraisal in a constructive manner which reinforces positive and progressive behavior; encouraging self-appraisal; openness to being appraised in turn.

5. Sanction of his or her professional conduct, through such academic and professional mechanisms as grades, peer review, credentials, memberships, privileges and rewards.

6. Collaboration in collegial manner in learning, practice, research or other professional endeavors, through joint activities as well as recognition of and support for his or her individual accomplishments.

7. Sponsorship, that is, presentation and certification to the professional community and to client populations through contacts, joint publication and other activities.

8. Acculturation, that is, acquaintance with the formal and informal mechanisms and the tacit and explicit values of the work environment and assistance with an adjustment that preserves mutual professional values. (pp. 204–207)

EXAMPLES OF SOCIALIZATION ACTIVITIES

Goal	Socialization Activity	Person Responsible
Knowledge of status, structure of organization	Discussion of organizational characteristics and formal organization	Inservice educator
	Discussion of implementation of formal organization on assigned unit	Head nurse
	Discussion of informal structure	Head nurse/Team leader
Expected role behavior	Discussion of job description	Inservice educator
	Discussion of how job description is implemented on assigned unit	Head nurse
	Discussion of actual expected role	Head nurse/Team leader
Acquisition of specialized language	Discussion of forms, records, reports	Inservice educator
	Discussion of use of forms, records, and reports on assigned unit	Head nurse
	Discussion of specific abbreviations, and so on	Head nurse/Team leader
Development of self-image as member of organization	Provision of name tag, parking, locker: tour of phsyical plant	Inservice educator

Goal	Socialization Activity	Person Responsible
	Tour of assigned unit and provision of personal space	Head nurse
	Assignments as functional member of team	Head nurse/Team leader
Development of interpersonal competence	Introduction to persons in support departments; that is, dietary, central supply, and so on	Inservice educator
	Introduction to staff on assigned unit	Head nurse
	Introduction to specific colleagues on assigned unit.	Head nurse/Team leader

These components stress the active participation of both the nurse leader and the person moving to a new role. Some elements, such as instruction, appraisal, and sanction may occur in large group settings. Others, such as identification, exemplification, and collaboration may require a one-to-one or only a small group to be effective. The extent to which all eight elements are incorporated into programs of socialization will determine the extent to which the goals of socialization can be achieved.

Evaluation Strategies

Evaluation of the extent to which socialization has occurred can be based on both verbalized attitudes and behavior.

The specific outcomes of the socialization process should be stated as measureable objectives that can then be used for evaluation of both role acceptance by the individual and overall success of socialization activities. Performance appraisal methods can be applied to socialization goals as well as work performance objectives. Effective socialization into the specific setting will result in a high degree of consequence between individual goals and organizational goals.

SUMMARY

Socialization is the process by which people gain skills, attitudes, and knowledge that enables them to become functional members of society. Through the family and other groups, a person acquires behaviors that are expected by that group. Childhood socialization is insufficient preparation for all expected adult roles. The process of socialization from infancy, however, develops the self-image of what it means to be masculine or feminine. Adult socialization is particularly concerned with overt behavior, synthesis of knowledge, realism, dealing with conflict among expectations, and role-specific expectations. Formal socialization for the role of a nurse begins in the first nursing education experience although expectations and ideas of the role may have been developed much earlier.

Before the nurse leader can successfully socialize a new employee into the appropriate role behaviors expected by the organization, a thorough assessment of the role expectations, the individual, and the leader must be done. Using the situational leadership theory, the nurse leader can assess the new employee in relation to both job maturity and psychological maturity.

Planning socialization strategies begins with the identification of expected outcomes. Among these outcomes are knowledge of the status structure of the organization, expected behaviors of the role, acquisition of the specialized language, development of the self-image, and development of interpersonal competence. It must also be kept in mind that the process of socialization into a new role is an interactive process.

REFERENCES

Andruskiw, O. Women administrators in higher education. In M. E. Conway & O. Andruskiw (Eds.), *Administrative theory and practice: Issues in higher education*. Norwalk, Conn.: Appleton-Century-Crofts, 1983.

Arter, M. H. The role of women in administration in state universities and land-grant colleges (Doctoral dissertation, Arizona State University, 1972). *Dissertation Abstracts International*, 1972, 5559-A. (University Microfilms No. 73-13, 006).

Brim, O. G., Jr. Socialization through the life cycle. In O. B. Brim, Jr. & S. Wheeler (Eds.), *Socialization after childhood: Two Essays*. New York: Wiley, 1966.

Cohen, H. Authoritarianism and dependency: Problems in nursing socialization. In B. C. Flynn & M. H. Miller (Eds.), *Current perspectives in nursing: Social issues and trends*. St. Louis: Mosby, 1980.

Dean, K.,& Emsweller, T. Explorations of successful performance on sex-linked task: What's skill for the male is luck for the female. *Journal of Personality and Social Psychology*, 1974, *29*, 80–85.

Diggary, J. *Self-evaluation: Concepts and studies*. New York: Wiley, 1966.

Elder, P. Women in higher education, qualified except for sex. *NASPA Journal*, Fall 1975, 9–17.

Epstein, C. F. Institutional barriers: What keeps women out of the executive suite? In F. E. Gordon & M. H. Strober (Eds.), *Bringing women into management*. New York: McGraw-Hill, 1975.

Flexner, A. Is social work a profession? *Proceedings of the National Conference of Charities and Corrections*, 1915.

Frieze, I. H. Psychological barriers for women in science: Internal and external. In J. A. Ramaley (Ed.), *Covert discrimination and women in the sciences*. Boulder, Colo.: Westview, 1978.

Group, T. M., & Roberts, J. I. Exorcising the ghosts of the Crimea. *Nursing Outlook*, 1974, *22*, 368–372.

Hennig, M., & Jardim, A. *The managerial woman*. Garden City, N.Y.: Anchor, 1977.

Hurley, B. A. Socialization for roles. In M. E. Hardy (Ed.), *Role theory: Perspectives for health professionals*. New York: Appleton-Century-Crofts, 1978.

Jacox, A. Professional socialization of nurses. In N. L. Chaska (Ed.), *The nursing profession: Views through the mist*. New York: McGraw-Hill, 1978.

Katz, D., & Kahn, R. *The social psychology of organizations*. New York: Wiley, 1978.

Kennedy, D. B., & Kerber, A. *Resocialization: An American experiment*. New York: Behavioral Publications, 1973.

Kramer, M. *Reality shock: Why nurses leave nursing*. St. Louis: Mosby, 1974.

Mauksch, I. Paradox of risk. *AORN Journal*, 1977, *25*, 1289–1312.

Mead, G. H. *On social psychology*. A. Strauss (Ed.). Chicago: University of Chicago Press, 1964.

Montager, A. *The natural superiority of women*. New York: Collier, 1974.

Moore, W. E. *The professions: Roles and rules*. New York: Russell Sage Foundation, 1970.

Raabe, M. S. *Diploma school socialization: Survival and defense*. In N. L. Chaska (Ed.), *The nursing profession: Views through the mist*. New York: McGraw-Hill, 1978.

Ramaley, J. A. (Ed.). *Covert discrimination and women in the sciences*. Boulder, Colo.: Westview, 1978.

Schlossberg, N. K. The right to be wrong is gone: Women in academe. *Educational Record*, 1974, *55* 257–263.

Styles, M. M. *On nursing: Toward a new endowment*. St. Louis: Mosby, 1982.

Tyler, B .B. Expectancy for eventual success as a factor in problem-solving behavior. *Journal of Educational Psychology* 1958, *49*, 166–172.

Valle, J. A., & Frieze, I. H. The stability of casual attribution as a mediator in changing expectations for success. *Journal of Personality and Social Psychology*, 1976, *33*, 579–587.

White, M. Women in the professions: Psychological and social barriers to women in science. In J. Freeman (Ed.), *Women: A feminist perspective*. Palo Alto, Calif.: Mayfield, 1975.

Williamson, J. The conflict-producing role of the professionally socialized nurse-faculty member. *Nursing Forum,* 1972, *11*, 356–373.

Yeaworth, R. C. Feminism and the nursing profession. In N. L. Chaska (Ed.), *The nursing profession: Views through the mist*. New York: McGraw-Hill, 1978.

Yura, H., Ozimek, D., Walsh, M. *Nursing leadership: Theory and process*. New York: Appleton-Century-Crofts, 1976.

CHAPTER 16
POWER: NATURE, ACQUISITION, AND USE

Constructive growth promoting use of power can lead to desirable consequences. This means using power judiciously and ethically with a clear notion of one's intended goals and the potential consequences for all affected. Through the use of power, the nurse manager can control and gain desired resources, implement new ideas, bring about change, block destructive actions, facilitate work group goals, and thus attain organizational goals. Collective use of power by nurses can lead to desired patient care practices, quality curricula and teaching methods, and desired growth and progress of the nursing profession.

Until recently, the use of power and involvement in politics had not been considered very professional by many nurses. Using power was perceived, and still is to some extent, as manipulative, not quite respectable, and even corrupt. In fact, "to many professionals, 'power' is an undesirable word, connoting dominance and submission, control and acquiescence, or one person's will over another's" (McFarland & Shiflett, 1979, p. 1).

Power can indeed be used maliciously. Nurses' careers can be jeopardized and lives negatively affected. Power can be used inappropriately. Too much of it can be stifling, thwart work group initiative, destroy potential, and lead to other dysfunctional behavior. The unbridled struggle for power can obscure the purposes for its intended use (Conway, 1978). Counter movements can be triggered to block the use of power. On the other hand, too little use of power can lead to the maintenance of the status quo, no change, and confusion among work group members.

Nothing in the nature of power, its acquisition, or its use is inherently unethical or Machiavellian. But, it can become so, if abused. Thus, it becomes important to examine one's use of power strategies to detect any undesirable behavior or potential negative consequences.

POWER, NURSES, AND THE NURSING PROFESSION

The need for nurses to exercise individual and collective power ethically is stressed by nurse leaders and authors on power (Ashley, 1979, 1980; Capuzzi, 1980; Claus & Bailey, 1977; Dieziger, 1980; Leininger, 1979; Mauksch, 1980; McFarland & Shiflett, 1979; Miller, 1980; Parsek, 1978; Peterson, 1979; Phippen, 1981; Sanford, 1980; Stevens 1980a, 1980b; Ver Steeg, 1979). Legitimate use of power by nurses is needed to influence national health policy decisions that impact on the accessibility and availability of cost-effective health care to all citizens. Power is needed by nursing in order to relate from a position of strength with other health care professional groups. Those professional groups with the most power tend to be those that are heeded when national health policy decisions are made by legislators. As McFarland and Shiflett (1979) note, "Nursing can serve both society and its members well, provided that it exercises legitimate power with appropriate ethics and competent practices" (p. 11).

Collective nurse power is needed for shaping and developing the scope and direction of the nursing profession. The danger exists for nursing to have tasks and responsibilities assigned to it that are not congruent with its evolution.

> There has to be rapid movement toward a role for nurses for which the prerequisites and characteristics have been set by the nursing profession and not by other groups. (Phillips, 1979, p. 739)

The work on identifying and developing nursing diagnoses and a taxonomy for the classification of nursing diagnoses by the North American Nursing Diagnoses Association is a step in this direction. So is that of the American Nurses' Association Steering Committee on the Classification for Nursing Practice Phenomena which is involved in identifying "phenomena of concern" to nurses.

There are other issues for which the exercise of collective nurse power is essential. Unequal reimbursement policies exist for nurses today. If nurses are to bring about change in current reimbursement practices, collective group power is needed.

The importance and use of power extends to the midlevel nurse leader and manager. For it is at this level that essential human resources need to be utilized in such a way as to attain quality patient care for patients as well as quality educational programs for nursing students. Power is important in order to achieve organizational goals, to facilitate adaption of the subsystem and system to its environment, and to contribute to necessary system maintenance functions.

The Use of Nurse Power

Many of the same nurse leaders and authors already mentioned attest that nurses have not acquired enough power nor learned to use individual or group power strategies effectively. Mauksch (1980), for example, claims that nursing is unique and essential, but that it is powerless. One could quibble with whether nurses are powerless or whether they give away their power. In any case, many nurses *feel* powerless.

What are some of the factors that have contributed to the evolution and perpetuation of this feeling of powerlessness? Miller (1980) suggests that nursing has not achieved a power base because (a) power has not been traditionally accorded to nurses, (b) nurse leaders have not generated a sufficient power base through personal influence, and (c) nurses have been unable to gain passage of legislation that would enable nurses to have increased control over their professional activities.

Nursing is now developing its own theories of nursing and attempting to delineate the phenomena of concern to nurses. Throughout the past, however, nurses have permitted other professionals, especially physicians, to assign them responsibilities and tasks. This has often contributed to a sense of powerlessness and/or an escape from direct confrontation through what Stevens (1980b) labels "a flight into uncontested turfs." Nurses have tended to cling to the myth of believing "in collegial and team relations with those who do not recognize us as colleagues and who only want team participation if they are captains" (Stevens, 1980b, p. 9). Whereas, in fact,

> medical efforts to undermine the confidence of nurses and their power to effect change has been a long-standing source of frustration for nurses. Out of an expression of class interest the medical profession has, up to the present, supported the view that nurses exist to serve physicians and their work in hospitals and elsewhere. . . . Physicians have encouraged the public to believe that the separate and distinct contributions of nursing really can be attributed to medical skill. (Ashley, 1979, p. 30)

Parallel to this is the fact that the majority of nurses are women, and women have historically had to fight many battles in order to gain the level of equality in society which they now possess. With the defeat of the Equal Rights Amendment, however, women have yet to gain full equality.

Compounding this source of powerlessness has been the discord and lack of unity among nurses themselves, as well as the frequent disrespect nurses display for each other. An example of this casual disrespect among nurses is "reflected in ambivalence toward nursing orders and failure to follow care regimens designed by fellow nurses" (Stevens, 1980b, p. 10). "If nurses would begin to care for other nurses, the profession would have more than enough power necessary for controlling its practice and its destiny" (Ashley, 1980, p. 21).

Until recently, the attitudinal change that is necessary in order to recognize and accept the importance of power has not been given a great deal of attention in nursing curricula, especially at the undergraduate level. Neither has much curricular focus been on the acquisition and constructive use of power, another variable that contributes to lack of power.

Nurse leaders and managers need a strong knowledge base in order to be able to acquire power and to use it constructively. To develop a power base for nursing, nurses must also become responsible and accountable for their actions. In addition, nurses must systematically acquire the prerequisites of power—"identity as a profession, unity in purpose, unity for our public, and visibility in the public domain"—as well as acquire the means to power, for example, positional power (Stevens, 1980b, p. 10). Most critically, sight must not be lost of nursing's ultimate goal—that of contributing to quality health care through the unique and essential contributions this profession has to offer society.

POWER AND RELATED TERMS DEFINED

Power

Power can be conceptualized as the generalized capacity or potential to get others to do something one wants them to do and which they would not ordinarily do otherwise (Dahl, 1957; Kotter, 1979). Power can refer to the capacity to mobilize others to achieve and maintain subsystem and system goals. Power is also the capacity or potential to avoid changing one's own behavior in response to others' attempts to force one to do what they want.

The extent of power one actor has over another (whether that actor is an individual, group, or organization) is based in part on the imbalance in dependency of one actor on another. That is, actor A possesses power over actor B, if B is dependent to some extent on A for goal attainment. For example, Mrs. Jones, head nurse, may have control of resources as staff that are needed by Mrs. White, team leader. Mrs. Jones may also have access and control of vital information or have the right to apply certain sanctions or offer certain rewards. Mrs. Jones's power over Mrs. White is dependent too on the availability of other resources to Mrs. White that will meet Mrs. White's needs and goals. For example, even though Mrs. Jones possesses information that is vital to Mrs. White, if Mrs. White can obtain that information from other sources, Mrs. Jones's power in relation to Mrs. White (which is based upon this possession of information) is lessened.

The power of A with respect to B is also based on the extent to which B *perceives* A as useful or instrumental in achieving B's own goals (Tedeschi, 1974). For example, in order for Mrs. Jones to utilize power in relation to Mrs. White, Mrs. White must accept its use as both appropriate and legitimate. If Mrs. White rejects being influenced by Mrs. Jones's use of power, then Mrs. White must accept the resulting consequences. "Power, no matter how arbitrary or absolute, has little hold on those who have no fear of death or unpopularity or public disgrace" (Harward, 1979, p. 8).

Authority and Power Differentiated

While power is the potential to get others to do what you want them to do based upon any one of a number of different factors or sources, *authority* is the *right* to do so solely by virtue of one's formal position in the organizational hierarchy. Authority can be seen as one type of power (McFarland & Shiflett, 1979). Because of a given status role in a hierarchy, the incumbent has the authority, or the right to expect certain behaviors from other persons, especially subordinates. Such rights and obligations are seen as part of the legitimate and sanctioned bureaucratic structure (Cumming & Cumming, 1979). Thus, authority often defines vertical relationships in an organization such as between managers or supervisors and their subordinates.

Power-Oriented Behavior and Politics

Power-oriented behavior refers to the actions of individuals, groups, or organizations aimed at acquiring and utilizing power (Kotter, 1979). *Politics* is defined as the process or manner of exercising control or influence over others in order to promote or protect vested goals or interests, that is, the art of achieving one's own ends (Leininger, 1979; Stevens, 1980a). Power has been defined previously as the capacity or potential to modify another's behavior. Stevens (1980a) sees a reciprocal relationship between the two, that is, power and politics. She states that "effective use of process (politics) is one source of power. Conversely, the state of holding power provides one with certain resources that make for effective politicking" (p. 208).

THEORETICAL FRAMEWORKS, SOURCES, AND TYPES OF POWER

Three overall and general elements characterize modern concepts of power (Votaw, 1979). First, although power can be abused, power has a positive side. Second, power exists and is utilized within the context of a relationship between individuals, groups, and/or organizations. Power is based, to an extent, on empowering responses, interpersonal expectations, and interpersonal attitudes. Third, power is dynamic and not static. Power is not destroyed: it is continuously transformed.

Field Theory Perspective

From a field theory perspective, French and Raven (1959) identified five bases of social power. These sources of social power, or of influence in a relationship, are expert, reward, referent, legitimate, and coercive power. The following descriptions are based on French and Raven's conceptualizations.

Expert Power

Expert power is power based upon a person's knowledge or skill. That is, person A possesses social power in relation to person B, if B perceives A to possess expertise in a specific area. The strength of A's expert power is related to the extent of knowledge B attributes to A.

A new staff nurse on a cardiovascular unit, for example, perceives the cardiovascular clinical nurse specialist as an expert who possesses a great deal of knowledge and skill in cardiovascular nursing. The clinical nurse specialist has the capacity or potential to bring about selected change in the staff nurse because of expert power.

Reward Power

The basis for reward power is the ability to give positive rewards to others who value them. The strength of reward power relates to the extent or rewards B *perceives* that A can provide, A's *actual* ability to *administer* positive sanctions and remove negative ones, and A's *actual* ability to *mediate* the rewards as perceived by B.

For example, a faculty chairperson has reward power in relation to a faculty member who highly values being able to attend a nursing conference. The chairperson has the ability to reward—for example, grant permission to attend the nursing conference—which is the basis of the reward power.

Referent Power

Referent power is based on B's identification with A. ("A" can refer to a person as well as a group, a concept that is also true for reward, coercive, expert, and legitimate bases of power.) B values and is attracted to A. Because B identifies with A, B will begin to assume the attitudes, beliefs, and behaviors of A. Thus, A has the potential or capacity to influence and change B's behavior. The more B is attracted to A, the stronger will be the identification, and the greater will be A's referent power over B.

For example, a public health nurse admires the nurse supervisor as a competent professional and identifies with this person. The public health nurse seeks association with the nurse supervisor and begins to adopt similar beliefs, behaviors, and attitudes. The supervisor's influence on the nurse's behavior is based on referent power. If the supervisor, on the other hand, uses positive or negative sanctions to influence the nurse, the basis for power is reward or coercive power, respectively. Similarly, if the nurse perceives the nurse supervisor to possess expertise and skill in a specific area, but does not identify with the supervisor, then the basis for the supervisor's power is expert power. To the extent, however, that the nurse gains satisfaction or avoids discomfort based on identification, regardless of the supervisor's response, the basis for power is referent power.

Legitimate Power

Legitimate power is based on B's internalized values that lead B to perceive A's *right* to influence B, as well as to B's sense of obligation to yield to this influence. Legitimate power always involves a standard or code of behavior that is accepted by person B, by virtue of which A, the external agent, can assert power.

The basis for legitimate power stems from such sources as cultural values, social structures, or designation by a legitimizing agent. Cultural values, for example, may sanction the right of persons with certain characteristics, such as age or royalty, to influence other persons who do not possess those characteristics. In formal organizations, A's legitimate power over B stems from the fact that A holds a superior office in the hierarchy, that is, the roles played by the participants in a power relationship in a formal organization are understood and the resulting legitimate power is accepted. Finally, a legitimizing agent, whom B accepts, can grant legitimate power to A. For example, the dean of a nursing school delegates responsibility together with authority to a faculty coordinator who then possesses legitimate power in relation to a faculty member.

Coercive Power

Coercive power is based upon B's perception of A's ability to administer punishment or to remove rewards. A's coercive power can be used to influence B's behavior since B expects punishment if conformity to the influence attempt does not occur. Coercive power stems from the fact that A is in a position of situational advantage over B, in which A has the ability to administer punishment or withdraw rewards.

Coercive power tends to decrease the attraction of B for A. On the other hand, reward power tends to increase this attraction. The change in behavior influenced by reward power tends to become internalized and a part of B's usual behavior pattern. In contrast, the results of behavioral change in B stemming from coercive power tends to remain dependent on A's use of punishment or withdrawal of rewards.

These bases of power are not necessarily mutually exclusive. In other words, several sources of power may be operant at the same time.

Social Exchange Theory Perspective

In addition to field theory, another major theoretical orientation of social power is social exchange theory as proposed by such theorists as Emerson (Busch, 1980). In this theory, power is perceived as a property of a social relation and the focus is on the characteristics of the relation among actors where actors might be a group–group, group–person, or person–person relation. That is, social relations are viewed as characterized by ties of mutual dependence between actors.

> A *depends* upon B if he aspires to goals or gratifications whose achievement is facilitated by appropriate actions on B's part. . . . These ties of mutual dependence imply that each party is in a position, to some degree, to grant or deny, facilitate or hinder, the other's gratification. . . . The power to control or influence the other resides in control over the things he values. . . . In short, *power resides implicitly in the other's dependency.* (Emerson, 1962, p. 32)

In social exchange theory as proposed by Emerson (1962),

> the dependence of actor A upon actor B is (1) directly proportional to A's *motivational investment* in goals mediated by B and (2) inversely proportional to the *availability* of those goals to A outside of the A–B relation. (p. 32)

These goals refer to gratifications consciously sought through the relationship.

For example, Mr. O'Brien, a staff nurse, is motivationally invested in being involved in increasingly complex professional job responsibilities. Miss Mabry, the head nurse, perceives the staff nurse role in a limited, circumscribed, and nonexpanding fashion.

Mr. O'Brien is highly dependent on Miss Mabry to meet desired career goals. This dependence diminishes when Mr. O'Brien turns to professional nursing activities outside the job in order to meet desired career goals. In other words, Miss Mabry's power is diminished.

As has been stated, power resides in the other's dependency. "The power of actor A over actor B is the amount of resistance on the part of B which can be potentially overcome by A" (Emerson, 1962, p. 32). The power of A over B will be evident when A makes a demand of B that runs against B's desire, that is, encountering resistance. The effect of the use of power is observable when there is a change in B's behavior that is attributable to the demands made by A.

In the previous example, Miss Mabry decides to grant Mr. O'Brien several expanded job responsibilities. At the same time, Miss Mabry demands that Mr. O'Brien work more afternoon and night shifts. The day shift is highly valued by Mr. O'Brien; therefore, this demand meets with some degree of resistance.

There is a "cost" involved for one actor, in this example Mr. O'Brien, to meet the demands made by the other actor, Miss Mabry. Emerson (1962) proposes several mechanisms to reduce this cost. B can reduce emotional investment in goals mediated by A, that is, there exists the option of withdrawal. B can find alternative sources to meet important goals. Or, the more dependent member in the relationship—B—can control the more powerful member through increasing the more powerful person's investment in the relationship. For example, B can give A ego gratification by acknowledging A's status and recognition to others. Finally, the strategy of forming coalitions against the stronger actor can be utilized, thus increasing the power of the weaker actors through coalition formation.

In an interesting treatment of power, Kotter (1979) describes the extensive dependence on the activities of other people that exists for managers. Although poor management structures or practices can increase dependence, dependence is still inherent in any managerial job because of the division of labor and limited resources in an organization.

> Because the work in organizations is divided into specialized divisions, departments, and jobs, managers are always made directly or indirectly dependent on many others for information, staff services, and cooperation in general. Because of their organization's limited resources, managers are also dependent on their external environments for support. Without some minimum degree of cooperation from suppliers of goods and services, from competitors, unions, regulatory agencies, and customers, managers cannot achieve their objectives and help their organizations prosper. (Kotter, 1979, pp. 11–12)

Dealing with the vulnerability from this dependence is an important part of a manager's job.

The director of a continuing education (CE) department in a school of nursing is dependent upon many other persons for information, staff services, and cooperation. Instructors from a variety of specialty areas in the school of nursing, as well as from other departments and the community, are relied upon to teach the various CE programs. The publications unit is relied upon for printing the brochures to be mailed to prospective applicants. Another department in the college maintains computerized records of all CE participants and awards Continuing Education Units. The director is equally dependent upon his secretarial staff to type the program schedule and correspondence. Likewise, the director is dependent on the external environment for support. The Continuing Education Advisory Committee is relied upon for feedback from the community, for the identification of potential resources, and for input in program planning and implementation. Some collaboration takes place with other CE providers in the area in order to develop a yearly schedule of programs. Cooperation is also needed from the professional Continuing Education Approval Committee in reviewing program applications and approving the continuing education programs for Continuing Education Units.

Nurse managers can cope with this dependence by eliminating nonessential dependence, being aware and sensitive to the dependence related to one's job, utilizing sound communication skills, and establishing counterveiling power over those others upon whom one is dependent.

> Without sufficient power, a manager is at the mercy of those he or she is dependent upon and will never be able to effectively plan, organize, control, motivate, and evaluate. (Kotter, 1979, p. 21)

Power-oriented behaviors—actions designed to acquire and utilize power—are needed by nurse managers to cope with the dependence in their jobs.

Strategic Contingencies Theory of Power

In the strategic contingencies theory of intraorganizational power, organizations are perceived as containing subsystems, each with interdependent and interrelated tasks that contribute to overall organizational goals and responsibilites. The subsystem becomes the basic source of power within the organization (Hickson, Hinings, Lee, Schneck, & Pennings, 1971). Each subsystem has a boundary that clearly differentiates one subsystem from another. The gatekeeper or manager for each subsystem helps to maintain those boundaries.

The theory proposes that the subsystem in the organization derives its power from its relationship with other subsystems in the organization.

> The division of labour in the organization is seen to provide the functional interrelationship of an organizational system of interdepartmental sub-units. The theory ascribes power relations to imbalances in this interdependency. (Clegg, 1975, p. 44)

One of the major task elements for the subsystem is coping with uncertainty. Each subsystem in the organization is responsible for attaining specific goals and achieving related tasks. This division of labor contributes to an interdependency among the subsystems. "Imbalance of this reciprocal interdependence . . . among the parts gives rise to power relations" (Hickson et al. 1971, p. 217).

The extent of the power of one subsystem over another subsystem is determined by the degree of imbalance in the interdependency and by how the subsystems respond to their environment. That is, in

> organizations, subunit B will have more power than other subunits to the extent that (1) B has the capacity to fulfill the requirements of the other subunits and (2) B monopolizes this ability. (Hickson et al. 1971, p. 218).

From the perspective of the strategic contingencies theory, power is defined as the ability of subsystem B to get subsystem A to do something the latter would not usually do. The extent of power is related to the degree of dependency of A on B. If ward B can do something for ward A that A can not do for itself, then ward A becomes dependent on ward B which increases the latter's power over the former.

Hickson et al. (1971) identify several important variables in the strategic contingencies theory of intraorganizational power. One is *uncertainty*. This refers to the absence of data about the future, which makes the selection of alternatives and a projection of their outcomes unpredictable.

Social systems, and the subsystems that comprise them, must deal with uncertainties in the external environment, that is, with variability in the sources and composition of inputs. For example, dramatic shifts in the economy can effect patients' decisions to undergo elective surgery. This, in turn, can decrease admissions to a hospital.

Social systems and subsystems must also deal with uncertainties in the throughput process. The quality of care rendered to patients in a hospital, as a case in point, can be adversely affected by a high staff turnover rate and the resultant staff shortage.

Uncertainty can also occur in the feedback process. For instance, there can be uncertainty in the speed, specificity, or accuracy of patient care audits. Then there are the uncertainites of the disposal of organizational outputs. Again using the hospital as an example, there are uncertainties that must be faced in dealing with patient discharge or appropriate referrals and placement in other health care agencies.

What gives a subsystem within a given social organization power is its ability to cope with uncertainty. Tasks allocated to the various subsystems in an organization vary in degree of uncertainty. Hickson et al. (1971) state that those subsystems that can cope most effectively with the most uncertainty will, in general, develop the most power because this coping reduces the adverse impact of uncertainty on other activities in the organization, thus contributing to the survival of the organization as a whole.

Another important variable in the strategic contingencies theory of power is *substitutability*. What this means is that the power residing in a subsystem is inversely proportional to the number of other subsystems that are capable of performing the functions of that subsystem. "The lower the substitutability of the activities of a subunit, the greater the power within the organization" (Hickson et al. 1971, p. 221).

A subsystem's power can be reduced if other subsystems within the organization begin to assume some of the tasks of that subsystem. The subsystem's power can, on the other hand, be increased if the subsystem withholds information that would permit other subsystems in the organization to do what it does. An intensive care unit may possess considerable power because the number of other units in a hospital capable of assuming the care of very critically ill patients is limited.

The other major concept in the theory is *centrality*. Centrality means, in part, the extent to which a subsystem and its activities are interlinked into the total system. In other words, centrality refers to the degree to which the work activities or tasks connect or interact with the work activities or tasks of other subsystems in the organization. A recovery room, for example, has a high degree of centrality in the hospital, as its activities connect with a number of other subunits, such as the operating room and any number of surgical units. As Hickson et al. (1971) hypothesize, "the higher the pervasiveness of the workflows of a subunit, the greater its power within the organization" (p.222).

Centrality also means that the tasks or activities of a given subsystem are essential to the total organization to the extent that if these activities were to stop, the primary workflow of the overall system would be impeded. The operating room has a high degree of power based upon the notion of centrality. If no more operations were to be performed in a hospital that has numerous surgical beds, this would have a serious effect upon the hospital as a whole. The workload of the admissions department would decline, the recovery room would most likely be closed down, and the patient census on the surgical units would gradually drop. As Hickson et al. (1971) hypothesize, "the higher the immediacy of the workflows of a subunit, the greater its power within the organization" (p. 222).

Finally, Hickson et al. (1971) hypothesize that "the more contingencies are controlled by a subunit, the greater its power within the organization" (p. 222). *Contingencies* in a social system are tangible resources such as nursing personnel, the nursing budget, equipment, supplies, and space. A subsystem has power to the extent that these contingencies are controlled. As a result of dealing with uncertainty, contingencies can be controlled. This, in turn, develops a power base for the subsystem if, at the same time, the subsystem possesses some degree of centrality and low substitutability. The intensive care unit can develop a considerable power base if uncertainty and contingencies are controlled since it usually possesses a certain degree of centrality and generally has low substitutability.

ASSESSING POWER IN SOCIAL SYSTEMS

The importance of assessing power in an organization should not be underestimated and is discussed by a number of authors (Butterfield & Posner, 1979; Drake & Mitchell, 1977; Dunne, Stahl, & Melhart, 1978; Kotter, 1978, 1979; Leininger, 1979; McFarland & Shiflett, 1979; Pfeffer, 1981; Stevens, 1980a; Ver Steeg, 1979; Zaleznik, 1979). The nurse leader, manager, or supervisor must be aware of personal sources of power and the bases of power for organizational subsystems. This knowledge facilitates the constructive use of power to achieve specific goals. From assessment, it may be determined whether one's source of power is sufficient to overcome opposition to one's goal. Assessment of power can also identify gaps in one's personal power base. Action can then be taken to increase power in these areas. A clinical nurse specialist, for instance, may discover that personal bases for reward power are rather limited given the present job description. Steps are then taken by the clinical nurse specialist to develop a process whereby input is routinely provided to the clinical coordinator when the performance evaluations are given to staff nurses on those units mutually shared by the clinical nurse specialist and the clinical coordinator.

It should be kept in mind, however, that power is relative and variable. Expert power may be possessed by actor A in relation to actor B but not in relation to actor C. Expert power may also vary in relation to actor B, since the latter may take courses and become as proficient in a given area of expertise as A and no longer perceive actor A as "the expert." Equally important is the fact that assessing one's bases of personal power as well as the power among subsystems in an organization is not an easy task.

Assessing the Personal Bases of Power

It is necessary to determine awareness of power sources and patterns of using these sources. Situations should be analyzed that result in behavior that would not have occurred without the use of power. Discussing the usual mode of confronting others and negotiating for power with a trusted colleague can help to clarify recurring patterns. A similar result can be achieved by documenting recent power-oriented behaviors.

In either method, ask and attempt to answer such general questions about the power-oriented behavior as:

1. Who are you really dependent upon in your position as nurse manager or supervisor? From a social exchange theory perspective, analyze the formal and informal structure of the organization, your position description, your job objectives, and

subsystem and organizational goals. Determine upon whom you are really dependent in order to perform your managerial or supervisory responsibilities. Analyze each of the identified dependencies. Are these dependencies *really* important to you? Are the dependencies functional? Dysfunctional?

2. Are you aware of your personal bases of power in general—as for example, from a field theory perspective, your expert, reward, coercive, referent, or legitimate power?

3. What is the degree of formal authority vested in your position relative to other positions in the organization? Does your job permit autonomy, visibility, and a chance to work on problems relevant to your organization? Research has shown that persons in powerful positions have jobs that permit them autonomy and discretion, make them visible, and allow them to work on problems that are important as well as relevant to their organization (Beatty, 1979).

4. Have you developed supportive relationships with others in order to augment your power base? Mentorships? Sponsorships? Peer network?

5. In how much power-oriented behavior do you engage? Enough to cope with the dependencies of your managerial position?

6. What is your usual pattern of using power sources? Do you, for example, rely heavily on coercive power to influence others?

7. Do you possess any psychosocial or culturally bound traits that deter you in gaining and using power constructively?

8. Before engaging in a power move, ask: What is the real issue? Who is involved? Is the issue important enough to me to engage in power-oriented behavior? Are my power resources superior to that of the opposition?

9. Finally, before engaging in power-oriented behavior, attempt to forecast the consequences to you if you win *or* lose. In other words, assess the consequences of your power-oriented behavior. Short-term gains may not outweigh the long-term effects of creating enemies or destroying valuable lines of communication.

Assessing Power in the Organization

Personal use of power is facilitated by an accurate diagnosis of power within the subsystem and organization as a whole. First, groupings of actors must be identified in a meaningful way in order to begin with a relevant unit for analysis of power within the organization. People should be clustered together to maximize their homogeneity in preferences, values, and opinions about relevant political or other salient issues of importance in the organization at the time of the assessment (Pfeffer, 1981). It is generally a good idea to begin the analysis using the various subunits that are designated by the organization.

In a school of nursing, the subsystems for analysis might be the undergraduate nursing department, the graduate nursing department, and the continuing education department. In a hospital, the units for consideration might be surgical ward A, ward B, and ward C and medical wards D, E, and F.

Once the groupings of actors have been identified for purposes of analysis, assess their relative power in order to identify "the powerful." Try to determine the preferences of the actors about a given issue. To assess power-oriented behavior between subunits, it is best to analyze those instances in which preferences between actors about a given issue truly conflict. As Pfeffer (1981) states, "if one knows the initial preferences, the attempts at influence undertaken, and then the final decision, power can be more reliably diagnosed" (p. 45).

Pfeffer has also identified five methods of assessing power between social actors or units of analysis in an organization: assessing power by its determinants, assessing power by its consequences, assessing power by its symbols, reputational indicators of organizational power, and representational indicators.

Assessing Power by Its Determinants

This is one strategy of assessing the power distribution in the organization. Keep in mind the determinants of power among subsystems in the organization. From a strategic contingencies theory of power, these include (a) the degree to which an imbalance exists in the interdependency among subsystems and (b) how the subsystem responds to its environment. Pfeffer (1981) points out that it is "necessary to be able to assess how much of each determinant or source of power each of the various social actors in the situation possesses" (p. 48). The accompanying chart illustrates how one can determine the sources of power of actors in a system.

DETERMINING THE SOURCES OF POWER OF THE ACTORS IN A SYSTEM

Question	Example
1. Does a subsystem or actor control its contingencies?	1. Nursing personnel, budget, supplies, equipment, and space of a surgical unit
2. Is a subsystem able to cope with uncertainties?	2. A surgical unit's capability to handle a dramatic increase in patient admissions
3. Does the subsystem possess a low degree of substitutability?	3. Few other units in the hospital providing adequate and safe care to surgical patients
4. What degree of centrality is possessed by the subsystem?	4. The activities of the surgical unit are interlinked with other units in the hospitals. The workflow of the entire hospital would be affected if the work flow of the surgical unit ceases

Since more than one determinant may be operating at any one given time in a situation, try to assess which source of power was the most important. Assessing power by its determinants does require skill but can give the nurse manager data essential to understanding power distributions among the subsystems in the organization.

Assessing Power by Its Consequences

Power distribution among actors or subsystems of an organization can also be assessed by determining the outcomes of power-oriented behavior among actors. Since power is used to affect choices and decisions, determine which subsystems benefit in contested decisions and to what extent.

In the example of a school of nursing, power distribution among the units in this social system can be assessed by examining the consequences of situations in which the units possess conflicting perspectives. Which unit receives the most resources in proportion to the other units, such as operational dollars for staffing, staff development, travel, space, awards, and allocation of additional staff positions?

Although rational decision-making is often employed in the allocation of such resources, it may not be empirically descriptive. Yet, the social actors frequently behave after the outcome of such a process of resource allocation as if everyone shared in the myth of rational choice—that decisions are made rationally rather than based, at least in part, on power-oriented behavior (Pfeffer, 1981). Those actors who fared well as a result of power-oriented behavior are not likely to advertise this fact widely. Likewise, those who did not fare so well tend to act as if they did better than hoped. In this fashion, "the belief in rational choice processes will be more easily maintained and the norm of rationality preserved as a socially shared myth" (Pfeffer, 1981, p. 50).

Assessing Power by Its Symbols

Symbols of social power are positively correlated with the distribution of power among actors and are visible evidence of this distribution of power within an organization (Pfeffer, 1981). Symbols of power refer to such things as office space, type of office furniture, carpeting, view from office, location of office (distance away from the ground floor), special parking spaces, name plates, special restrooms, and use of company automobiles. The distribution of power among actors in a social system can be assessed to some extent by identifying such symbols. Although these symbols generally differentiate power among actors who are located at different vertical levels in the organizational hierarchy, they may also differentiate among subunits that are supposedly on the same hierarchical level (Pfeffer, 1981). As Pfeffer states,

> The provisions of social actors with the symbols of power both ratifies their power position within the organization and provides them with power because of the symbols. (1981, p. 54)

In a school of nursing, the dean's office is generally more plush than that of the average nurse faculty member. It is generally larger, may have more windows and a better view, better quality furniture, and carpeting. The dean's secretary, too, generally has a larger and more pleasant office than the secretaries assigned to the faculty. Special parking privileges may be extended not only to the dean but to section chairs. Further observations may reveal differences in symbols of power between subunits other than administrative and nonadministrative staff. The department of nursing research, if very highly valued in a school, may have visible symbols of power that set it apart from other departments within a college of nursing.

Reputational Indicators of Organizational Power

The technique used in this strategy is to assess the distribution of power by obtaining information from actors within the organization. A questionnaire is developed and administered to selected actors in the organization. An interview guide can be developed and interviews conducted with actors in the organization.

Although this method might work for conducting formal research, especially in another organization, it would present much resistance if attempted within one's own organization. Although there is evidence that "there are socially shared judgments within organizations concerning influence distributions," it is extremely difficult to convince informants to share this information (Pfeffer, 1981, p. 56). Pfeffer continues,

> Those who do know the distribution of influence and are skilled in political strategies have nothing to gain by sharing this knowledge, and, in fact, are probably more effective because this knowledge is not widely shared within the organization. (1981, p. 56).

Representational Indicators

In this method of assessing the distribution of power, it is important to determine the membership of social actors on major committees, boards, or occupancy of key administrative posts. Important committees provide power to their members because the committee has responsibility for important decisions, allocation of resources, or controls essential organizational information. Key administrative positions are often given to powerful persons who, in turn, gain additional power from the information, decisions, and responsibilities that are within the scope of the position. Membership on major committees can serve as an indicator of power and powerful units or departments often have larger representation on such committees as a direct consequence of their power (Pfeffer, 1981).

STRATEGIES FOR ACQUIRING AND USING POWER IN SOCIAL SYSTEMS

The data base resulting from assessing personal and organizational power sources and power-oriented behavior is critical in arriving at a diagnosis for the nurse manager and for the subsystem. What are the strengths and limitations in power-oriented behavior? If limitations are identified, the manager can use strategies to increase personal bases of power in these areas, and can seek ways to enhance those personal power bases already possessed. It is not generally beneficial to discuss diagnosing and enhancing personal bases of power with subordinates, but, a trusted colleague or mentor can be an invaluable resource in analyzing personal power-oriented behavior.

On the other hand, the nurse manager may want to involve the work group in analyzing the subsystem's bases of power in the organization. The nursing team can assist in formulating diagnoses about uncertainty, substitutability, centrality, and control of contingencies. Strategies can then be selected to reduce limitations and augment already existing sources of power. This takes a great deal of trust, self-disclosure, and loyalty among group members and leader. In groups without these traits, such risk taking can be politically damaging to either group member or leader.

Keep in mind that strong bases of personal power help deal with the dependencies of the managerial position as well as being useful in developing the bases of power in the subsystem.

Sources of Personal Power

Psychological

Basic to developing one's psychological source of power is self-awareness—knowledge of personal strengths and limitations. Assistance must be sought, for example, in the orientation in which power is primarily sought and drawn from more powerful others (McClelland, 1975). Awareness of one's own values and goals is equally important. The nurse manager may perceive and use power as a force to achieve organizational goals in a constructive manner, a value subordinates can generally appreciate. On the other hand, the nurse manager who utilizes power strictly for personal gains and "empire building" often leaves a trail of destruction behind. A psychological source of power also stems from a clear notion of one's professional role as a nurse and a belief in and commitment to that role. Internalized professional nursing values and beliefs can become translated into action when the manager is faced with conflicting situations.

Critical to a psychological power base for nurse leadership, management, or supervision is a strong self-concept. Having assessed personal strengths and limitations, identify areas of desired personal growth. For example, the personal basis of expert power can be increased by more knowledge about cancer nursing since additional patients with a diagnosis of cancer are being admitted to the clinical unit. Plan a program of action to achieve this goal. Reward yourself when major steps have been achieved.

Developing a strong self-concept is critical to successful and constructive power-oriented behavior. Strive to grow personally. Seek appropriate outlets for stress. Reward yourself for job responsibilities well done and learn to accept praise graciously.

Finally, claiming psychological power involves excellent communication skills so an accurate presentation of the self can be conveyed to others (De Joseph & O'Riordan, 1981). Communication skills, discussed elsewhere in this volume, are important to utilize in interacting with others in general, and in power-oriented behavior in particular.

Kalisch and Kalisch (1982a, b) point out some interesting verbal and nonverbal communication characteristics of a person who possesses power. The power holder is generally addressed more formally by others, rather than on a first-name basis. The power holder can control and impose silence more readily, interrupts more frequently, contradicts more often, and talks more than persons with less power. The power holder talks with more confidence, orients, gives commands, conveys information, and uses more direct messages and less qualifiers in the conversation. Self-disclosure is carefully monitored, but self-disclosure from the less powerful is frequently expected. Nonverbal expressions of power by the powerful take the form of more desirable space, more spatial freedom, sitting at the head of a table, and controlling one's distance from others. In relation to the use of time, the more powerful take up more time and request time at their convenience from the less powerful. In turn, less time is generally granted to the less powerful with careful determination of the time to be allocated. Other activities may be engaged in while interacting with the less powerful. Appointments may be required and barriers to access may be erected. The power holder uses direct eye contact, stares more frequently, and seeks greater visual information. Touch may be used but others are not permitted to touch the power holder. The facial expression is frequently characterized by frowns, raised chin, raised eyebrow, wide-open eyes, jutting neck posture, and a stern masklike expression.

Interpersonal

Personal power can be enchanced through mentorships and sponsorships. Likewise, one can engage in strategies to increase one's expert, reward, referent, legitimate, and coercive bases of power.

Mentorships and sponsorships. A *mentor* is a person in the organization who has a vested interest in your job performance and career progress. The mentor possesses enough power to facilitate your way through the organizational maze. The mentor frequently counsels and provides help. A mentor can thus augment one's personal power-oriented behavior in the organization.

A sponsorship, on the other hand, is a less consuming relationship but can, nevertheless, augment personal power-oriented behavior. A *sponsor* is someone who

gives you early information about what's going on, who gives you some guidelines to the ways the organization functions, who perhaps puts in a good word for you during performance appraisal time or when your name comes up at a meeting. (Beatty, 1979, p. 3)

One should strive to establish at least one mentorship or sponsorship with a superior in the organization. At the same time, there may be a competent subordinate who can be groomed by your being a mentor or sponsor.

Networking. Other selected members from one's network of personal colleagues can assist in analyzing and improving power-oriented behavior. "Know who's who. Act assertively. Do favors for other powerful persons, and start accumulating those psychological debts to be paid when you need them" (Stevens, 1980a, p. 211). Develop communication networks, nurture them, and keep them open. At professional meetings, for example, one should strive to meet colleagues and keep a liberal supply of personal professional business cards available. Mutually supportive relationships can be developed in this fashion, relationships that can help work through power-based situations. A nurse practitioner, for example, can call on his or her network of practitioner colleagues to discuss ways to increase his or her sources of power in order to deal with opposition to her role.

Networking can also be useful when forming peer coalitions and are essential as a political strategy. In research conducted by Archer and Goehner (1981), nurse administrators, in fact, reported that building peer coalitions was the second most important and successful political strategy. Networking can increase collective power in policy making arenas relevant to health care and to the profession.

The work group. Last but not least, relate to and treat members of the nursing team or group in such a way that they will be supportive in attaining organizational goals. A cohesive, highly functional, and supportive group of nurses can be an invaluable source of power when they rally behind the nurse manager on an important issue. Interpersonal relations with subordinates are essential—enhance them and the personal bases of power are likewise enhanced.

Expert power. As has been discussed, a sound knowledge base can be an important source of power in relation to another person who values that knowledge. First, develop competence in leadership, managerial, or supervisory processes and skills. If in the clinical setting, enhance nursing expertise in the specialty area through continuing education. If in the educational setting, strive also for expertise in areas such as curriculum development or instructional technology. For example, computer technology and knowledge in developing computer-assisted instructional modules are in high demand and can serve as a considerable source of power.

As a nurse manager and supervisor, also acquire power through the control of useful information and channels of information. In a complex organization, "information can be even more important than traditional tangible resources, because rational problem solving and influence by persuasion are essential in complex settings" (Kotter, 1979, p. 27). Information is power.

Reward power. The ability to grant a reward to a subordinate is an important basis of power. In order to be able to grant such rewards, however, a constructive relationship with higher sources of authority in the organization is needed. In addition, direct control over some of the tangible resources such as budgets for staff development, travel, and so forth, "clearly put a manager in a better position to influence others and to acquire other types of power" (Kotter, 1979, p. 26).

Control over tangible resources can be gained in a number of ways. Doing a good job and pleasing one's supervisor is a way of gaining desired resources that can be used to reward subordinates. Another strategy is to select a managerial or supervisory position that has the potential for control over a wide variety of resources. Finally, be sensitive to those resources already possessed and do not inadvertently give them away.

Referent power. Identification can be fostered in a number of ways. Some nurse leaders naturally possess a charismatic personality. Even if not the most naturally blest, the nurse manager's personality will be respected if an atmosphere of trust, honesty, mutual respect, and openness is created. In addition, develop a good professional reputation through visible achievement and assertive behavior.

Legitimate power. As Claus and Bailey (1977) state, "Much of the power derived from the formal authority of the organization is engendered in the managerial position" (pp. 119–120). Be familiar with and seek to enhance formal power to make decisions and initiate actions, to control and gain important information, to control human and nonhuman resources, to formulate and enforce policies and procedures, and to have access to key leaders in the organization. Be keenly aware of the legitimate base of power connected with the position and how it compares with other positions in the organization.

Coercive power. The use of coercive power is not favored, although it can get quick, short-term results. Frequent reliance on coercive power tends to increase employee resistance and hostility, to lower morale and enthusiasm, and to contribute to absenteeism and job turnover in the long-run. It can likewise destroy the respect a nurse may have had for the manager, supervisor, or leader who uses coercion as a bases of power to change subordinates' behaviors.

Gaining Power by Managing Dependence

As has been reviewed previously, the nurse manager, supervisor, or leader may be dependent on a number of persons to accomplish subsystem and organizational goals. Analyze job responsibilities, find out who is really important in getting the job done. Eliminate any unnecessary dependencies. The psychological and interpersonal power strategies outlined previously can be used as counterveiling sources of power. Finally, explore other avenues for meeting dependence needs when any one resource becomes particularly problematic.

Mr. O'Neil, head nurse on a surgical unit, for example, is dependent upon the staff development department to provide staff orientation and in-service programs for his staff. An inexperienced and autocratic recently employed director of the staff development department is meeting resistance from nurse educators employed by this department. Consequently, Mr. O'Neil finds the educational services sporadic, not well planned, and of questionable quality. To deal with his managerial dependence on the staff development department, Mr. O'Neil mobilizes his power sources and arranges with sanctions from his supervisor, the assistant director of surgical services, to develop and implement his own staff orientation and in-service programs. In the process, he uses some of his more experienced staff as well as receiving part-time assistance from the surgical clinical nurse specialist. Mr. O'Neil agrees to use the staff development educators once nursing administration has worked through the difficulties experienced with the staff development director.

Developing Sources of Power in Subsystems

Developing and maintaining sources of power in the subsystem is part of managerial responsibilities. Psychological and interpersonal sources of power, as well as the ability to deal with the dependency inherent in the position, are important variables as the input, throughput, feedback, and maintenance processes of the subsystem are managed. Attention should be directed toward building a strong and viable subunit that is viewed as a relevant, respected, and contributing part of the larger organization.

As pointed out in the strategic contingencies theory of power, the power of any given subsystem in an organization stems from the extent of its ability to meet the requirements of other subsystems, to monopolize the ability to meet these requirements, and to respond to its environment. As gatekeeper of the subsystem's boundaries, power can be gained by managing resources, uncertainty, substitutability, and centrality.

Power Through Resources

Resources/inputs include personnel, technology, equipment, supplies, money, and nonmaterial resources as expertise/prestige and rewards/sanctions. Any subsystem is in continuous interaction with its environment. As gatekeeper, the manager is responsible for securing an adequate supply of resources to enable the subunit to carry on its functions. A formal budget request is generally demanded yearly. Keep in mind, however, that power-oriented behavior does enter the decision-making process regarding some of the resources being distributed. Personal sources of power can be used to obtain the needed resources for the subunit.

At the same time, recognize that those subunits "within the organization that can provide the most critical and difficult to obtain resources come to have power in the organization" (Pfeffer, 1981, p. 101). A subunit successful in obtaining funding through grants and contracts tends to develop power within the total organization, such as a school of nursing. The funding can expand the nursing education program, increase student enrollment (thus generating more income for the school), and increase instructional technology. In addition, a successful grant project or contract can develop a school's reputation and prestige. Likewise, a hospital-based nursing research unit that obtains external sources of funding can gain considerable power. The ability of bringing outside resources into the organization, in general, enhances the power of that subsystem within the total organization.

Coping with Uncertainty

As discussed, coping with uncertainty can contribute to a subsystem's bases of power. Uncertainties confronting an organization arise basically from three different sources (Thompson, 1967). First, there is a generalized uncertainty arising from a lack of understanding of cause-and-effect relationships in the environment. This source of uncertainty makes selection of alternatives and evaluation of outcomes very difficult. Second, uncertainty may arise from an environment where understanding of cause and effect is present but which may be uncooperative in relation to an organization's goals, needs, and outputs. Third, uncertainty for the organization can stem from the internal interdependency of its component parts. Galbraith (1973) adds task uncertainty meaning "the difference between the amount of information required to perform the task and the amount of information already possessed by the organization" (p. 5). Pfeffer (1981) further points out that as decision-making contexts vary, so does the uncertainty faced by the subsystem. A subunit's power source increases when considerable capabilities are possessed/gained in coping with a particular type of uncertainty faced by the organization.

What strategies can a midlevel nurse manager use to cope with these uncertainties, thus developing a subsystem's bases of power? To cope with generalized environmental uncertainty, participate when possible in organizational efforts to evaluate the external environment in forecasting and in planning. Develop a plan to gather relevant information about the environment for the operation of the subunit. Staff members can be given assignments to assist the manager in this information gathering activity. Analyze the information. Forecast and attempt to make predictions about, and plans for, subunit goals and activities that will contribute maximally to the overall organization. Evaluate the results, including a determination of whether the efforts have added to the subunit's bases of power.

Managing subsystem boundaries becomes critical when coping with uncertainties arising from an uncooperative environment. Use personal sources of power to negotiate for resources or for resolving issues affecting the subunit's input, throughput, output, and feedback processes. Strive to buffer the subsystem from uncooperative and damaging environmental elements. Finally, at times it may be necessary to vary subsystem activities in order to match the demands of an uncooperative environment more closely.

Even though on a smaller scale, the midlevel manager may need to cope with some degree of uncertainty arising from interdependencies among subsystem parts. If the continuing education brochures can suddenly not be printed in the usual manner, the CE nursing director will need to cope with this uncertainty, perhaps by having CE flyers typed and photocopied for distribution instead.

Finally, the nurse manager will need to cope with task uncertainty. Such strategies as improving data management and record keeping, increasing staff abilities through educational experiences, and utilizing experts, such as clinical nurse specialists, can be useful in coping with task uncertainty. In summary, coping with uncertainty contributes to the development of a subsystem's power base.

Being Irreplaceable and Assuring Centrality

Being irreplaceable contributes to the source of power of a subsystem. Pfeffer (1981) mentions four strategies for increasing a subunit's source of power by being irreplaceable: documentation, specialized language, centralization of expertise, and controlling externally based sources of expertise. Documentation refers to the process of not writing information down so that expertise is not so readily available to others. Specialized phrases and words keep subspecialty knowledge from being readily obtained by others. Centralization of expertise means keeping a given body of expertise within a subsystem. Controlling consultants to that subsystem would reduce the threat from other subunits gaining this specialized expertise.

Using the cardiac surgical intensive care unit (ICU) as an example, the head nurse can continue to provide substantial justification for the maintenance of this separate ICU along with its separate staff of cardiovascular nurse experts. This strategy keeps the specialized body of nursing knowledge centered in this ICU and the hospital continues to depend on this ICU for the care of its surgical cardiovascular patients.

The basis of power is also increased for a subsystem if its activities are essential to the central goal of the organization and are linked to the tasks of other subsystems. By maintaining a separate ICU, the head nurse in the example derives subsystem power through the concept of centrality. The ICU remains both essential to the hospital and its activities are linked to other subsystems as the operating room and the postsurgical wards.

SUMMARY

Power can be used as a constructive force by the nurse leader, manager, or supervisor. Power can be used to gain needed resources, to bring about desired change or block destructive actions in the throughput process, and to create subsystem outputs important and valued by the total organization. Individual and/or collective power used wisely can improve patient care, enhance the quality of nursing education, facilitate the development of the nursing profession, and bring about desired change in the health care delivery system.

Power is the generalized capacity or potential to get others to do something one wants them to do that they ordinarily would not do otherwise. Several theoretical frameworks for understanding power are discussed: the psychological orientation, field theory, social exchange theory, political science theory, and the strategic contingencies theory of power.

Assessing sources of power facilitates the constructive use of power in achieving specific goals. Personal sources of power, as well as the bases of organizational/subunit power, should be analyzed. Strengths and limitations in power-oriented behavior can thus be identified. Action plans can then be formulated to augment power in essential areas. Finally, strategies for acquiring and using power in social systems that are useful in developing such action plans are reviewed.

REFERENCES

Archer, S., & Goehner, P. Acquiring political clout: Guidelines for nurse administrators. *The Journal of Nursing Administration*, November–December 1981, *11* (11–12), 49–55.

Ashley, J. This I believe about power in nursing. *Nursing Dimensions*, 1979, *7*(2) 28–32.

Ashley, J. Power in structured misogyny: Implications for the politics of care. *Advances in Nursing Science*, 1980, *2*, 3–22.

Beatty, N. (Ed.) *Women and power: An exploratory view*. Cambridge: Radcliffe College, 1979.

Busch, P. The sales manager's bases of social power and influence upon the sales force. *Journal of Marketing*, 1980, *44*, 91–101.

Butterfield, D., & Posner, B. Task-relevant control in organizations. *Personnel Psychology*, 1979, *32*, 725–740.

Capuzzi, C. Power and interest groups: A study of ANA and AMA. *Nursing Outlook*. 1980, *28*, 478–482.

Claus, K., & Bailey, J. *Power and influence in health care. A new approach to leadership*. St. Louis: Mosby, 1977.

Clegg, S. *Power, rule, and domination: A critical and empirical understanding of power in sociological theory and organizational life*. Boston: Routledge & Kegan Paul, 1975.

Conway, M. The acquisition and use of power in academia: A dean's perspective. *Nursing Administration Quarterly*, 1978, 2, 83–90.

Cumming, E., & Cumming, J. The locus of power in a large mental hospital. *Nursing Dimensions*, 1979, 7(2), 43–49.

Dahl, R. The concept of power. *Behavioral Science*, 1957, 2(3), 201–218.

De Joseph, J., & O'Riordan, E. Claiming power: A strategy for change. *Nursing Administrative Quarterly*, 1981, 5(2), 24–26.

Dieziger, S. Power–politics–problems. In National League for Nursing, *Raising your political blood pressure* (Pub. No. 52–1827). New York: National League for Nursing, 1980.

Drake, B., & Mitchell, T. The effects of vertical and horizontal power on individual motivation and satisfaction. *Academy of Management Journal*, 1977, 20(4), 573–591.

Dunne, E., Stahl, M., & Melhart, L. Influence sources of project and functional managers in matrix organizations. *Academy of Management Journal*, 1978, 21(1), 135–140.

Emerson, R. Power-dependence relations. *American Sociological Review*, 1962, 27(1), 31–41.

French, J., & Raven, B. The bases of social power. In D. Cartwright (Ed.), *Studies in social power*. Ann Arbor: The University of Michigan, 1959.

Galbraith, J. *Designing complex organizations*. Reading: Addison-Wesley, 1973.

Harward, D. *Power: Its nature, its use, and its limits*. Boston: Schenkman, 1979.

Hickson, D., Hinings, C., Lee, C., Schneck, R., & Pennings, J. A strategic contingencies theory of intraorganizational power. *Administrative Science Quarterly*, 1971, 16(2), 216–227.

Kalisch, B., & Kalisch, P. *Politics of nursing*. Philadelphia: J. B. Lippincott, 1982. (a)

Kalisch, B., & Kalisch, P. *The power and politics of nursing*. Lectureship, George Mason University, 1982. (b)

Kotter, J. Power, success, and organizational effectiveness. *Organizational Dynamics*, 1978, 6, 27–40.

Kotter, J. *Power in management*. New York: AMACOM, 1979.

Leininger, M. Territoriality, power, and creative leadership in administrative nursing contexts. *Nursing Dimensions*, 1979, 7(2), 33–42.

Mauksch, I. Nursing is unique and essential, but powerless. *Texas Nursing*, 1980, 54, 7,13.

McClelland, D. *Power: The inner experience*. New York: Irvington, 1975.

McFarland, D., & Shiflett, N. The role of power in the nursing profession. *Nursing Dimensions*, 1979, 7(2), 1–13.

Miller, M. Nurse power: A reality now. *Georgia Nursing*, 1980, 40(5), 1, 6.

Parsek, J. Politics and conflict: Some thoughts. *Nursing Administration Quarterly*, 1978, 2(2), 66–68.

Peterson, G. Power: A perspective for the nurse administrator. *Journal of Nursing Administration*, 1979, 9(7), 7–10.

Pfeffer, J. *Power in organizations*. Marshfield: Pitman, 1981.

Phillips, J. Health care provider relationships: A matter of reciprocity. *Nursing Outlook*, 1979, 27(11), 738–741.

Phippen M. Power: What nursing school never taught. *AORN Journal*, 1981, 33(4), 650–656.

Sanford, N. Power for the OR nurse. *AORN Journal*, 1980, 31(5), 787–794.

Stevens, B. Power and politics for the nurse executive. *Nursing and Health Care*, November 1980, 1(4), 208–212. (a)

Stevens, B. Development and use of power in nursing. In National League for Nursing, *Assuring a goal-directed future for nursing* (Pub. No. 52–1814). New York: National League for Nursing, 1980. (b)

Tedeschi, J. *Perspectives on social power*. Chicago: Aldine, 1974.

Thompson, J. *Organizations in action: Social science bases of administrative theory.* New York: McGraw-Hill, 1967.

Ver Steeg, D. The political process, or, the power and the glory. *Nursing Dimensions,* 1979, 7(2), 20–27.

Votaw, D. What do we believe about power? *Nursing Dimensions,* 1979, 7(2), 50–63.

Zaleznik, A. Power and politics in organizational life. *Nursing Dimensions,* 1979, 7(2), 64–74.

BIBLIOGRAPHY

Baker, C. Role conflicts of middle managers in baccalaureate and higher degree nursing programs in the United States. In American Nurses Association, *Power: Nursing's challenge for change.* (Pub. No. G-1355M). Kansas City: The American Nurses Association, 1979.

Cartwright, D. (Ed.) *Studies in social power.* Ann Arbor: The University of Michigan, 1979.

Cobb, A. Informal influences in the formal organization: Perceived sources of power among work unit peers. *Academy of Management Journal,* 1980, 23(1), 155–161.

Craig, J. *Synergic power: Beyond domination, beyond permissiveness.* Berkeley: Pro Active Press, 1979.

Day, C. Creating power in powerless positions. *Medical Laboratory Observer,* 1981, 13, 51–52, 55–57.

Dubrin, A. *Winning at office politics.* New York: Van Nostrand Reinhold, 1978.

Kennedy, M. *Office politics.* New York: Warner Books, 1980.

Martin, N., & Simms, J. Thinking ahead: Power tactics. *Harvard Business Review,* 1956, 34(6), 25–36 +.

McNeil, K. Understanding organizational power: Building on the Weberian legacy. *Administrative Science Quarterly,* 1978, 23, 65–90.

Mowday, R. The exercise of upward influence in organizations. *Administrative Science Quarterly,* 1978, 23, 137–156.

Perez, T., & Perez, A. Power—an essential need for effective managers: Part I. *Contemporary Pharmacy Practice,* 1981, 4(3), 137–141.

Roos, L., & Hall, R. Influence diagrams and organizational power. *Administrative Science Quarterly,* 1980, 25(1), 57–71.

Salmin, D. The concept of authority and power. *The ANPHI Papers,* 1977, 12, 3–13.

Sanford, N. Identification and explanation of strategies to develop power for nursing. In American Nurses' Association, *Power: Nursing's challenge for change.* (Pub. No. G-1355M). Kansas City: The American Nurses' Association, 1979.

Schuldt, S. Supervision and the informal organization. *The Journal of Nursing Administration,* 1978, 8(7), 21–25.

Shaw, M., & Heyman, B. Constructs of relationships and issues of authority in nursing. *Journal of Advanced Nursing,* March 1980, 5, 187–198.

Stead, A. *Women in management.* Englewood Cliffs, N.J.: Prentice-Hall, 1978.

Stern, W. *The game of office politics.* Chicago: Henry Regnery, 1976.

Wrong, D. *Power: Its forms, bases, and uses.* New York: Harper & Row, 1979.

CHAPTER 17
TEAM BUILDING

This chapter introduces a number of team-building strategies that have been developed for intervention in a wide variety of organizations, both nationally and internationally. A review of team and group dynamics in nursing provides the conceptual foundation for much of this chapter. In addition, other chapters in Part III contain valuable ideas for team-building activities.

In most cases, examples of a particular type of team-building activity are presented and refer the reader to more comprehensive volumes treating activities of that genre. A number of excellent books and handbooks that provide hundreds of team-building activities, ideas, and suggestions are available.

DIAGNOSING THE SYSTEM

Simpleminded as it may seem, it is often necessary for the nurse manager/supervisor to determine whether he or she is leading or supervising a team or simply a group of employees. Remember, in a true team all members share a common mission and task *and* are expected and required to work cooperatively with each other in order to be successful.

If a particular group does not have both of these characteristics, then it does not require *teamwork* and team-building efforts may have little effect upon group performance. Some group environments are inherently competitive (e.g., tennis "teams") and unsuited for team building. In the vast majority of situations in nursing, however, cooperation is *vital* to team effectiveness.

Differentiating Type A and B Teams

Most nursing groups are true teams and require teamwork. Still to be determined is whether a particular team is type A or B. A fuller discussion of type A and B teams has been presented previously. Briefly, type A teams have a shared mission, expect and require cooperation *and* have tasks which are relatively routinized. Type B teams, on the other hand, have a shared mission, expect and require cooperation, but have tasks that are not easily routinized and require extensive problem-solving skills. Few nursing teams are pure type A or B teams and the nurse manager/supervisor must assess the predominant character of her or his team. If the success of a team depends primarily upon the efficiency with which members carry out prescribed tasks, then the team is probably best characterized as type A. If a team's success depends largely upon diagnostic skills, development of new state-of-the-art procedures, innovation in training, planning, or budgeting, it is probably best characterized as type B.

Proper diagnosis of the team will help the nurse manager/supervisor select the proper forms of team building. Type A team-building programs will focus on issues of team member role definition and clarification, supervision and authority, effective communication, interpersonal conflict management, goal setting, time management, team health and stress management, socialization and team culture, and measurement and evaluation of team effectiveness. Type B team-building programs will focus on issues of effective problem-solving, decision-making, and follow-through processes. Within the context of these processes will be interwoven issues of communication, conflict resolution, creativity and innovation, time management, leadership and power, goal setting, and evaluation.

TEAM-BUILDING METHODS

The Organization Development Approach

Organization development (OD) as a generic term refers to a collection of interventions for organizations that has deep philosophic and theoretical roots in the laboratory education approach to social and organizational change pioneered by Kurt Lewin and the National Training Laboratories (NTL). No single author or practitioner is credited with starting OD. Rather, a number of consultants and trainers of the T-group tradition began applying small group training methods directly in organizations.

T-group proponents recognized that the transition from off-site T-groups to the work site was critical to the method's success. Unfortunately, the structural and social obstacles to this linkage proved very difficult to overcome. T-groups continued to be recognized as excellent environments for management training and professional development, but were considered ineffective vehicles for specific team building.

The conservative or restraining forces inherent in *any* social system easily overwhelmed the driving forces for change mobilized by one or two members of a team even if these members were team leaders. Planned and gradual change brought about by careful and respectful consideration of resistance to change and stewarded by managers and team-building consultants proved to be the only reliable method for bringing about needed organizational change.

This approach required much more structure and discipline than in T-groups where experimentation and spontaneity were highly encouraged. Concerns about personal, interpersonal, and team security became highly relevant. Teams have a much longer life cycle than T-groups and the consequences of any action are much longer lasting.

The barriers to open and honest communication are greater in intact teams than in "stranger" T-groups. Past experiences with each other may also make the development of trust more difficult in intact teams than in T-groups.

Three OD team-building activities are presented briefly: (a) an "icebreaker" exercise, (b) a survey feedback activity, and (c) a communications exercise. These activities are but a small sample of team-building activities available. (The reader should refer to the references and bibliography of this chapter for more detailed descriptions of team-building activities.) Each activity is presented with detailed instructions for the team-building leader concerning the goals, ideal group size, time requirements, materials, and physical setting. While most team-building exercises can be conducted by team leaders themselves, it is highly recommended that they have first-hand experience as a participant or co-leader in team-building programs.

The leader's confidence in conducting team-building activities is crucial to success. Since team-building activities typically are highly structured, there is little danger that serious psychological problems will develop for any of the team members. The inexperienced team-building leader will more likely encounter problems in proper timing of activities and resistance, overt and covert, from team members toward the program.

OD practitioners skilled in assessing and dealing with team and group dynamics will be very helpful to the nurse manager/supervisor who is conducting OD team-building activities for the first time. Many team-building books and handbooks (e.g., Francis & Young, 1979) give instructions for locating and using OD team-building consultants.

An Icebreaker Exercise

In most cases, leaders and participants experience anxiety, fear, and some dread at the start of a team-building program. Many have heard rumors about the new program based upon other peoples' experiences in "groups." Some participants are fearful that the numerous "hidden agendas" between team members will be discussed openly, causing embarrassment, or worse, harm to interpersonal relationships. Other team members have a general fear of group meetings and of participation in groups based upon unpleasant experiences in the past. The team-building leader(s) will likely experience anxiety and worry about the ultimate success of the program or about their performance in a new role.

The following ice breaker activity allows a group to address these concerns while learning about the communication process of the team. This exercise is especially useful for teams that feel reluctant or even hostile about the team-building program.

A COMMUNICATION ANALYSIS: A GETTING-ACQUAINTED ACTIVITY

GOALS

I. To establish a laboratory or learning climate in the initial stages of a group composed of hostile or reluctant participants

II. To experience openness in exploring positive and negative feelings in a nonthreatening atmosphere

III. To examine how affective elements (especially negative feelings) influence the results of communications

GROUP SIZE

Twelve or more participants

TIME REQUIREMENTS

Approximately 1 hour

MATERIALS

I. Eight sheets of newsprint (medium that can be purchased in 3′ × 4′ pads or 24″ rolls), each of which bears a different heading from the Communication Analysis Work Sheet

II. Felt-tipped markers and masking tape

III. A copy of the Communication Analysis Work Sheet and a pencil for each participant

PHYSICAL SETTING

A room large enough to accommodate all participants comfortably. A long wall should be available for posting the data on newsprint.

PROCESS

I. The facilitator posts the sheets of newsprint, each containing one heading from the Communication Analysis Work Sheet. The facilitator indicates that she or he is interested in the communication that each received as inducement to attend the session, since the participant's feelings about the message, the person who sent the message, and so on, can clearly affect his or her feeling about participating in the event. The facilitator tells the group members, "Rather than just telling you about the effects that various styles and methods of communication have on us, I would like to examine them with you so that we can learn from each other."

II. The facilitator asks the participants to share with the group the messages or communications that brought them to the session. Each volunteered message is recorded on the first sheet, "message received."

III. The facilitator continues to elicit information from each participant concerning each heading on the Communication Analysis Work Sheet (10 minutes).

IV. The facilitator selects a few (three to six) examples that are representative of good and poor communication (resulting in support or antagonism from the group) and lists each of these examples on a sheet of newsprint.

V. The facilitator then discusses the similarities and differences between good and poor communications and lists his or her major points on the newsprint.

VI. Subgroups of five or six participants each are formed. Each group member is given a copy of the Communication Analysis Work Sheet and a pencil.

VII. Each participant is instructed to complete a worksheet concerning his or her own communications regarding the workshop (10 minutes) and then to discuss his or her responses with other members of the small group (20 minutes).

VIII. The entire group reconvenes. Each small group reports on its discussion and what they learned. The facilitator then summarizes the knowledge gained from the experience.

COMMUNICATIONS ANALYSIS WORK SHEET

Message received:
The following questions are spaced evenly on an 8½" × 11" sheet of paper:

- How did you understand the message?
- What did you judge the quality of the message to be?
- How was the message given?
- Who gave the message?
- Type and quality of relationship with giver:
- Other influences that affected your feelings about the message:
- Feelings and motivation toward session (or workshop):

SOURCE: Adapted from Jorgensen, R. Communications analysis: A getting-acquainted activity. Reprinted from John E. Jones and J.W. Pfeiffer (Eds.). *The 1977 Annual Handbook for Group Facilitators*. San Diego: University Associates, 1977. Used with permission.

A Survey Feedback Activity

This activity may be used as an icebreaker activity when teams begin team-building programs in a positive and open manner. In teams that have reservations about the program or in teams where there are significant interpersonal conflicts, it is best to use an icebreaking activity to reduce tension before beginning this feedback activity.

THE TEAM-REVIEW QUESTIONNAIRE

GOALS

I. To help a work team address its strengths and weaknesses
II. To determine whether the group has the desire and the energy to begin a team-building program
III. To help a team understand the characteristics of effective teamwork

GROUP SIZE

Six to fifteen team members per group, three to four groups of teams may work together

TIME REQUIREMENTS

A minimum of 2 hours

MATERIALS

I. A copy of the Team-Review Questionnaire, the Team-Review Questionnaire Answer Sheet, the Team-Review Questionnaire Interpretation Sheet, and a pencil for each participant

II. Blank paper for each participant

III. A large pad of paper to use as a blank flip chart (newsprint is handy), masking tape and a felt-tipped marking pen, or a chalkboard and chalk

PHYSICAL SETTING

A quiet room where team members can sit and write comfortably

PROCESS

I. One person in the team, often the manager/supervisor, takes an hour prior to the meeting to become familiar with the method described in "Analyzing the Team-Review Questionnaire," which follows the questionnaire. This person acts as coordinator and discussion leader for the session.

II. The session begins with a brief explanation by the coordinator about the process the team is about to undertake. He or she emphasizes that voluntary involvement is essential and invites people to express their concerns. Only if there is full agreement should the questionnaire materials be distributed and the activity continued (10 minutes).

III. Team members complete the questionnaire, including the interpretation sheet (20 minutes).

IV. Using the information given in "Analyzing the Team-Review Questionnaire," the coordinator guides the team in charting the reactions (15 minutes).

V. Now comes the most significant part of the activity. The coordinator introduces a discussion of the results, and the team members discuss the following questions for approximately 20 minutes each.
1. How valid are the Team-Review Questionnaire results?
2. What are the significant strengths and weaknesses of the team?
3. What resources are we prepared to devote to strengthening our team and working through blocks?
It is important to be very specific about the last question. One way of measuring the team's commitment is to allocate money to the project. If a team is willing to spend scarce resources on self-development, then it is clearly committed and action is more likely to follow.

VI. When the discussion has been concluded, the team as a whole should make the decision whether to proceed with team building. Sometimes it is useful to allow a few days for reflection before the final decision is made. Once this is done, if the team wishes to proceed, it can begin by planning other team-building activities to address the blocks to effective teamwork identified in the survey-feedback activity.

VII. Even if the team does not proceed with formal team-building activities it may wish to discuss the issues and blocks identified in the survey-feedback activity in traditional staff and team meetings.

THE QUESTIONNAIRE

Instructions

Part 1
Write in the following space a precise definition of the team under review. Either write the names of all those included or a designation that is unmistakable.
The team under review is

```
┌─────────────────────────────────────────────────────────┐
│                                                           │
│                                                           │
│                                                           │
│                                                           │
└─────────────────────────────────────────────────────────┘
```

Part 2
You will find 108 statements listed below. Think about each statement in relation to the identified team. Use the Team-Review Questionnaire Answer Sheet to respond to the statements. If you feel that a statement is broadly true, mark an X on the appropriate number in the answer sheet grid. If you feel that a statement is not broadly true, then leave that number blank.

Work methodically through the questionnaire, answering each question. There may be times when you find it difficult to answer a particular question; come to the best answer you can. It might be useful to note in the margin the numbers of these difficult questions.

Remember that the quality of the result is directly related to your openness when answering the questions. This is not meant to be a scientific survey, but rather it serves as a tool to provoke thought and discussion.

1. The team's manager and members spend little time in clarifying what they expect and need from one another.
2. The work of the team would improve if members upgraded their technical qualifications.
3. Most of the members feel that the aims of the team are hardly worthwhile.
4. People in this team often are not really frank and open with each other.
5. The objectives of our team are not really clear.
6. Team members are unsure about the team's contribution to the wider organization.
7. We rarely achieve much progress in team meetings.
8. The objectives of some individual team members do not gel with those of other members.
9. When team members are criticized, they often feel that they have lost face.

10. New members often are just left to find their own place in the team.
11. Not many new ideas are generated by the team.
12. Conflicts between our team and other groups are quite common.
13. The team manager/administrator rarely tolerates leadership efforts by other team members.
14. Some team members are unable to handle the current requirements of their work.
15. Team members are not really committed to the success of the team.
16. In group discussion, team members often hide their real motives.
17. In practice, the team rarely achieves its objectives.
18. Our team's contribution is not clearly understood by other parts of the organization.
19. When the team is having a meeting, we do not listen to each other.
20. Team members are uncertain about their individual roles in relation to the team.
21. Members often restrain their critical remarks to avoid "rocking the boat."
22. The potential of some team members is not being developed.
23. Team members are wary about suggesting new ideas.
24. Our team does not have constructive relationships with some of the other teams within the organization.
25. Team members are uncertain where they stand with the team manager.
26. Our mix of skills is inappropriate to the work we are doing.
27. I do not feel a strong sense of belonging to the team.
28. It would be helpful if the team could have "clear-the-air" sessions more often.
29. In practice, low levels of achievement are accepted.
30. If the team were disbanded, the organization would not feel the loss.
31. The team meetings often seem to lack a methodical approach.
32. There is no regular review of individual objectives and priorities.
33. The team is not good at learning from its mistakes.
34. Team members tend not to show initiative in keeping up-to-date or in developing themselves.
35. We have the reputation of being stick-in-the-muds.
36. The team does not respond sufficiently to the needs of other teams in the organization.
37. The team manager/administrator gets little information about how the team sees his performance.
38. People outside the team consider us as unqualified to meet work requirements.
39. I am not prepared to put myself out for the team.
40. Important issues often are "swept under the carpet" and not worked through.
41. Individuals are given few incentives to stretch themselves.
42. There is confusion between the work of this team and the work of others.

43. Team members rarely plan or prepare for meetings.
44. If team members are missing, their work just does not get done.
45. Attempts to review events critically are seen as negative and harmful.
46. Little time and effort are spent on individual development and training.
47. This team seldom innovates anything.
48. We do not actively seek to develop our working relationships with other teams.
49. The team would get better quality decisions if the team members took the initiative.
50. The team's total level of ability is too low.
51. Some team members find it difficult to commit themselves to doing the job well.
52. There is too much stress placed on conformity.
53. Energy is absorbed in unproductive ways and does not go into getting results.
54. The role of our team is not clearly identified within the organization.
55. The team does not set aside time to consider and review how it tackles problems.
56. Much improvement is needed in communication between team members.
57. We would benefit from an impartial assessment of how we work.
58. Most team members have been trained only in their technical discipline.
59. Good ideas seem to get lost.
60. Some significant mistakes would have been avoided if we had better communication with other teams.
61. The team manager/administrator often makes decisions without talking them through with the team.
62. We need an input of new knowledge and skills to make the team complete.
63. I wish I could feel more motivated by working in this team.
64. Differences between team members rarely are properly worked through.
65. No time is devoted to questioning whether our efforts have been worthwhile.
66. We do not have an adequate way to establish our team's objectives and strategy.
67. We often seem to get bogged down when a difficult problem is being discussed in team meetings.
68. The team does not have adequate administrative resources and procedures.
69. We lack the skills to review our effectiveness constructively.
70. The team does not take steps to develop its members.
71. New ideas from outside the team are seldom accepted.
72. In this organization, teams and departments tend to compete rather than collaborate.
73. The team manager/administrator does not adapt his or her style to changing circumstances.
74. New people coming into the team sometime lack the necessary qualifications.
75. No one is trying hard to make this a winning team.
76. Individuals in this team do not really get to know each other as people.

77. We seem more concerned about giving a good appearance than achieving results.

78. The organization does not use the vision and skills that the team has to offer.

79. We have team meetings, but do not examine their purpose properly.

80. We function in rather a rigid manner and are not sufficiently flexible in using team resources.

81 Performance would improve if constructive criticism were encouraged.

82. Individuals who are retiring or uncertain often are overridden.

83. It would be fair to say that the team has little vision.

84. Some of the other teams/departments seem to have a low opinion of us.

85. The team manager/administrator is not sufficiently sensitive to the different needs of each member.

86. Some team members are not adapting to the needs of the team, despite efforts to help them.

87. If a team member gets into difficulties, he or she usually is left to cope with them alone.

88. There are cliques and political maneuvering in the team.

89. Nothing that we do could be described as excellent.

90. The team's objectives have not been systematically related to the objectives of the whole organization.

91. Decisions made at meetings are not properly recorded or activated.

92. Team members could collaborate much more if they examined the possibilities of doing so on a person-to-person basis.

93. Little time is spent on reviewing what the team does, how it works, and how to improve it.

94. A person who questions the established practices in the team probably will be smartly put back in place.

95. Only a few members suggest new ideas.

96. We do not get to know the people working in other teams in the organization.

97. I do not know whether our team is adequately represented at higher levels.

98. Some team members need considerable development to do their work effectively.

99. Team members are committed to individual goals at the expense of the team.

100. Disagreements between team members are seldom worked through thoroughly and individual viewpoints are not fully heard.

101. We often fail to finish things satisfactorily.

102. We do not work within clear strategic guidelines.

103. Our meetings do not properly resolve all the issues with which we should deal.

104. We do not examine how the team spends its time and energy.

105. We make resolutions but, basically, we do not learn from our mistakes.

106. Individuals are not encouraged to go outside the team to widen their personal knowledge and skills.

107. Creative ideas often are not followed through to definite action.

108. If we worked better with other teams, it would help us all to be more effective.

TEAM REVIEW QUESTIONNAIRE ANSWER SHEET

1. Follow the instructions at the beginning of the questionnaire.
2. In the grid shown here there are 108 spaces numbered to correspond to the statements on the questionnaire.
3. If you think a statement is broadly true about your team, mark an X through the number. If you feel a statement is not broadly true, then leave the space blank.
4. Fill in the top line first, working from left to right; then fill in the second line, and so on.
5. Be careful to respond to each statement, but mark an asterisk next to the numbers of statements that you find especially significant or difficult to answer. These can be explored later.

1	2	3	4	5	6	7	8	9	10	11	12
13	14	15	16	17	18	19	20	21	22	23	24
25	26	27	28	29	30	31	32	33	34	35	36
37	38	39	40	41	42	43	44	45	46	47	48
49	50	51	52	53	54	55	56	57	58	59	60
61	62	63	64	65	66	67	68	69	70	71	72
73	74	75	76	77	78	79	80	81	82	83	84
85	86	87_	88	89	90	91	92	93	94	95	96
97	98	99	100	101	102	103	104	105	106	107	108

Totals

| I | II | III | IV | V | VI | VII | VIII | IX | X | XI | XII |

When you have responded to all 108 statements, total the number of X's in each vertical column, then use this information to fill out the Team Review Questionnaire Interpretation Sheet below.

TEAM REVIEW QUESTIONNAIRE INTERPRETATION SHEET

When you have totaled all the X's in each of the 12 vertical columns of the answer grid, copy these totals next to the appropriate roman numerals on the chart shown here.

	Your Score	Your Ranking	Team Average	Team Ranking	
I.					Inappropriate leadership
II.					Unqualified membership

234

III. _____ Insufficient group commitment

IV. _____ Unconstructive climate

V. _____ Low achievement orientation

VI. _____ Undeveloped corporate role

VII. _____ Ineffective work methods

VIII. _____ Inadequate team organization

IX. _____ Soft critiquing

X. _____ Stunted individual development

XI. _____ Lack of creative capacity

XII. _____ Negative intergroup relations

List below the three highest scores for yourself and the team average.

Personal Highest Scores	Block Title	Team Average Highest Scores	Block Title
1.			
2.			
3.			

ANALYZING THE TEAM-REVIEW QUESTIONNAIRE

Now that the questionnaire has been completed, further explanation of the framework of analysis is helpful. Team members usually want to compare and contrast each other's scores directly after the completion of the questionnaire or, if it was completed prior to the meeting, at an early stage in the session. The following procedure quickly brings out key points and provides a reliable bank of reference information. You will need a large newsprint pad.

First, find out whether each team member is willing to share his or her scores. Depending on the decision of the team, scores may be reported anonymously or each member may announce his or her scores. These scores are posted on a master chart and they are totaled both horizontally and vertically. Experiment with the materials, while allowing time to discuss the results both at the levels of thinking and feelings.

SOURCE: Reprinted from Francis, D., & Young, D. *Improving work groups: A practical manual for team Building*. San Diego: University Associates, 1979. Used with permission.

A Communications Exercise

This exercise is an example of an activity which may be chosen by the team-building leaders to address a problem identified in a diagnosis exercise such as described previously.

DEFENSIVE AND SUPPORTIVE COMMUNICATION: A DYADIC ROLE PLAY

GOALS

I. To examine the dynamics of defensive and supportive communication in supervisor/subordinate relationships

II. To develop skills in listening to and understanding a contrasting point of view

III. To explore the concept of synergy in dyadic communications

IV. To examine the expectations that defensive communication creates for a continuing relationship

GROUP SIZE

Any number of dyads preferably with an equal balance between the sexes

TIME REQUIREMENTS

Approximately 1½ hours

MATERIALS

I. A copy of the appropriate Defensive and Supportive Communication Background and Role-Description Sheet for each participant

II. Two copies of the Defensive and Supportive Communication Discussion Guide for each participant

III. A pencil for each participant

PHYSICAL SETTING

A room large enough to allow dyads to interact without disturbing one another

PROCESS

I. The facilitator introduces the experience by presenting a short lecture on defensive and supportive communication, covering the following points:

1. Communication becomes defensive when the sender's goal is to persuade the receiver to agree with his or her opinions, ideas, facts, or information.

2. Defensive communication is characterized by evaluation, control, strategy, superiority, and certainty.

3. Communication becomes supportive when the goal is to actively hear and understand the other's opinions, thoughts, or feelings.

4. Supportive communication is characterized by empathy and spontaneity; it promotes problem solving and synergy.

II. The facilitator divides the participants into dyads and announces that there will be four rounds of dyadic role-play to enable participants to experience the two forms of communication and to understand how the dynamics of each form emerge. The facilitator explains that during rounds 1 and 2, one member of the dyad will role-play a supervisor and the other a subordinate and that their roles will be reversed during rounds 3 and 4. Dyads are instructed to determine who will role play the supervisor and subordinate for rounds 1 and 2.

III. A Defensive and Supportive Communication Background and Role-Description Sheet is given to each participant. The facilitator notes that specific instructions for each round are described on the role-description sheet. Players are given time to study their roles.

IV. The facilitator initiates round 1. The participants role play their respective roles.

V. After stopping the role play, the facilitator distributes one copy of the Defensive and Supportive Communication Discussion Guide and pencil to each participant. Each participant fills out the form by placing a "1" in the spaces provided to indicate his or her feelings about round 1 (3 minutes). The round is then discussed by the partners (5 minutes).

VI. The facilitator initiates round 2. At the conclusion of the round, participants once again fill out the same Defensive and Supportive Communication Discussion Guide, this time by placing a "2" in the appropriate places. They then discuss round 2 with their partners. They are told to focus on the differences between rounds 1 and 2.

VII. For rounds 3 and 4, the pairs of participants reverse roles using the same role-play situation. Steps IV through VI are repeated with new role-play situations. Following round 3, another copy of the Defensive and Supportive Communication Discussion Guide is distributed to each participant. It is filled out (3 minutes) and discussed (5 minutes) as before.

VIII. At the conclusion of round 4, participants once again fill out their discussion guides and briefly discuss the differences between rounds 3 and 4.

IX. The facilitator assembles the total group and leads a discussion of the different modes of communication. He or she may ask the group:

1. What were the differences between the defensive and supportive modes of communication? (Reactions to questions on the Defensive and Supportive Communication Discussion Guide can be reviewed at this point.)

2. What were the differences between sending and receiving the two types of communication?

3. How did the power relationship of the supervisor and subordinate roles affect the communication processes?

4. How were the outcomes of rounds 1 and 2 different? To what degree were the outcomes of round 2 synergistic? (The facilitator explains the concept of synergy.)

5. What are the implications of the two modes of communication in real-life settings?

DEFENSIVE AND SUPPORTIVE COMMUNICATION
BACKGROUND AND ROLE-DESCRIPTION SHEET

Background

This case focuses on the development of a system to appraise employee performance. Dale Clark, personnel director, has asked to meet this afternoon with Robin Smith, director of administrative services, to discuss Robin's proposal for such a system. They are meeting at 2 P.M.

Role-Description Sheet (Supervisor)

Robin Smith: You are director of administrative services for an organization that has tripled its size since its creation 2 years ago. This rapid growth has led to a need to develop an appraisal system that will foster the development of employees for managerial positions and furnish data for maintaining an inventory of employee talent and for making promotion and transfer decisions.

Early last week, you wrote a memo to the company personnel director, Dale Clark, who is your subordinate, describing the need for such a system and outlining your thoughts for its design. As soon as a design is agreed upon, you expect Clark to implement and administer the system.

Under your plan, supervisors would use a standard form to appraise employees every 12 months. The appraisal would be discussed with the employee and signed by both the supervisor and employee. Copies of the appraisal would be retained by the personnel department, the supervisor making the appraisal, and the employee.

Your proposed system is based on the assumption that it is important for supervisors to let employees know those areas in which they need to develop. For purposes of record keeping, you also feel that it is important that a standardized form be used for performance appraisal. Two days ago, Dale Clark requested a meeting to discuss your proposal and, you think, probably to raise some questions about your design.

Round 1. Your goal is to get Dale Clark to agree with the tenets of your design. You should explain as best you can the rationale supporting the design. You are determined that your way shall prevail.

Round 2. Your goal is to create a climate to explore the differences between yourself and your personnel director. You should encourage Clark to express her position and search for a resolution that achieves your objectives as well as those of the personnel director.

Role-Description Sheet (Subordinate)

Dale Clark: You are the personnel director for an organization that has tripled its activity since its creation 2 years ago. Last week you received a memo from your boss, Robin Smith, director of administrative services, noting that the organization's growth has led to a need to develop a performance-appraisal system. The purpose of the system is to foster the development of employees for managerial positions, furnish data for maintaining an inventory of employee talent, and aid in making promotion and transfer decisions.

Under the plan outlined in Smith's memo, supervisors would use a standardized form to appraise employees every 12 months. The appraisal would be discussed with the employee and signed by both the supervisor and employee. Copies of the appraisal would be retained by the personnel department, the appraising supervisor, and the employee.

You believe that this approach is detrimental to employee development. It places the supervisor in the role of judge and tends to bring about a defensive reaction from subordinates. You favor a problem-solving approach in which the supervisor initiates interviews with the employees regarding their own ideas for job improvement. Under this system, the supervisor stimulates employees to self-diagnose their needs for development. Interviews are not initiated by a written appraisal. Problems not addressed by subordinates can be brought up by the supervisor after the employees have had a chance to voice their concerns. Such problems can be introduced by asking for a subordinate's help.

You feel that this method of appraisal is superior to the traditional one suggested by Robin Smith because it develops a climate of mutual interest and almost always leads to new ideas and improved performance. The employee is motivated to think constructively rather than defensively.

Two days ago, you requested a meeting with Robin Smith to discuss your ideas. You hope to achieve some modifications in your supervisor's design.

Both Rounds: You are to interact with Smith, explaining your approach and its rationale.

DEFENSIVE AND SUPPORTIVE COMMUNICATION DISCUSSION GUIDE

Use these scales to guide your discussion after each round of interaction. Place a "1" on each of the scales to indicate your experience in round 1, a "2" on each scale at the end of round 2, and so forth.

1. How well did you listen to the other person's point of view?

   Not well _____ _____ _____ _____ _____ _____ _____ Very well

2. What kind of feeling climate was stimulated by the interaction?

   Competitive _____ _____ _____ _____ _____ _____ _____ Cooperative

   Judging of the _____ _____ _____ _____ _____ _____ _____ Empathetic
   other person

   Controlling _____ _____ _____ _____ _____ _____ _____ Problem-
   oriented

   Superior _____ _____ _____ _____ _____ _____ _____ Equal

   Positive _____ _____ _____ _____ _____ _____ _____ Provisional

   Defensive _____ _____ _____ _____ _____ _____ _____ Supportive

3. How satisfied are you with the interaction?

Very ____ ____ ____ ____ ____ ____ ____ Very
dissatisfied   satisfied

4. How satisified are you with the outcome or product of the discussion?

Very ____ ____ ____ ____ ____ ____ ____ Very
dissatisfied   satisfied

SOURCE: Adapted from Combs, G. Defensive and supportive communication: A Dyadic role play. Reprinted from John E. Jones and J.W. Pfeiffer (Eds.) *The 1979 Annual Handbook for Group Facilitators*. San Diego: University Associates, 1979. Used with permission.

Effectiveness Circles

In addition to the three OD team-building activities described—an icebreaker exercise, a survey-feedback activity, and a communication exercise—there are other team-building strategies. One such example is the effectiveness circle. The *effectiveness circle* is an adaptation of the quality circle that has been enormously successful in business and industry in the 1970s and 1980s. The name has been changed from "quality" to "effectiveness" in order to emphasize an essential difference between product-oriented and service-oriented organizations.

It is much more difficult to measure quality in human service professions, such as nursing, than in a product industry such as automobile production. Quality in production can be measured by the percentage of flawed or rejected finished products or by a comparison of one product with another competitive product. Such figures are very difficult to assess, however, in the health care field. In assessing the success rate of a particular surgical procedure, for example, one must consider the preoperative condition of the patient, the surgical complications beyond the control of the surgical operating team, and the quality and age of the operating instruments and the technological support equipment.

Nurses working in hospital and community settings, as well as in university and college settings, would have similar problems of comparability and measurement. In general, measurement of quality is more discrete and quantifiable in product-oriented organizations and more qualitative and nondiscrete in service-oriented organizations.

The concept of effectiveness, however, is useful in nursing practice. Nurses in all areas of service who are already, by necessity and professional pride providing high-quality care, can use the techniques discussed here to further increase their team's effectiveness.

The History of Quality Circles

Although the quality circle movement is associated with Japanese management, its philosophical roots are in the same tradition as progressive American management science and the general systems theory approach presented in this volume.

Kaorii Ishikawa is credited with conceiving and developing the quality circle concept in 1961 as an engineering professor at Tokyo University. He was greatly influenced by Abraham Maslow, Douglas McGregor, and Frederick Herzberg, men who have also had a tremendous impact upon American management theory. Ishikawa and his developing team undoubtedly were familiar with the T-group movement of the late 1950s and early 1960s. Quality circles borrow many of the group techniques found to be so useful in small group methods in this country. In fact, quality circles may have more in common with T-group methodology than OD team-building techniques. Both quality circles and OD team-building programs utilize more structure than their common ancestor, the T-group.

The Structure of Effectiveness Circles
An adaptation of the quality circle (the effectiveness circle) to nursing will be discussed. Only minor adaptations in methodology have been made and the interested reader may consult the recommended readings on quality circles for many additional useful ideas.

Each quality circle potentially consists of all the individuals in a team. Ideally, each team should be no larger than seven or eight individuals, although the actual size may vary from five to twelve members. Larger teams may be divided into several smaller effectiveness circles. Each member must have joined the team voluntarily. Attendance is voluntary since extensive experience with quality circles and T-groups indicates that compulsory attendance requirements have destructive consequences for team effectiveness. If conducted properly, effectiveness circles will have little difficulty attaining high levels of commitment and attendance by team members.

Frequency, Length, and Site of Meetings
Most teams will find that weekly 1-hour meetings are best. However, this is a guideline and not a hard-and-fast rule. Some teams have found biweekly meetings of ½ hour or bimonthly meetings of 2 hours more appropriate for their teams. In general, shorter, more frequent meetings will be content-oriented while longer, less-frequent meetings will raise interpersonal process issues as well. The team leader must evaluate the content-versus-process needs of their team as well as the work group maturity before recommending a frequency and length of meeting for a circle.

The circle meetings are held on "company time" to show the organization's commitment to the circle and its evaluation of the importance of its work. This policy also reduces the resistance of many team members to participation since they are not being asked to sacrifice family or personal time for company interests. The circle must be seen as a joint venture in which both the individual's and organization's interests are protected. Again, this is fully in keeping with our philosophy.

Effectiveness Circle Roles
The roles (covered more fully in chapter 18)—facilitator, recorder, gatekeeper, and process observer—are well-suited for conducting a circle meeting. While the formal team leader may wish to be facilitator initially, it is a good policy to rotate roles throughout the circle to reduce role-lock and to increase everyone's range of contributions to group work.

Most of the recommendations presented in the chapter on conducting effective meetings apply to circles. (Indeed, most of the concepts come from the same research and theory.) Consensus decision rules are preferable to majority rule or autocratic decision rules and the collaboration-encouraging procedures are to be preferred over strict adherence to conflict-oriented Roberts' Rules (i.e., parliamentary procedure). A young, immature, or conflict-laden group may need to fall back on Roberts' Rules, majority, or autocratic decision rules. If this happens, however, the team leader must press for resolving the interpersonal issues that cause the conflicted climate and encourage growth in team maturity.

The Steering Committee: A Link to the Organization

An important innovation developed by quality circle practitioners is the steering committee. If any change is to be effectively implemented by a circle, it must be consistent and congruent with organizational goals and operating policies and procedures. A weakness in earlier organizational change methods was a tendency to leave management hierarchy out of the process unintentionally or sometimes by design (believing that management would be unsympathetic if it knew what was being planned and discussed). Many sound and well-intentioned plans were self-sabotaged by this omission in the overall change design. There is a rule of thumb in organizational change practice that states that you need the support of at least two levels of management above the site of a change intervention in order to be successful.

The *steering committee* is a formal structure designed to set the goals and objectives of the circles so that they are consistent with organizational goals and objectives. The steering committee includes circle facilitators and management representatives from the major departments of the organization. Formal meetings with the steering committee help circles to set priorities and prevent them from wasting their time on projects that have little support throughout the rest of the organization.

Management Presentations

Periodically (usually every 3 months or whenever the circle is ready to present a major change in policy or procedure) the circle, including facilitator and members, makes a formal presentation to management regarding their activities. This formal activity provides a forum for direct communication between management and teams. The circles receive recognition for their contributions and get first-hand feedback concerning management reaction to their ideas. Morale can be greatly increased through this form of participative management.

The Effectiveness Circle Process

The effectiveness circle method provides new problem-solving skills to circle members as well as providing a conducive structure for change. In effect, members are given practical instruction in the scientific method taught in the sciences. Besides using problem-solving methods discussed elsewhere, circle members are taught data collection techniques (e.g., selecting an unbiased sample), data analysis methods (checklists, charts, graphs, and cause-and effect problem analysis), and decision analysis using Pareto charts.

The first circle meetings are largely devoted to training members in effective problem-solving methods and are therefore quite structured. This structure allows members to become acquainted with each other in this new context with a minimum of anxiety. Dewar (1980) has presented a 10-session training module that covers most relevant topics and methods for beginning an effectiveness circle.

Many of the methods used in effectiveness circles will be familiar to nurses who have received instruction in research methodology in their academic preparation. Other innovative methods have been presented in other chapters.

After completing the initial training that teaches circle members effective problem-solving skills, the circle is ready to begin work on problems that currently face a particular team. The problems selected may be proposed by the steering committee or may be proposed by the team itself and endorsed by the steering committee. In any case, the circle must agree that it is a real problem that they want to tackle. The problem cannot be dictated by the steering committee or management. Any recommendation resulting from the problem-solving process is ultimately presented in management presentations by the circle for approval, revision, and implementation.

The effectiveness circle approach to team building is excellent for encouraging innovation and improvement in technology-intensive work settings because of its logical, cause-and-effect approach that utilizes a scientific/engineering methodology and terminology. Problems that involve human relationships, however, generally do not follow linear, cause-and-effect logical rules (Watzlawick, Beavin, & Jackson, 1967) and are not as amenable to solution using this approach. OD team-building programs are more suitable for solving interpersonal problems of human resource management because they rely more on a contextual and analogical view of problematic situations and permit nonlinear and circular logical analysis.

An ideal mix of team-building activities might be an ongoing, on-site effectiveness circle program for teams to deal with technical and everyday policy and procedure problems and annual or semiannual OD team-building retreats to make more holistic evaluations of team and organizational problems and provide an environment conducive to solving complex interpersonal problems. When problems prove to be insoluble by these "self-help" approaches, a third team-building option is available.

General Systems Consultation

General systems consultation shares theoretical roots with OD team building, effectiveness circles, and general systems theory but not the tradition in small group theory and practice. Rather, this approach borrows heavily from family systems theory and the intervention style of family therapy. As discussed earlier, many management science theorists are turning to the family or clan as a more adequate conceptual model for organizations than the small, unstructured group (Ball, 1982; Leonard & McGuaghey, 1980; Ouchi, 1981).

A full description of this approach is beyond the scope of this volume and requires skills and knowledge not commonly taught in nursing curriculum. Further, it is not easily learned and mastered without close supervision and training. While the approach is logically consistent with the principles discussed in this volume, application of the principles does not always lead to straight forward and commonsense solutions. In many different situations involving human relations, however, paradoxical solutions have often been far more effective than direct and commonsense approaches (Haley, 1976; Minuchin, 1974; Leonard & McGaughey, 1980; Selvini Palazzoli, Boscoli, Cecchin, & Prata, 1978; Weeks & L'Abate, 1982.)

In brief, the general systems consultation approach sends a consultation team directly into the problematic situation to observe how the team is working together to produce a service or product. Based upon its observations and experimentation, a prescription is given to the team, which involves behaving in certain specified ways. Sometimes they are asked to behave differently and at other times they are asked to behave in the same way but more intensely. The aim of the experimentation and prescription is to learn the rules of the team's interactions so that basic and fundamental changes may be effected to improve team effectiveness. A schedule of consultation visits is arranged following the same pattern of direct observation, experimentation, and prescription. The consultation continues until the problem is solved or the contracted number of consultations has been been fulfilled. Some teams need a time-limited approach to reduce procrastination. Needless to say, this approach requires an experienced and skilled professional consultant and should not be attempted without adequate supervision.

SUMMARY

This chapter presented the various team-building strategies available to the nurse manager/supervisor. Before setting up a team-building program one must assess whether the team is a true team, and if it is a true team, whether it is of type A or B. Proper diagnosis at this point will assist the team-building leader in choosing the proper approach and activities.

The organization development (OD) approach to team building utilizes structured activities tailored to the diagnosis of team problems. An entire team engages in these activities, usually off-site, with the goal of translating resultant learnings and improvement in team functioning into behavior on the job. Three sample team-building activities were described to give the reader a small sample of available OD team-building activities.

A second approach, the effectiveness circle, was presented as an adaptation of the quality circle programs that originated in Japan. This is also a structured approach to team building in which an entire team meets regularly, on-site, to engage in problem-solving activities aimed at improving the team's effectiveness. Team members are instructed in a simplified form of the scientific method and develop skills in sampling, experimenting, analyzing, and presenting results to the organization. Both the OD and effectiveness circle approaches to team building are seen as stemming from the same management science philosophies as presented in the text.

Finally, a general systems consultation approach to team building was presented. This approach requires an outside consultant who is well versed in general systems theory and who also has a knowledge and appreciation of family dynamics and therapy. These strategies consider the family system as a better model for understanding team dynamics than the small unstructured group, although group dynamics concepts are also applied when relevant.

REFERENCES

Ball, K. *Man's inhumanity to man revisited—the Industrial Revolution*. Paper presented at American Psychological Association Annual Convention, Washington, D.C., 1982.

Combs, G. Defensive and supportive communication: A dyadic role play. In J. Jones & J. Pfeiffer (Eds.), *The 1979 annual handbook for group facilitators*. La Jolla, Calif.: University Associates, 1979.

Dewar, D. *Quality circle: Leader manual and instructional guide*. Red Bluff, Calif.: Quality Circle Institute, 1980.

Francis, D., & Young, D. *Improving work groups: a practical manual for team building*. La Jolla, Calif.: Quality Circle Insititute, 1979.

Haley, J. *Problem-solving therapy*. San Francisco, Calif.: Jossey-Bass, 1976.

Jorgenson, R. Communication analysis: A getting-acquainted activity. In J. Jones & J. Pfeiffer (Eds.) *The 1977 annual handbook for group facilitators*. La Jolla, Calif.: University Associates, 1977.

Leonard, H., & McGaughey, T. *Consulting to difficult and "near impossible" systems*. Paper presented at American Psychological Association Annual Convention, Montreal, Canada, 1980.

Minuchin, S. *Families and family therapy*. Cambridge, Mass.; Harvard University Press, 1974.

Ouchi, W. *Theory Z: How American business can meet the Japanese challange*. New York: Avon, 1981.

Selvini Palazzoli, M., Boscolo, L., Cecchin, G., & Prata, G. *Paradox and counterparadox.* New York: Jason Aronson, 1978.

Watzlawick, P., Beavin, J., & Jackson, D. *Pragmatics of human communication.* New York: Norton, 1967.

Weeks, G., & L'Abate, L. *Paradoxical psychotherapy: Theory and practice with individuals, couples, and families.* New York: Brunner/Mazel, 1982.

BIBLIOGRAPHY

Austin, M. *Management simulations for mental health and human services administrations.* New York: Haworth, 1978.

Gryna, F. *Quality circles: A team approach to problem solving.* New York: AMACOM, 1981.

Ingle, S. *Quality circle master guide: Increasing productivity with people power.* New York, New York: AMACOM, 1982.

Pfeiffer, J., & Jones, J. (Eds.) *The annual handbook for group facilitators.* La Jolla, Calif.: University Associates, 1972–(published yearly).

Pfeiffer, J., & Jones, J. *A handbook of structured experiences for human relations training:* La Jolla, Calif.: University Associates, 1972–(published yearly).

Ross, J. *Japanese quality circles and productivity.* Reston, Va.: Reston, 1982.

Thompson, P. *Quality circles: How to make them work in America.* New York: AMACOM, 1982.

Vaughan, J., & Deep, S. *Program of exercises for management and organizational behavior.* Beverly Hills, Calif.: Glencoe, 1975.

CHAPTER 18
FORMAL NURSING MEETINGS

Formal meetings are characterized by most of the organizational processes discussed so far. Meetings have a structure or recurring cycle of events; have primary and subsidiary purposes; require strict management of time, place, and membership boundaries; require formal and informal roles and norms; develop hierarchies of power, status, and prestige; have developmental patterns; require problem solving and decision making; and exhibit productive and nonproductive group processes. The complexity of the formal meeting process is matched by the opportunity to apply sound social systems principles to achieve results that are far superior to those normally achieved by individual problem solvers and decision makers.

In this chapter, typical problems encountered in formal nursing meetings will be described. Principles of effective social system management will be applied to conducting and facilitating effective formal nursing meetings. Other elements of effective group meeting behavior are presented elsewhere in this volume. These principles are applicable to such nursing meetings as faculty meetings, change of shift reports, clinical unit meetings, nursing care planning meetings, peer review committees, and so forth.

TYPICAL PROBLEMS IN MEETINGS

Unfortunately, some experiences in group meetings are unpleasant. Despite the fact that typical organizations spend 7–15% of their personnel budget directly on meetings (Doyle & Straus, 1976, p. 4), meetings often gain negative reputations. As a result, attendance becomes a chronic problem for many voluntary meetings. In addition, commitment is lacking in many compulsory meetings. Meetings can be quite wasteful of the time of professional nurses if ineffectively run. The following section discusses a few of the major problems contributing to ineffective formal nursing meetings.

Poor Boundary Maintenance

Ineffective meetings typically begin late and continue beyond the planned ending time. At these meetings, either key members are missing or there are those present who have no useful role or who inhibit the process while contributing little. In many cases, those conducting the meeting fail to appreciate the importance of firmly managing the critical boundaries of the meeting.

Agenda Problems

Agenda problems include four types: (a) the meeting begins without a clear agenda that is understood by everyone; (b) the priority for each agenda item is not clear and time limits are not recommended for each agenda item; (c) members have no role or input into constructing the agenda; (d) the agreed-upon agenda is not followed. The results of these agenda problems have been described as the "multi-headed animal syndrome" by Doyle and Straus (1976).

Failure to Specify Both Content and Process for Meetings

Failure to specify content and process for meetings undermines group effectiveness. An example follows.

Ms. Jones, RN, BSN, psychiatric nursing team leader, has called a meeting of her nursing staff to discuss discharge treatment planning for patient X.

MS. JONES: Mr. X is being discharged on Monday and needs a discharge plan to be sent to the Outpatient Department.

MS. HARPER: He needs a place to stay.

MR. DONALLY: Why can't he live with his parents?

MS. HARPER: (*heatedly*) They're the reason he's in the hospital in the first place!

MR. DONALLY: (*defending his idea*) That's not how I see it! They sent him here because they really care for him.

MS. FERGUSON: (*a friend of Ms. Harper*) The mother is a cool cucumber. I think he'll end up back here in a week if he goes home.

MR. DONALLY: (*feeling threatened*) Nobody else cares about him. Have you got any better ideas?

Ms. Jones now encounters difficulties. The major agenda item for the meeting is to develop a treatment plan for Mr. X. The agenda is the *content* for the meeting. The *process* for discussing the agenda, however, is not specified by Ms. Jones. Consequently, typical and predictably debilitating group dynamics begin to develop that deflect the team from its mission, promote hidden agendas, and threaten to split the team into camps supporting or critiquing the patient's parents. A lack of an agreed-upon process to cover content, risks unleashing the destructive group dynamics discussed in other chapters.

Inability to Regulate Communication

Undoubtedly Ms. Jones, in the example just cited, felt the need to intervene to keep the meeting on task, to prevent destructive interpersonal conflict, and to encourage other team members to contribute to the meeting. Doyle and Straus (1976, p. 28) discuss the difficulties in keeping an open and balanced communications flow:

A human system of regulating flow is almost always more responsive than a mechanical one. Have you ever had to sit at a red light when there was a lot of traffic on your street and none on the cross street? A policeman would immediately see the situation and adjust the directional flow to meet the momentary need. The same applies to rigid rules in a meeting, like speaking in a fixed order. It is hard to get a constructive dialogue going. A human system—a sensitive moderator—could adjust to the moment-by-moment needs of the individuals in the group without letting anyone dominate the meeting for long.

A solution to this problem is to include a role of "traffic cop" in Doyle and Straus's (1976) terminology, in the responsibilities of the leader for the meeting.

Asymmetrical Communications in Hierarchies

It has been observed that power differentials distort the communication process in hierarchies. Information downward from authority figures is often overvalued in importance by subordinates, and information reported upward is frequently "sanitized" to give the most favorable impression of subordinates (Nord, 1976).

The same dynamic occurs in meetings between members of differing power, status or prestige. Low-power members are hesitant to speak forcefully or honestly for fear of jeopardizing their position or standing in the organization. High-power members may complain in meetings, but may pull rank in handling disputes or in controlling the process of discussion. For instance, nurse managers/supervisors may give more recognition to members who give vocal or tacit support for their positions or may ignore low-status members with unpopular views.

Role-Lock Problems

When members of a group, that meets frequently, have the same roles for every meeting, they tend to limit their behavior to be consistent with their prescribed roles. For instance, group members serving as recording secretaries typically play limited roles in policy debates because they are concentrating on constructing a record of the agenda, discussion, and decisions. On the other hand, assuming the same role in every meeting prevents members from experiencing the problems as well as advantages of other necessary roles, tends to typecast individuals, and hardens destructive coalitions and alliances. The "company critic" can be easily "disconnected" if he or she is always seen as disagreeing with suggestions. Others who have objections may remain silent, trusting that the "critic" will forcefully voice opposition to most proposals. Shifting the "critic" periodically into a role that requires the use of other aspects of his or her personality serves to give a new perspective to the "critic" and allows other members the experience of voicing their negative as well as positive concerns on issues.

Inflexible Decision-Making Processes

Most teams or committees develop rigid formal or tacit agreements concerning the decision rules they utilize. Many teams and committees agree that all decisions, large or small, simple or complex, will be made by majority rule. Even teams or committees that are sophisticated in their knowledge of group and organizational dynamics, such as social science faculties, respectfully defer to Roberts' Rules for parliamentary procedure for all decisions.

In the chapter on decision-making processes (Chapter 13), the advantages and disadvantages of alternative decision rules were presented. It is not necessarily "un-American" to choose an autocratic decision rule in *certain* situations, if the advantages outweigh the disadvantages. The well-documented benefits of consensus decision making may easily justify the additional time for debate and negotiations required for this method. There is no one "best way" to make decisions for all situations. Time is well spent in discussing decision rules for different types of issues and problems.

Misuse of Power, Personal Attack, and Scapegoating

The misuse of power, personal attack, and scapegoating represent a few of the typical and debilitating group dynamics that can ruin formal nursing meetings. These problems are actually combinations of the difficulties already identified: inability to regulate communication, asymmetrical communications in hierarchies, role-lock and failure to specify content and process.

Without appropriate structure, meetings, like any unstructured and unregulated group, will tend to be controlled by the powerful, will lead to the personalization of issues, and will select scapegoats for its failures and uncomfortable impulses.

The results of these processes are equally predictable. Authority figures are told what they want to hear and do not receive important negative feedback. Low-power members contribute less than higher-power members. All members are cautious and less spontaneous for fear of "group rape." Problem solving will not occur.

REQUISITES FOR EFFECTIVE MEETINGS

In summary, the following requisites for successful meetings are proposed: (a) development of an agenda specifying content, time, and membership boundaries for the meeting including specific agenda items; (b) agreement on the process for disseminating information, problem solving, and decision making; and (c) development of clear roles for each meeting to regulate communication, to protect individuals from personal attack, to regulate time, membership, and space boundaries, and to record the work of the meeting for future use.

CONDUCTING EFFECTIVE FORMAL NURSING MEETINGS

Having identified many of the problems and pitfalls in meetings, methods and procedures for conducting formal nursing meetings will be presented.

Recognizing Power Differentials in Meetings

Virtually all meetings can be classified as hierarchical or horizontal with regard to formal power, status, and prestige (Doyle & Straus, 1976). Many nursing meetings are clearly hierarchial with a head or charge nurse being ultimately responsible for decisions. A manager's performance is evaluated, in large part, by the quality of team decisions, and the acceptance of this decision through behavior by the team. It is fruitless for a team to deny this fundamental reality and insist that the team, rather than the team leader, have the final decision. On the other hand, the nurse manager/supervisor must recognize that good decisions, without team follow-through, will not result in positive evaluations.

Certain decision rules, such as majority rule, are impractical in hierarchial meetings. A nurse manager cannot allow a decision to be made if she or he believes it will be ineffective. Their inevitable veto makes a majority decision rule seem a sham to team members.

In other situations, nurses may find themselves in horizontally organized meetings in which everyone has equal formally authorized power. Task forces, committees, and boards of directors are examples of horizontally organized meetings in which authority and responsibility for making decisions rests with the group as a whole, rather than with a particular individual.

In order to accomplish its work, horizontally organized meetings must develop their own internal structure by selecting a chair, secretary, and other roles. Resulting decisions are seen as reflecting group, rather than individual, views. In this case, majority decision rules are feasible, if not optimal.

Even though formal power may be equal, informal power inevitably develops, based upon position and power outside of the meeting. This will have a bearing upon meeting dynamics. For this reason, the structure of these meetings must also include methods for reducing power hierarchies. In both hierarchical and horizontal meetings, efforts may be made to reduce or "flatten" formal or informal power hierarchies, but, it is neither possible or advisable to eliminate power hierarchies altogether.

Selection of Facilitator

A facilitator is necessary for effective meetings. This does not mean, however, that the designated authority for a team or work group is the ideal person to serve as facilitator in all situations. Every task group needs leadership, but choosing the recognized authority for a team or work group as permanent group facilitator can be problematic.

In formal meetings, the objective is to choose the best solutions to problems, regardless of who suggested them or how they were developed. This requires neutrality on the part of the facilitator throughout the problem-solving process. Many formally authorized leaders find it difficult to be, or appear to be, impartial in discussions because of their large investment in a project or their real power in the team. Authority figures can, at times, have constricting effects on the perceptions and behaviors of group members.

A second reason for not designating the formal leader as permanent facilitator is to free him or her to contribute in ways that are not possible if he or she becomes locked into the role of facilitator. The facilitator's role is taxing, and is related primarily to regulating the process of a meeting, rather than its content. The neutral and non-manipulative stance required for good facilitation inhibits the formal leader from contributing fully to the discussion of agenda items. Since the formal leader's feelings and opinions are critical for selecting and implementing any decision, it is often best to free him or her from the responsibility of facilitating the process as well.

Combining the formal authority and power of a group leader with the facilitator role places everybody in a bind. The leader may feel inhibited in expressing his or her feelings and opinions for fear that he or she will disrupt effective group process. Members may have difficulty separating the power and process roles of the formal leader-as-facilitator and even look for nonverbal clues that would identify the facilitator's feelings or opinions. A scowl, voice inflection, or body posture can be just as an effective communication as a word of praise or disapproval. In short, the leader has difficulty remaining neutral and process-oriented and the membership is overly vigilant in trying to read their leader's feelings and opinions.

There are a number of alternative ways to select a facilitator for formal meetings. The facilitator role can be rotated through the membership by alphabetical order or other similar technique, or, four or five members may volunteer to rotate the facilitator role among themselves. This method is often chosen by teams with members who feel unsure of their capabilities as facilitator. While selection of facilitators must be on a voluntary basis, selecting a few members as permanent rotating facilitators poses the danger that higher power and status members will be selected for the role, creating many of the problems inherent in having the formal leader as facilitator.

One solution to this problem is to negotiate with an outside facilitator to assume this role. Independent organizational and group consultants or specialists are ideal since they have no formal connection with the rest of the organization and have training and experience as facilitators. However, while members can observe and respond to proper facilitation and can use the outside facilitator as a role model, at some point the group needs to take over this role for itself in order to avoid becoming permanently dependent upon outside consultation.

Facilitator Role Behavior

The primary task that the facilitator must attend to is to manage and regulate the *process* of the meeting. This does *not* mean ignoring the content of a meeting. On the contrary, the facilitator must ensure that all relevant content is submitted for consideration, that a public agenda is developed and agreed upon, that priority is given to the consideration of specific agenda items, and that recommended time boundaries are set for specific discussion of each agenda item.

What is required is that the facilitator maintains a neutral and nonevaluative attitude toward the content of a meeting. It is the membership's role to evaluate the content. If a facilitator feels too heavily invested in an agenda item to the point that he or she is unable to remain neutral and nonjudgmental, then it is wise for that person to step down from the facilitator role and ask someone less invested to take over.

The facilitator also manages the time, place, and membership boundaries of a meeting. That is, the facilitator ensures that the meeting starts on time, stays on schedule, ends on time, has an appropriate place to meet, and has appropriate membership or a quorum.

The facilitator regulates communication flow: encouraging low-power members to participate, limiting members who tend to monopolize meeting time, helping less-articulate members to clarify their views, moving discussion along when time boundaries are being exceeded, and calling for a decision when the members seem to be avoiding one. It should be clear now why the facilitator must maintain neutrality: The trust and cooperation of all members are crucial in conducting this regulatory aspect of the facilitator role.

As process guardian, the facilitator also needs to be on guard for personal attacks and scapegoating. The facilitator in his or her neutral and nonevaluative manner is able to depersonalize debate and protect members from being verbally attacked.

When the meeting is "on task," sticking with the agenda, problem solving effectively, making decisions, identifying implementation steps, and so forth, the facilitator may need to play little or no direct role in the process. The facilitator is there, however, when process problems that require attention arise. Using the traffic cop analogy, as long as traffic is running smoothly, little action is required. When traffic builds up from many directions, motorists cannot decide who has the right of way. Accidents impede traffic or make it dangerous. The traffic cop is there to "facilitate" traffic. Ideally, the cop is only there to assist, not to control or aggravate the motorist. So it should be with the facilitator. The accompanying list presents typical roles and responsiblities for the effective meeting facilitator.

How to Build an Agenda

Meetings may have prepared agendas that have been carefully prepared prior to the start of the meeting, or they may have only rough and vague agendas that need to be developed by members at the beginning of meetings.

RESPONSIBILITIES OF AN EFFECTIVE MEETING FACILITATOR

1. Identify recorder and make arrangements to coordinate and support each other
2. Clearly define roles for group—facilitator, recorder, gatekeeper, and so on
3. Clearly define boundaries for the group—time, place, agenda, membership
4. Introduce or develop common agenda. Look for hidden as well as open agendas
5. Obtain agreement on the methods to be used to accomplish tasks identified in the agenda: problem-solving techniques, decision-rules, and so on
6. Focus energy of group on common task
7. During work of group:
   - Encourage participation
   - Protect individuals and their ideas from attack
   - Reinforce group for task behavior
   - Encourage diversity of discussion early in the problem-solving process that reflects the concerns of all individuals and subgroups
   - Encourage group to consider their own questions instead of deferring to facilitator
   - Limit conversation of facilitator to efforts to keep process on track and progressing; otherwise keep a low profile
   - Make sure necessary decisions are made. Call for decisions and keep group on task until resolution of an agenda item is ensured
   - Make sure decisions are clearly understood and recorded
   - Make sure follow-up plans for decisions are made—who, what, when, where, and how
   - Manage time boundaries so that the meeting starts and stops on time

If the agenda topics have been determined prior to the meeting, this agenda should be distributed to the members with enough lead time to allow them to prepare for the meeting. This is a major advantage of previously prepared agendas. A major weakness, however, is that it may not reflect the perceptions other members have for an appropriate agenda. Asking members to submit agenda items by a certain date compensates for this weakness in prepared agendas. Another solution is to prepare an agenda with the flexibility of adding new agenda items at the start of the meeting.

In many cases, however, it is not possible to prepare a detailed agenda prior to the meeting. For example, agendas for weekly clinical nursing team meetings may contain a mixture of issues that may have developed only hours before the meeting. In this case, the facilitators should make up a list of agenda items contributed by members at the start of the meeting. The members are then asked to rank them in order of priority for discussion. This is an extremely important step, since members in formal meetings will often latch onto the first item presented whether or not it is the most important. Entire meetings have been conducted on trivial or less important agenda items, particularly if they are controversial in nature. With support from the facilitator, however, the group may decide to cover brief and noncontroversial items first, as they may be completed quickly, leaving the majority of the meeting to discuss the larger and more difficult topics.

As always, the facilitator must maintain a neutral position while facilitating the construction of the agenda. He or she must also make certain that powerful and high-status members do not push an agenda item into discussion without the groups' approval nor suppress an item contributed by less-influential members. Above all, the facilitator must be sure that a clear agenda has been constructed, is approved, and is understood by the members before proceeding.

This simple guideline is most often broken in informal meetings, where the purpose for meeting is not well understood by members. Even though the agenda may consist of one problem, the facilitator can create an agenda containing the problem-solving step that the group needs to go through (i.e., problem definition, acceptance, analysis, generating solutions, selecting solutions, implementing solutions, and evaluating results).

Recording Meetings

In many formal meetings, this function is carried out by the secretary for the meeting. The term recorder is used because it avoids the pejorative connotations of submissiveness and sexism frequently associated with the title secretary. The recorder role is an active and essential one for any meeting.

Just as individuals have developed short- and long-term memory-storage capabilities, formal meetings also need to have short-term memory capacity as well as a long-term record of ongoing issues, planning processes, and decisions. It is known, however, that short-term memory is quite limited. People have great difficulty remembering or considering more than seven "bits" of information at a time (Miller, 1956). More information overloads the mind's capacity, with the result of confused collapsing of "bits" into fewer categories, or ignoring some "bits" of information.

People's long-term memory capabilities are impressive, but it is often difficult to retrieve necessary information quickly and efficiently. Values, attitudes, psychological defenses, and current demands and stresses frequently distort our recall so that a group of people will have significant differences in their memory of a common event 1 week later.

Long-term records of meetings have traditionally been kept in the form of written minutes. This may provide an adequate record of meeting process. These minutes are frequently flawed, however, by being composed by one person from their particular perspective. These minutes are often not monitored for accuracy or neutrality by anyone else in the group when they are being composed. By the time the minutes are reviewed by the meeting members, the events are generally a week to a month old and memories of specific meeting behavior is dulled by time.

Short-term memory needs for formal meetings are even less well met than long-term memory needs. Typically, meetings rely mainly upon individual note-taking and individual short-term memory for this purpose. The limitations of mental capacity (seven "bits" or less) and distortion have serious consequences. When a recording device such as a chalkboard, is used, its capacity is rapidly reached requiring erasures resulting in lost information. The presenter needs to be able to write and talk at the same time, a difficult and time-consuming task.

The solution to this problem is a "group memory" method that serves as a short-term recording device and a basis for long-term record keeping. Such a technique should: (a) save all relevant information, problem-solving and decision-making processes, and so forth; (b) be relatively neutral as to personal bias and distortion; (c) free individuals from relying heavily upon personal memory or having to keep personal notes; and (d) should promote, rather than hinder, spontaneous creative processes.

A common solution to "group short-term memory" is to have the recorder write on-going meeting business upon large sheets of newsprint (Doyle & Straus, 1976). As one sheet is filled, it may be removed and placed on the walls of the meeting room with masking tape, so that a permanent, visual record of meeting process is always available. In addition, the short-term process notes can be used to compose the long-term record or minutes for the meeting, if this is desired.

Newsprint is a cost-efficient medium that can be purchased in large pads (3' × 4') or in 24"-wide rolls. Masking tape may be used to attach filled sheets of newsprint to painted walls without damaging them when they are removed. Felt-tip markers (water soluble, if possible) are ideal for printing purposes. Several colors may be employed for visual emphasis.

Recorder Role Behavior

Like the facilitator, the recorder should be a mental servant of the group. While the facilitator's job is managing the meeting, the recorder's job is to provide an accurate, understandable, and neutral visual record of meeting events. It is an active, demanding job that requires continuous feedback behavior between the group and recorder to ensure that an idea or thought has been recorded accurately, has not been missed, or under- or overemphasized. The recorder may have to ask brief questions for clarification, when unsure of an idea or thought, or if group process happens more rapidly than it is physically possible to record. These questions, however, should not be used as an indirect way to support or criticize an idea or thought. When recording, speaker's exact words, if possible, should be used. Paraphrasing and editing should be avoided and the names of those contributing ideas or thoughts should be left off. In this way, the recorder is able to capture many of the key aspects of the ideas or thoughts expressed so that they can be evaluated separately from the group's feelings and thoughts about the contributing member.

Because of the need for neutrality and the demanding physical nature of the role, the recorder should remain essentially silent, avoiding debates with members or contributing to problem-solving or decision-making activity. If a member objects to the way their ideas are recorded, the words should be changed to suit the contributor without objecting or being defensive. Remember, the recorder is a "servant" of the group.

The accompanying list presents helpful suggestions to those taking on the role of the recorder.

GUIDELINES FOR EFFECTIVE MEETING RECORDING

- Listen for key words
- Do not attach contributor's names to ideas
- Capture basic ideas, the essence
- Use contributor's own words, but do not write down every word, only the essence
- Write legibly

- Do not be afraid to misspell
- Abbreviate words
- Circle key ideas, statements, or decisions
- Vary colors; use colors to highlight and divide ideas
- Underline
- Use stars, arrows, numbers
- Number all sheets

SOURCE: Reprinted by permission of Berkeley Publishing Group. From *How to make meetings work* by Michael Doyle and David Straus. © 1976 by Michael Doyle & David Straus.

Additional Roles: Gatekeeper and Process Observer

Two additional roles are often appropriate and needed for meetings. Since many nursing meetings are held in nursing stations where in-coming telephone calls and interruptions due to other hospital personnel entering the room are frequent, one member of the meeting can be given the role of gatekeeper.

The responsibilities and authority of the gatekeeper are to answer the phone, tend the door, and take messages for other members. When disruption does occur, the group can continue to work, knowing that someone will handle outside interruptions for the group.

One additional role, that of process observer, may be desirable in some situations. The task of the process observer is to follow the undercurrent or covert group processes that occur in any group. When the group feels stalemated and unproductive, the process observer may be called upon to point out possible blocks to more effective performance. Group behaviors such as scapegoating, secret coalitions, hidden agendas, and basic assumptions may be addressed by the process observer.

This role requires a fair degree of sophistication in group dynamics and a great deal of trust and respect among group members. Many nurses, especially psychiatric nurses, are receiving training in group dynamics and group facilitation and would be able to assist the group in the capacity of process observer. Meetings that have members who know each other well, respect each other, and whose task requires creative problem-solving behavior would profit by selecting a process observer.

Additional Techniques for Conducting Effective Formal Nursing Meetings

Many techniques have been developed over the years to prepare members for formal meetings, to keep meetings productive and on-task, and to eliminate oversights and slip-ups. Schindler-Rainman, Lippitt, and Cole (1975) and Doyle and Straus (1976) have compiled many of these techniques that would be useful resources for any meeting. Some of the most useful techniques will be described briefly.

Schindler-Rainman, et al. (1975) have devised a number of planning forms that are useful to leaders planning meetings. The meeting planner(s) consider responses to the following issues: (a) thinking about the members (e.g., how many, subgroups and individual differences, needs, readiness, interests, expectations); (b) some desirable outcomes of the meeting (e.g., skills, information, values, concepts, actions, plans, recommendations, decisions); and (c) ideas for activities, experiences, and resources to facilitate the outcomes (e.g., exercises, projects, resources, facilities, work groups). Priorities are then set for the responses made within each category. As the next step, a chart is designed indicating the timing, flow, assignments, and arrangements for each phase of the meeting. Using both of these charts and agenda items submitted from group members, a preliminary agenda can be constructed and circulated. This agenda gives time estimates, role assignments, premeeting activities for members, and outside resources that will be utilized in the meeting. For complex meetings and conferences, Schindler-Rainman, et al. (1975) have devised the following checklist.

CHECKLIST FOR MEETINGS AND CONFERENCES

	Who Responsible	*By When*
1. PUBLICITY/PROMOTION/NOTIFYING		
_____ notices—to whom	_____	_____
_____ letters of invitation	_____	_____
_____ direction to meeting place	_____	_____
_____ phone calls	_____	_____
_____ news releases	_____	_____
_____ contact with the media	_____	_____
_____ copies of speeches	_____	_____
_____ copies of meeting plan	_____	_____
_____ pictures/photographs	_____	_____
_____ bulletin boards	_____	_____
_____ personal contacts	_____	_____
_____ other	_____	_____
2. AGENDA AND RESOURCE MATERIALS		
_____ copies of agenda	_____	_____
_____ contact people on the agenda	_____	_____
_____ materials needed (e.g., reprints)	_____	_____
_____ previous minutes	_____	_____
_____ committee reports	_____	_____
_____ previous agreement and time commitments	_____	_____
_____ others	_____	_____
3. RESPONSIBILITIES BEFORE THE MEETING		
_____ leadership assignments	_____	_____
_____ documentation or recording assignments	_____	_____
_____ resource persons?	_____	_____
_____ observers?	_____	_____
_____ "hosting" roles	_____	_____
_____ making reports	_____	_____
_____ trying out equipment	_____	_____
_____ test whether charts, posters are readable	_____	_____

_____ test electrical outlets
_____ preview films for timing & content   _____   _____
                                                             _____   _____

4. SPACE CHECK OUT
_____ size and shape of space   _____ access to meeting room (s)
_____ electrical outlets   _____ lighting
_____ mike outlets   _____ name of custodian/engineer-
_____ acoustics   ing, where to be reached
_____ doors   _____ telephone access for
_____ bathrooms (where, no. can   messages and calling out
                accommodate)   _____ exhibit space
_____ stairs   _____ wall space for newsprints, etc.
_____ elevators   _____ emotional impact (color,
_____ heat/cold regulation   aesthetics)
_____ ventilation   _____ others
_____ parking facilities: number &   _____
                access   _____
_____ registration area   _____
_____ location   _____
_____ transportation, access to facility   _____
_____ room set up arrangements   _____

5. EQUIPMENT FOR MEETING
_____ tables (number, size, shape)   _____ film projector
_____ chairs (comfort, number)   _____ chalkboard, chalk
_____ microphones   _____ typewriters
_____ audio tape recorder   _____ waste baskets
_____ audio tape cassettes   _____ bulletin boards
_____ video tape recorder   _____ pillows
_____ video tape cassettes   _____ chalkboard eraser
_____ extension cords   _____ projection table(s)
_____ overhead projector   _____ flannel board
_____ newsprint easel (chart stand)   _____ easel
_____ slide projector   _____ others
_____ screen   _____
_____ platform   _____
_____ record player   _____
_____ records   _____
_____ gavel   _____
_____ coffee, tea dispensers   _____
_____ water pitchers   _____
_____ cups   _____
_____ camera   _____
_____ film   _____
_____ transparencies & appropriate   _____
                pens & grease pencils   _____
_____ extension cords   _____
_____ ditto machine or other   _____
                duplication equipment

6. MATERIALS AND SUPPLIES FOR THE MEETING

_____ name tags/tents	_____ pamphlets
_____ small tip felt pens	_____ display materials
_____ large tip felt pens	_____ flowers or flower arrange-
_____ masking tape	ments
_____ paper clips	_____ decorations
_____ crayons	_____ posters
_____ pins	_____ instruction sheets
_____ scissors	_____ resumes of resource
_____ stapler	people
_____ glue	_____ directional signs (to meeting)
_____ newsprint paper	_____ chalk (various colors)
_____ scratch paper	_____ file folders
_____ pencils	_____ others
_____ dittopaper and ditto masters	_____
_____ fluid for ditto masters	_____
_____ self carbon paper	_____
_____ reprints of articles	_____
_____ copies of previous minutes	_____
_____ copies of reports	_____
_____ books	_____
_____ visual aids	_____
_____ puppets	_____
_____ colored paper	

7. BUDGET*

Costs   Estimated Cost

_____ mailing and stamps		_____
_____ telephone calls		_____
_____ telephone conferences		_____
_____ rental of equipment		_____
_____ rental of space		_____
_____ paper materials		_____
	_____ name tags	_____
	_____ newsprint	_____
	_____ paper	_____
	_____ construction paper	_____
_____ writing materials		_____
	_____ pens	_____
	_____ crayons	_____
	_____ special pens for overhead	_____
	_____ grease pencils	_____
_____ secretarial time		_____
_____ transportation		_____
_____ meals		_____
_____ bar		_____
_____ coffee, tea, juice		_____

*Some of these will not be budget cost items for some planners.

_____ reproduction of
                materials   _____
_____ folders   _____
_____ tapes   _____
_____ operator of projection   _____
                equipment
_____ operator of P. A.   _____
                equipment
_____ speaker fees   _____
_____ consultant fees   _____
_____ entertainment   _____
_____ flowers   _____
_____ film reproduction   _____
_____ tape reproduction   _____
_____ others   _____
_____   _____
_____   _____
_____   _____
_____   _____
_____   _____

Income   *Estimated Income*

_____ registration fees   _____
_____ sale of materials   _____
_____ grants   _____
_____ sale of meal tickets   _____
_____ donations   _____
_____ membership fees   _____
_____ coffee and tea charges   _____
_____ others   _____
_____   _____
_____   _____
_____   _____
_____   _____
_____   _____

8. JUST BEFORE THE MEETING   *Who Responsible*

_____ seating arrangements—general session   _____
                and subgroupings
_____ extra chairs   _____
_____ extra tables   _____
_____ P. A. system checkout   _____
_____ equipment (easels, screens, etc.)   _____
_____ materials (paper, pens, etc.)   _____
_____ ash trays   _____
_____ water, glasses   _____
_____ thermostat   _____

_____ opening and closing of windows _____

_____ refreshment set-up _____

_____ registration set-up _____

_____ check that charts, boards, screens can be _____
                     seen from everywhere

_____ agendas available _____

_____ other materials available for handouts _____

_____ name tags/tents _____

_____ table numbers _____

_____ coffee, tea, etc. _____

_____ evaluation forms ready _____

_____ reproduction equipment (e.g., ditto machine) _____

_____ audiovisual equipment ready _____

_____ others _____

_____ _____

_____ _____

_____ _____

_____ _____

9. AT THE MEETING   *Who Responsible*

_____ meeting, greeting, seating of participants _____
                     and guests

_____ documentation—recording _____

_____ greeting of latecomers _____

_____ evaluation activity _____

_____ handing out materials _____

_____ operation of equipment _____

_____ process review, stop sessions, and so on _____

_____ announcements _____

_____ others _____

_____ _____

_____ _____

_____ _____

10. END OF MEETING—AND AFTER

_____ collect unused materials _____

_____ return equipment _____

_____ clean up _____

_____ thank helpers _____

_____ read and analyze evaluation/feedback _____

_____ prepare feedback on feedback _____

_____ mail follow-up materials _____

_____ remind people of their follow-up _____
                     commitments—phone _____
                                  write _____

_____ lay plans for next meeting; dates _____
                     if there is to be one

_____ pay bills _____

260

_____ collect outstanding moneys
_____ others

SOURCE: Reprinted from Eva Schindler-Rainman and Ronald Lippitt with Jack Cole. *Taking your meetings out of the doldrums*. San Diego: University Associates, 1975. Used with permission.

Schindler-Rainman, et al., (1975) also have some useful suggestions for techniques that enable members to diagnose blockages to effective meeting behaviors and to prescribe changes to improve meeting process. When a meeting drifts from the announced agenda, loses the interest of its members, or is rife with tension from unknown causes, the facilitator may suggest that members turn to their neighbors for an organized "buzz" session. In a minute or two, members are to talk to one or two other members about their impressions of the meeting so far (e.g., how well is it going, what is blocking effectiveness, what are some unstated hidden agendas, and what ideas do they have for improving the meeting's productivity). At the end of the short "buzz session," the facilitator encourages members to share their perceptions and ideas for improving the meeting.

In a variation of this idea, the facilitator may plan a brief "stop session" into the agenda to allow the group to make midcourse corrections. Simple rating scales and check lists may be devised to aid in this process (Schindler-Rainman, et al., 1975). These scales and checklists may be expanded for use as end-of-meeting evaluations in order to help plan subsequent meetings.

Parliamentary Procedure: Roberts' Rules

Roberts' Rules of Order for Parliamentary Procedure are undoubtedly the best-known procedural methods for conducting formal meetings. The structure recommended by Roberts' Rules is usually taught in primary and secondary schools for conducting school councils, student meetings, and other formal meetings. In most cases, training and practice in Roberts' Rules obtained in this way represents the only formal basic training for running a meeting.

Roberts' Rules were developed to deal with the specific problems encountered in the British Parliament, a large, horizontally organized meeting whose primary purpose is to debate and decide upon prepared proposals. In contrast, many meetings in nursing involve small groups of team members. Sometimes these groups include several disciplines, include members with significant differences in status or hierarchical level, and have primary purposes of problem solving, information dispersal, coordination, or professional support.

Roberts' Rules were devised to contend with the inherent devisiveness of a two-party system and almost ensure a win/lose decision-making philosophy by using a majority-rule decision rule. Most meetings encountered in nursing, however, require a structure that promotes collaboration, conflict resolution, team acceptance of decisions, and creative problem solving.

In most cases, strict adherence to Roberts' Rules undermines these processes. Those who vote on prepackaged proposals are not involved in the necessary problem-solving steps. Members are forced to choose sides rather than develop synergistic solutions, and the spontaneous flow of ideas is restricted by clumsy, awkward, and elaborate procedures. While some situations and formal meeting requirements may call for use of Roberts' Rules, or a similar parliamentarian procedure, the typical nursing meeting will be more effectively conducted by using the procedures described earlier in this chapter.

SUMMARY

Meetings involve all of the processes characterized by organizations. Utilization of sound social systems management will avoid most of the pitfalls of ineffective meetings: poor boundary management, agenda problems, failure to specify both content and process for meetings, inability to regulate communication, asymmetrical communications in hierarchies, role-lock problems, an inflexible decision-making process, and misuse of power, personal attack, and scapegoating.

The requisites for effective meetings include: (a) development of an agenda specifying content, time, and membership boundaries for the meeting, as well as specific agenda items; (b) agreement on the process for disseminating information, problem solving, and decision making; and (c) development of clear roles of each meeting to regulate time, membership, and space boundaries, and to record the work of the meeting for future use.

Decision rules must take into account the power differentials between members. In vertical organizations, the power differentials are explicitly recognized in the structure of the meeting. In horizontal organizations, the power differentials evolve in informal ways, related to the personality of the individuals and their position and stature outside the meeting.

Roles are recommended for effective meetings. The facilitator, recorder, gatekeeper, and process observer are responsible for the process rather than content of the meeting. In major cases, it is desirable to separate the facilitator roles from the formal leader or authority role and to rotate the facilitator role throughout the group membership. The facilitator role focuses upon managing the critical boundaries for meetings (time, place, agenda, and membership) and guiding the group in the use of constructive rather than destructive group processes.

The recorder's role focuses on keeping short- and long-term records for the meeting. The short-term "memory" for the meeting is easily kept by using large newsprint sheets that can be filled and kept in view by attaching them to the walls of the meeting room. A permanent record of thoughts, decisions, and any assignment of responsibilities can be utilized to relieve members of the burden of keeping personal notes. This allows them to use their short-term memory and may serve as the basis for accurate long-term memory or meeting minutes.

Two additional roles may be desirable: gatekeeper and process observer. The gatekeeper controls the flow of people and communications into and out of the meeting. Sophisticated and experienced groups wishing to achieve maximum creativity in their meetings may designate a member to monitor the covert and "off-task" behavior in the meeting.

The strategies described in this chapter are designed to improve upon the formal meeting structure employed by Roberts' Rules of Order of Parliamentary Procedure. With these strategies, poor boundary maintenance, agenda problems, ineffective communication, role-lock, inflexible decision making, and misuse of power are minimized. Collaboration, creative problem solving, conflict resolution, and collegiality, are, on the other hand, encouraged.

REFERENCES

Doyle, M., & Straus, D. *How to make meetings work*. New York: Playboy Business Paperbacks, 1976.

Miller, G. The magical number seven, plus or minus two: Some limits on capacity for processing information. *Psychological review*, 1956, *63*, 81–97.

Nord, W. Communication. In W. Nord, (Ed.) *Concepts and controversy in organizational behavior* (2nd ed.). Santa Monica, Calif.: Goodyear, 1976.

Schindler-Rainman, E., Lippitt, R., & Cole, J. *Taking your meetings out of the doldrums*. La Jolla, Calif.: University Associates, 1975.

CHAPTER 19
TIME MANAGEMENT: EFFECTIVE AND EFFICIENT USE OF TIME

Time is one of the most valuable and unique resources for the nurse manager. Time cannot be stored and it is nonrenewable. Everyone possesses the same number of hours per week. If these hours are not managed wisely, time is lost forever. The way time is managed affects the degree to which jobs are managed and individual career and personal goals are achieved. Whether the goals of a health care agency or school of nursing are met, and how well, depends in part on whether or not the nursing staff or faculty utilize time effectively and efficiently. Nurse leaders are responsible not only for using their individual on-job time wisely but for bringing about corrective interventions within their organizations that contribute to time management.

WHAT IS TIME MANAGEMENT?

Time management means using time effectively and efficiently. It is a way of working more intelligently, rather than working harder or longer hours. Managing time at both the individual and organizational level involves using resources efficiently, engaging in activities selectively, and striving for the achievement of organizational goals in optimal time.

As a result of utilizing time management, the nurse manager has time enough to plan and organize individual job responsibilities and to properly plan, organize, delegate, and control the productive efforts of subordinates. Job performance—quantity, quality, timeliness, and cost effectiveness—can be improved through time management. Likewise, time management contributes to optimal flow of organizational input and through-put for effective organizational output and goal achievement.

The process involved in time management is similar to the process of action research. Data is systematically collected about individual and organizational time wasters. Time logs are kept or workload records are documented. Individual career goals and organizational goals and objectives are clarified or formulated. All resulting data is analyzed and feedback is given where appropriate. Diagnoses about major time wasters are formulated. Time management interventions are selected and implemented to alter factors at the individual, subsystem, or system level based on the data and the formulated diagnoses. The results are then evaluated.

TIME WASTERS

Time wasters are activities, tasks, or occurrences that require the use of the resource—time—but contribute neither toward achieving individual career or organizational goals. Time wasters are activities that keep the nurse leader, manager, or supervisor from doing things that are *more* important and have *more* value, cost considerable amounts of time, yet add little to the accomplishment of priority goals (Ferner, 1980). Time wasters interfere with the smooth flow of selecting resources and dealing with inputs; with utilizing those resources and inputs in the throughput process; with the output of some desired goal and service; and with the feedback mechanism necessary to keep any system viable.

LeBoeuf (1980) reported major time wasters selected by executives in a survey conducted in 14 countries:

> Telephone interruptions; drop-in visitors; meetings (scheduled and unscheduled); crises; lack of objectives, priorities, and deadlines; cluttered desk and personal disorganization; ineffective delegation and involvement in routine and detail; attempting too much at once and estimating time unrealistically; lack of, or unclear, communication or instruction; inadequate, inaccurate, or delayed information; indecision and procrastination; confused responsibility and authority; inability to say no; leaving tasks unfinished; and lack of self-discipline. (p. 41)

Those time wasters that are externally generated are often more readily identified than internally generated ones. Externally generated time wasters are those imposed by the environment, as for example, telephone interruptions. Internally generated time wasters are those that are self-imposed, as for example, personal disorganization. Internally generated time wasters appear to be more difficult to identify. Mackenzie (1975) reports that an initial list of time wasters identified by a group of managers included many externally generated ones, for example, outside activities, telephone interruptions, meetings, routine tasks, drop-in visitors. After viewing a film in which a manager's behavior displays time wasters, this same group of managers identified a second list of time wasters, many of which were internally generated ones, for example, not delegating tasks, procrastination, and personal disorganization such as cluttered desks, and not listening.

ASSESSMENT OF INDIVIDUAL AND ORGANIZATIONAL TIME WASTERS

Graphically depicting the process involved in time management described earlier, Step 1 is clearly the gathering of data (Figure 19-1). For an entire week, collect data on your use of time at both the individual and organizational level. Marriner (1979) states that ensuring maximization of time and effectiveness at the organizational level is accomplished through the activities of planning, organizing, staffing, directing, and controlling and that these activities be assessed for time wasters.

The initial assessment is made by keeping a record of activities while on the job at 15-minute intervals. An example of a time use data collection and analysis tool is provided in Figure 19-2. In column 1, record, at 15-minute intervals, all activities performed on the job. *Do not* wait until the end of the day to complete this part of the tool, otherwise the data collected will not be as accurate.

Although the emphasis here is on the way time is spent while officially on the job, the analysis can be extended to include all 24 hours of the day. Many nurse managers, supervisors, and leaders spend time on professionally related activities beyond the

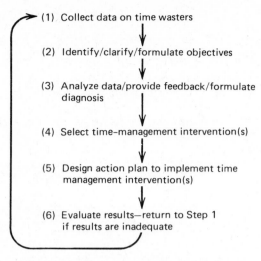

(1) Collect data on time wasters

(2) Identify/clarify/formulate objectives

(3) Analyze data/provide feedback/formulate diagnosis

(4) Select time-management intervention(s)

(5) Design action plan to implement time management intervention(s)

(6) Evaluate results—return to Step 1 if results are inadequate

FIGURE 19-1: THE TIME MANAGEMENT PROCESS.

officially designated work time. Analysis of this time is important in evaluating its contribution to personal career goals. In addition, including an analysis of "off-duty" time can provide a more holistic view of one's life style regardless of whether the activities are related to career or other personal goals.

Once activities have been recorded for one day, a time-use analysis should be done using the raw data collected in column 1 of the tool in Figure 19-2. The general analysis is recorded in column 2. This is an overall assessment of whether time was used effectively and efficiently. Assess each 15 minute record of activities and determine which statements in the accompanying list best described the activity. Record the selected numbers in column 2.

GENERAL ASSESSMENT OF TIME USE

1. The activity contributed greatly toward goal(s).
2. The activity contributed moderately toward goal(s).
3. The activity contributed minimally toward goal(s).
4. The activity contributed nothing toward goal(s).

5. You were the correct person to perform the activity.
6. You should have delegated the activity.

7. The activity was performed at the right time.
8. The activity had a different priority and should have been performed at another time.

9. The activity was clearly not a time waster.
10. The activity was, in part, a time waster.
11. The activity was entirely a time waster.

Time Use Data Collection and Analysis Tool		Name: _____ Date: _____	
Time	**Column 1** Specify and Briefly Describe Activities You Performed on the Job	**Column 2** General Analysis	**Column 3** Analysis of Time Wasters
8:15			
8:30			
8:45			
9:00			
9:15			
9:30			
9:45			
10:00			
10:15			
10:30			
10:45			
11:00			
11:15			
11:30			
11:45			
12:00			
12:15			
12:30			
12:45			
1:00			
1:15			
1:30			
1:45			
2:00			
2:15			
2:30			
2:45			
3:00			
3:15			
3:30			
3:45			
4:00			
4:15			
4:30			

FIGURE 19-2: TIME USE DATA COLLECTION AND ANALYSIS TOOL.

Adapted from Reynolds, H., & Tramel, M. *Executive time management.* Englewood Cliffs, N.J.: Prentice-Hall, 1979.

ANALYSIS OF DATA AND FORMULATION OF TIME-MANAGEMENT DIAGNOSES

The next step is to analyze the raw data in column 1 for specific time wasters to be recorded in column 3 (keep in mind the analysis already completed in column 2). Again at the end of each day, assess each 15-minute record of activities and determine which time wasters were used. Record the time waster in column 3 by the corresponding number and letter selected from the list of common time wasters which apprears below. Remember to differentiate between an activity that is an externally generated time waster from one that is really internally generated. For example, was the time waster really an interruption (phone, drop-in visitors) or primarily procrastination—that is, allowing an interruption because it was an excuse to keep from doing an unpleasant priority task? The time wasters in the following list are organized under major headings. These headings, except item 10, correspond to major components of the processes of leadership, management, and supervision.

COMMON TIME WASTERS

1. *Communicating*
   a. Nonassertive communication
   b. Interruptions (e.g., drop-in visitors, telephone calls)
   c. Insufficient, unclear, or lack of communication
   d. Junk mail or voluminous reading material
   e. Poor listening habits
   f. Excessive/inappropriate socializing
   g. Unproductive use of telephone (e.g., repeated calls to same person)
   h. Unnecessary meetings
   i. Unproductive meetings
   j. Excessive communication or overload
   k. Delayed information
   l. Writing memo or letter when phone call suffices
   m. Other (specify)

2. *Problem Solving*
   a. Indecision or delayed decision
   b. Snap decisions
   c. Collecting inappropriate data (too much, too little, nonrelevant)
   d. Failure to clarify and identify problem
   e. Failure to identify and examine alternative solutions
   f. Failure to select most appropriate solution

g.   Failure to examine consequences of selected solution(s)
h.   Failure to utilize evaluation of selected action to reformulate problem
i.   Using group decision-making inappropriately
j.   Acting without thinking
k.   Other (specify)

3.   *Delegating*
  a.   Ineffective or inappropriate delegation
  b.   Not matching task assignments with staff member's blend of skills and traits
  c.   Doing it by self
  d.   Delegating responsibility without appropriate authority
  e.   Unclear or insufficient instructions
  f.   Involvement in routine detail
  g.   Inadequate or inappropriate instructions
  h.   Not following through after delegation
  i.   Other (specify)

4.   *Directing, Controlling, Evaluating*
  a.   Incomplete or unclear directions
  b.   Lack of performance standards
  c.   Unclear or inappropriate performance standards
  d.   Not requesting progress reports and feedback on performance of job activity frequently enough
  e.   Not providing needed feedback on job performance
  f.   Discussing tangential issues while providing job guidance to subordinate
  g.   Failure to establish or maintain subsystem or system linkages
  h.   Not doing the job right
  i.   Inaccurate or inadequate information
  j.   Excessive review of performance
  k.   Too little review of performance
  l.   Inability to say "no"
  m.   Overly critical attitude
  n.   Rigid expectations and adherence to "the way things have been done"
  o.   Other (specify)

5.   *Fostering Constructive Human Interaction*
  a.   Poor conflict management

    b. Nonassertive communications

    c. Creating "bottleneck" for co-workers

    d. Not intervening in inappropriate interpersonal behavior

    e. Failure to assess personal traits creating interpersonal friction or conflict

    f. Failure to discuss interpersonal difficulties openly

    g. Engaging in group blocking behavior

    h. Not intervening in ripple effects of poor time management on others

    i. Other (specify)

6. *Motivating*

    a. Use of inappropriate change strategies

    b. Lack of motivation toward organizational goals

    c. Use of inappropriate rewards

    d. Excessive criticism or inappropriate use of negative feedback

    e. Assigning job tasks and activities inappropriately

    f. Not giving sufficient recognition for work well done

    g. Other (specify)

7. *Managing the Work Environment*

    a. Indiscriminate open-door policy

    b. Inadequate storage space for essential materials

    c. Inadequate work space

    d. Excessive or distracting noise

    e. Disorganization of work space

    f. Permitting unessential materials to accumulate

    g. Nonfunctional arrangement of furniture and materials needed for work

    h. Other (specify)

8. *Organizing*

    a. Nebulous job descriptions

    b. Resources for job performance not readily accessible

    c. Confused authority

    d. Frequent crisis situations

    e. Unclear lines of formal authority

    f. Underdefined or overdefined roles and responsibilities

    g. Duplication of tasks

    h. Focusing on unimportant or unessential tasks

    i. Failure to break complex tasks into component parts

j. Personal disorganization and clutter

k. Failure to use prime time for priority tasks

l. Red tape

m. Not doing the right job

n. Exclusive focus on component parts of complex tasks

9. *Personal Habits, Traits*

a. Procrastination

b. Perfectionism

c. Lack of self-discipline

d. Poor reading skills

e. Excessive need for recognition

f. Complaining

g. Boredom, inattention, "I don't care" attitude

h. Negative attitude, resentment

i. Carelessness

j. High state of tension

k. Lack of self-confidence in achieving goals

l. Loafing or daydreaming

m. Not assessing personal or group time wasters

n. Excessive attention to routine and detail

o. Inability to communicate assertively

p. Gathering or distributing gossip about co-workers

q. Failure to consider personal vulnerabilities and weaknesses

r. Setting unrealistic goals: expecting everything to be done immediately

s. Attitude that task can't be finished

t. Feeling "pulled in all directions"

u. Frequent absenteeism or tardiness

v. Making mistakes and producing poor quality work

w. Inability to say "no"

x. Mental blocks

10. *Goal Setting, Planning*

a. Absence of or unclear organizational and subsystem goals and objectives

b. Failure to set, plan, or schedule daily activities

c. Absence of or unclearly established priorities: treating all tasks as priorities

d. Unrealistic time frame (attempting too much or too little)

e. Failure to determine the who, what, when, where, how

f. Failure to identify viable alternatives

g. Failure to work on priority tasks

h. Immersion in detail and process without attention to objectives

i. Neglecting to plan because of pressure

j. Concentrating on staying busy while losing sight of objectives

k. Lack of contingency plans

l. Preoccupation with process

m. Leaving tasks unfinished

n. Trying to accomplish too many things at once

o. No self-imposed deadlines

p. Other (specify)

11. *Recording, Reporting*

a. Excessive record keeping

b. Unorganized files

c. Complicated reporting and recording system

d. Inadequate filing system

e. Failure to purge files of outdated materials

f. Failure to use standardized letters or memos where appropriate

g. Lack of periodic status reports

12. *Staffing, Staff Development*

a. Lack of adequately prepared staff

b. Inadequate staff development or continuing education

c. Inadequate direction and guidance

d. Inappropriate assignment of responsibilities

e. Poor assignment of number and type of personnel

f. High staff turnover or absenteeism

g. Lack of adequate number of personnel

h. Inadequate support staff

i. Tardiness

j. Inappropriate type of assignments

k. Failure of finding ways for involving staff in ways to expand their abilities

l. Other (specify)

13. *Utilizing Facilities and Nonhuman Resources; Budgeting*

a. Frequent ordering and obtaining supplies

b. Inadequate or improper supplies for work to be performed

c. Mechanical failures or nonusable supplies
d. Failure to project adequate facilities, resources, or budget
e. Inputs exceeding requirements for throughput and output
f. Not having appropriate resources available for job

SOURCE: Developed from observations and review of literature: Berlin (1980), Bliss (1976), Davidson (1978), Fanning & Fanning (1979), Ferner (1980), Lancaster (1981), LeBoeuf (1980), Love (1978), Marriner (1979), McCarthy (1981), McDougle (1979), Rader (1979), Reynolds & Tramel (1979), Schwartz & Mackenzie (1979), Smith & Besnette (1978), Wiley (1978).

Collect data for an entire week. At the end of the week, tabulate the sum of the frequencies of the statements selected from the general assessment of time use tool that are recorded in column 2 of the time use data collection and analysis tool (Figure 19-2). Calculate, as accurately as possible, the *total* actual time involved in each of these activities for the entire week.

Likewise, tabulate the sum of the frequencies of each time waster selected from the list of common time wasters that are recorded in column 3 of the time use data collection and analysis tool (Figure 19-2). Again, calculate as accurately as possible the total actual time spent in the week for each of these time wasters, as well as within each of the 14 categories as categorized in the list of common time wasters.

The week selected for keeping the time log should be as typical as possible. It may be useful, however, to select an additional typical week and keep a second time log. Data is again tabulated as above. The similarities and differences between the two weeks are noted and the results of the two sets of data are averaged for final results. From this data analysis, a pattern begins to emerge about the major time wasters in which you engage while on the job.

At this point, several questions should be raised. How does the nurse leader's, manager's, or supervisor's poor time management affect the subsystem for which she is responsible? How does the nurse leader affect the work group? How do subordinates or co-workers affect the nurse leader's ability to engage in good time-management habits? What effect do the members of the nursing team have on each other's ability to manage time wisely?

The first two questions can be answered, in part, by examining the data already collected. For example, is a large amount of time wasted in delegating? Does the nurse manager delegate effectively? Are many time wasters documented under the category, communicating, relating? Is time wasted for the nurse manager as well as for others by insufficient, unclear, or lack of communication; by excessive socializing; by unnecessary or unproductive meetings; or by the unproductive use of the telephone? Similar questions can be raised for the other processes of leadership, management, and super-vision. From the data available, the nurse leader or manager can then draw implications about the effect his or her unique combination of time wasters has on the subsystem, and the work group for which he or she is responsible.

The third question—How do subordinates or colleagues affect the nurse leader or manager's own ability to use time effectively and efficiently?—can also be answered in part, by analyzing the data recorded and tabulated on the time use data collection and analysis tool (Figure 19-2). "Our time problems are very much affected by the people around us, especially at work. One person's poor time management habits will have 'ripple' effects on everyone nearby'' (Ferner, 1980, p. 38). For example, are subordinates or colleagues constantly dropping by with questions, assistance with work, or just to chat?

The point that one person's pattern of time wasters has a ripple effect on colleagues in the work environment should be kept in mind by the nurse leader or manager. It is important for all nurses in the organization to become aware of personal time-management habits. Staff nurses should be assisted by their nurse supervisors in arriving at a personal assessment of time management through a process such as has been described previously. A modified data collection tool would need to be developed. The effect that members of the nursing team have on each other's ability to manage time wisely can be identified. Data analysis can determine how much a nurse's time management habits affect her or his co-workers. Through data analysis, major time wasters can be identified.

One method that can be used by the nurse supervisor in arriving at group data is to encourage nurses in the organizational subsystem to meet as a group. A collective group average of the data collected on time wasters by each group member can be tabulated and rank ordered prior to the meeting. Feedback on the major time wasters identified can then be provided to the group. The feedback data, along with each nurse's own individual time analysis data, can serve as a starting point for discussion about major time wasters for the group.

Perhaps the group average data and discussion reveals that the largest amount of time is wasted in the area of communication. Group analysis then centers on determining the exact nature of the problem(s) in this area. For example, are nursing meetings unproductive? By analyzing the data, the members of a nursing staff or faculty team can identify and diagnose major problems in time management. The group is then ready to identify and implement appropriate intervention strategies.

GOAL FORMULATION IN TIME MANAGEMENT

In order to (a) engage in a comprehensive analysis of time-management habits, (b) formulate accurate time-management diagnoses, and (c) select appropriate intervention strategies, at both the individual and subsystem or system level, organizational and personal career goals must be clearly identified, modified, or newly formulated. It is critical that nursing staff be made aware of organizational or system goals. Subsystem goals that mesh with system goals can then be formulated. If nurses are to analyze their use of time, system and subsystem goals must be considered in the analysis. The critical question can then be asked—Does this activity contribute to organizational goals? In our example of unproductive nursing meetings, the answer to this question may well alter the purpose of the meetings or even lead to their termination.

It is also important to have clearly formulated *personal* career goals. Successful time management means ''setting realistic goals, consistent with your strengths and weaknesses—goals which will satisfy your needs, including esteem and self-actualization'' (Ferner, 1980, p. 46). There are now two sets of goals—organizational and individual. If the two sets are compatible, there is no problem. For example, one of the individual goals may be to write two professional articles during the next year. At the same time, the unit's goals may include active nursing staff involvement in professional activities, including publications. However, if the two sets of goals are different, and in conflict, then a resolution must be attained. If the nurse leader cannot fulfill the priorities of the organization and has been unsuccessful in either changing those priorities or adjusting personal goals, then she or he might be more productive working in a situation where her or his own career goals and the goals of the organization are more closely matched (Davidson, 1978).

In this analysis, however, the nurse leader must be careful to consider personal resolution of reality shock. Kramer's (1974) research focused on the reality shock that is encountered by new nurse graduates as they enter the nursing work world. There they may encounter personal conflict between their own professional values and the bureaucratic values supported by the organization. How the nurse resolves this conflict over time affects her or his own career behavior and choices in the long run.

Suffice it to say that if system and/or subsystem goals are vague or nonexistent, it is critical to clarify or formulate them. Likewise, if the nurse is unclear about his or her own career goals, the formulation of them is essential. Only then can time-management habits be analyzed from a comprehensive perspective. The questions—Does this use of on-job time contribute to organizational goals? Does this use of time contribute to personal career goals?—can then be asked. Once time-management problems have been fully diagnosed, intervention strategies can be selected and implemented.

SELECTION AND IMPLEMENTATION OF TIME-MANAGEMENT STRATEGIES

Once the nurse leader and the team have formulated diagnoses about major time wasters in the subsystem, then the group can begin the process of selecting and implementing intervention strategies. Predictions about the best outcome should be made by the group when selecting intervention strategies from among a number of alternatives. Organizational constraints must obviously be kept in mind in the selection process. Again, group discussion can be utilized to select the most appropriate alternative and formulate the process for implementation.

The nurse leader may want to initiate personal change in time management before working with the entire group. In any case, the most appropriate intervention strategies must be selected. Suggestions appear in the following, and are organized by similar headings appearing in the list of common time wasters.

Communicating

Limit Interruptions

What are the major interruptions that disrupt work? The time a faculty team leader or coordinator sets aside for developing lesson plans or course schedules may be interrupted by drop-in visitors eager to chat, or by numerous trivial telephone calls. Nursing supervisors, head nurses, and clinical team leaders are even more prone to interruptions from subordinates, peers, interdisciplinary staff, visitors, or superiors. Schwartz and Mackenzie (1979) comment that the "average manager is interrupted every eight minutes all day long. Successful control of interruptions is essential" (p. 26).

Telephone interruptions can be reduced in a number of ways. When possible, have a secretary or ward clerk screen telephone calls and put through only those which require your expertise. If concentrating deeply when interrupted, write down a clue for the next thing that needs to be done after the telephone call. This will reduce start-up time when getting back to the job activity. A long-winded caller can be assisted in getting to the major point of the call if you steer the conversation to that point. In addition, the caller may be asked initially for an estimate of the time required to discuss some complex topic and then negotiate that time. Make a concerted effort to time personal calls and set realistic limits.

A system that is useful to some nurses is the consolidation of all telephone calls—except for emergency or other very important calls—into a specified block of time, by means of a call-back system. That is, the caller is informed by the secretary that the call will be returned between hours designated. The secretary is instructed to take messages. Prior to returning the calls, review these messages. Pertinent information or records can then be secured in preparation for the calls. A professional tone can be set at the beginning of the telephone call. Thus, time is saved by reducing the number of interruptions throughout the day.

Another means of consolidating phone calls is to assign staff members, on a rotating basis, the responsibility of responding to telephone calls. This is especially helpful where frequent general nursing information or consultation is requested by the public.

Be alert to telephone interruptions that keep repeating themselves. Some unnecessary calls may occur because of a lack of clear communication. For example, a subordinate may need a clearer set of instructions than those given initially. Finally, if most of the telephone interruptions

> come from your boss, don't assume that you must put up with them. Pick a judicious time . . . to explain that you are trying to get better control of your time, and ask if you could arrange mutually convenient times each day to check with each other on routine matters. (Bliss, 1976, p. 51)

Interruptions by drop-in visitors may need to be controlled. The nursing faculty coordinator can post office hours during which time he or she is available to faculty or students. Blocks of time for uninterrupted work can then likewise be set aside—time that will not be open to drop-in visitors. In a clinical setting, the nurse manager can clearly communicate to staff that, except for clinical emergencies, a given block of time is designated for uninterrupted individual staff counseling, planning for the clinical unit, or other relevant job responsibilities.

When unwanted drop-in visitors do occur, evaluate the overall benefits versus the loss of time. As a nurse leader, good judgment must be used. There are several actions that can be taken to limit the interruptions: a secretary can screen visitors; talk to the visitor outside the office. If the visitor is already in the office, be assertive, and learn to dismiss them tactfully. Volk-Tebbitt (1978) suggests that the manager should not even sit down with the unwanted guest. Remain standing and likewise do not invite the other person to sit. Indicate how much time is available and stick to the limit. Keep a clock in full sight. Expect the members of the work group to come as prepared as possible to any meeting. When ready to terminate, Reynolds and Tramel (1979) recommend phrases such as—"Before we finish, or Before we wrap it up, or Before I let you go" (p. 99).

General interruptions from nearby conversations and from other noise are particularly difficult to control in office settings that are characterized by open space. In such settings nurse leaders must set a personal example as well as encourage their team members to demonstrate sensitivity to each others' need for quiet time so that job responsibilities requiring concentration can be completed. When noise such as from required meetings, cannot be avoided, a quiet area removed from the open area should be available to other staff members. Assertive communication skills must be utilized by group members until a pattern develops that respects needs for quiet and privacy. Setting a specific block of time aside for the entire group to observe as a quiet time has been attempted in some office settings.

The arrangement of physical space can be utilized to control interruptions from others. A closed door generally connotes the "I'm busy" impression and tends to reduce interruptions. Desks can be placed so that they do not face colleagues at nearby desks or a busy hallway. Bookcases and cabinets can be utilized as artificial partitions in open space or shared offices.

In the clinical setting, it is difficult to control interruptions. In fact, certain interruptions are important to nurse leaders and are encouraged, such as the request from a staff nurse to discuss a complex clinical problem. However, there are unnecessary interruptions from others, that if controlled, would permit more time to be devoted to dealing with patient care problems or in providing leadership to staff. Continuous interruptions from subordinates about minor decisions or detail may point to a need for clearer communication, improved delegation, or basic staff training.

In rare instances, the other person's own perceptual distortions may put the nurse manager in an unfavorable light no matter the nature of reality. A professional and sincere commitment to do the best job possible, in most instances, conveys to others that work is taken seriously. Others will, in turn, tend to respond in a professional manner. Unnecessary interruptions from frequent social chitchat, gossip, and concern with trivia will tend to be minimized.

Manage Other Information Inputs/Outputs

Excessive communication or information overload should be avoided. Information overload occurs when the nurse manager can no longer process all the information inputs effectively. Work productivity is adversely affected and time is wasted. Effects of the strain show up in decreased productivity and increased rate of errors. Relevant data may no longer be retained for effective decision making. Excessive information can deter goal-related behavior and organizational goals can get lost. The nurse manager suffering from information overload can begin to exhibit symptoms of psychological stress and physical illness. As Rader (1979) points out, communication overload can affect entire organizations and lead to organizational decline.

What are some other strategies for managing communication inputs and managing time well? A secretary should sort all incoming mail and be taught some basic information about its disposition. If sorting must be done by the nurse manager, a wastebasket must be handy. Be generous in pitching nonessentials. Sort mail during nonprime productive hours. Handle each piece as few times as possible. In other words, take action where needed and possible. Review all requested reports and other communications from staff.

Avoid being caught up in the paper chain by using the most effective means of replying—which may be a quick telephone call. When sending written replies, utilize standardized form letters or forms for checking alternatives whenever possible. Bliss (1976) makes the interesting statement that

> when people are judged by how well they comply with directives, rather than by how well they meet the organization's objectives, paper work will multiply: a proliferation of memos and reports designed to prove that procedures are being followed. (p. 48)

Communicate clearly to subordinates what information is considered essential.

Since receiving and processing information is critical, but time is of essence to the nurse manager, excellent reading skills are essential. Rader (1979) suggests reading for structure, pattern, and thoughts, as well as reading with a clear goal. Enrolling in a course to improve reading skills is a wise investment. Love (1979b) makes several additional suggestions for saving time when obtaining input through reading. Select for reading those items that serve a purpose. Scanning material first may help to decide whether it should be read. Keep in mind objectives for reading an item and skip and scan, picking out the most important sections for more careful reading. Vary the speed according to your goals for reading and on the basis of the difficulty of the material.

Problem Solving

The nurse manager faces a variety of problems about which decisions are needed. Time is saved by utilizing the problem-solving process, but first ask who should solve this problem or make this decision. Behavior should be examined for patterns of indecision, delayed decision, making snap decisions, or acting without thinking. Try to eliminate these patterns and utilize the problem-solving process in order to manage time.

There are three types of managerial problems: "(1) deviation from what has happened to what is happening; (2) choosing between alternatives; and (3) deciding rank order" (Reynolds & Tramel, 1979, p. 55). Initially, additional clarity and identification of the problem may be needed. Collect data relevant to the problem area. This data can then be utilized to identify and clarify the problem more succinctly, if needed, and as a baseline for formulating alternative solutions.

Time can be wasted if too much, too little, or irrelevant data is collected. Problem analysis may be strengthened by seeking input from your nursing staff or faculty. However, this too can be a time-costly endeavor unless opposing viewpoints are used as a strategy by the nurse manager to examine all aspects of the problems and potential alternative solutions.

Delegating

Are there too many job responsibilities to be accomplished during the time available? In addition to other time-management strategies, delegation can be used wisely by the nurse manager or supervisor. Some tasks to consider delegating are (a) routine tasks, for example, coordinating patient treatment schedules or scheduling classroom space for lectures; (b) challenging tasks for a nursing staff or faculty member, for example, preparing patient educational materials or preparing a presentation for students interested in entering nursing; (c) preparation of preliminary drafts of policies, procedures, or reports, for example, unit policy and procedure on visiting hours or a report on student course evaluations during the past two years; and (d) data collections, for example, literature review in order to implement active use of nursing diagnoses in patient care planning or data to determine the most appropriate clinical placement for students.

In summary, proper delegation has several time-saving advantages. Delegation releases nursing

> supervisors for more important work. It helps to develop initiative in subordinates. Delegation extends your capabilities from doing, to coordinating and controlling. Successful delegation leads to good time management primarily because it allows personnel to handle higher priority tasks. (Smith & Besnette, 1978, p. 37)

Directing, Controlling, Evaluating

The time-wise nurse manager directs, controls, and evaluates in a manner that increases motivation among employees and enhances staff's commitment to doing the best job possible. Excessive review of performance or an overly critical attitude can result in wasted time. Likewise, not setting clear or appropriate performance standards or reviewing performance too little can also result in wasted time.

Fostering Constructive Interpersonal Interactions

Staggering amounts of time can be wasted through nonconstructive interpersonal interactions (Davidson, 1978). A nurse who is a "spontaneity seeker" or "fun-loving clown" attempts to place aspects of the job into a humorous vein, but often inappropriately. Other examples of these nonconstructive interpersonal interactions are the chronic complainer, attention seeker, I'll-show-you type, fear-ridden type, and junior psychiatrist. Assess personal behavior and have staff participate in assessing theirs. Wasted time is reduced if the nurse leader takes constructive steps to intervene in such nonproductive behaviors.

Creating a work atmosphere where open communications are permitted, encouraged, and supported is an important role for the time-conscious nurse leader or manager. When nursing staff can openly and assertively express their viewpoints and reactions to one another, conflicts can be resolved openly. Personal traits that create interpersonal friction can be examined and changed. Interpersonal difficulties can be discussed openly and a resolution can be sought. In particular, the leader should point out when the group is engaging in basic nonproductive assumptions rather than work. Of prime importance, an open system encourages assertive communication and supports the analysis of, and intervention in, nursing work group interaction with the goal of time management.

Motivating

Nursing staff or faculty members who experience job dissatisfaction and lack of motivation often engage in time wasters. Consider job aspects such as the type of supervision received; organizational patient care, and personnel policies and procedures; working conditions; and salary. The nurse leader or manager can then implement change to improve major job conditions. Seek consultation from a trusted colleague or enroll in seminars to improve leadership or management style. A nursing team that is worth retaining deserves the very best leadership capabilities.

Managing the Work Environment

If time wasters stem from the work environment itself, brainstorm with other staff for ways to increase individual and group efficiency. Unit or office furniture or supplies can be arranged so that the materials needed to get the job done are conveniently located. Supplies should be ordered on a regular basis and both properly and conveniently stored in an organized fashion.

Do not permit unessential materials and papers to accumulate. Dispose of nonessential materials unless there is a legal requirement to keep them. Streamline written input. Remove yourself from lists for materials that no longer contribute to your subsystem goals. If possible, train an assistant to triage the mail. Have a place for everything and keep everything organized accordingly. Remember, however,

> excessive record-keeping is a symptom of insecurity and defensive thinking. It indicates that you are less concerned with attaining objectives than you are with documentation, and that your thinking is oriented to the past, and not the present. (Bliss, 1976, p. 37)

Organizing

Developing an organizational structure that facilitates goal achievement saves time. Job descriptions should be understood by the nursing staff; roles and responsibilities clearly delineated; and duplication of tasks eliminated. Lines of authority should be clarified so that time does not have to be spent solving these conflicts nor wasted through the duplication of tasks.

Organize your workload by assigning priorities to all the tasks that need to be accomplished. Setting priorities is obviously easier to do in a nonclinical setting. Even though there is less control over one's time in the clinical area, especially for those nurses providing direct patient care, choices among professional job responsibilities must be made. Time is managed effectively if job responsibilities and tasks are prioritized according to importance.

How much does each task contribute to organizational goals or professional goals? Rank order the tasks into three groups—very important, moderately important, and minimally important. Remember the Pareto principle: 80% of the results or outcome of your work are related to only 20% of the tasks completed (Bliss, 1976). Therefore, it is very important to identify those important tasks.

List the tasks in the order in which they need to be accomplished, considering not only their *importance* but also their *urgency*, that is, take into consideration deadlines or specific time parameters set by your own supervisor. Complete those responsibilities that are the most important, get the most results, and are urgent first, that is, select the right job to be done. Identify personal prime working time. Work on the top-priority tasks during this time. Do less important tasks when no longer in "top condition."

Do not become tyrannized by tasks that are primarily urgent:

> Responding unwittingly to the endless pressures of the moment. . . . we leave ourselves open to the onslaught of the consequences of having left the more important task undone. The result is . . . a full blown crisis waiting to strike, and no telling where and when it is going to hit. (McCarthy, 1981, p. 62)

Time and energy are expended in dealing with crisis situations. Time is conserved if a crisis is averted.

> Many of the crises that arise in business or in personal life result from failure to act until a matter becomes urgent, with a result that more time is required to do the job. (Bliss, 1976, p. 25)

To prevent crises in management, allocate a reasonable time frame to a project. Provide follow-up after delegation and request periodic status reports. If a crises does occur, analyze contributing factors and seek preventive measures in order to prevent a similar situation.

Organize the work area into a functional and efficient space. Have adequate resources available. When possible avoid red tape: assist team members in working through a complex bureaucratic structure.

Personal Habits, Traits, Skills

Specifically identify and list those job tasks that are chronically put off. For each of the tasks listed, examine and document the reasons for the procrastination. Determine the consequences of the procrastination. Are there positive payoffs? What are the negative results of the procrastination? Would it be appropriate to delegate the responsibility?

If you must perform the task, acknowledge the fact that you do not like doing it, then decide that you are in control of yourself and have the power to make the decision to complete the responsibility (Davidson, 1978). Develop an action plan to complete the task. For example, large tasks can be broken down into smaller more manageable components. Finally, implement your plan. Some time can be set aside to work on the task at regular intervals.

Personal behaviors, such as gathering and distributing gossip about co-workers, excessive socialization, attention getting, complaining, carelessness, and lack of self-discipline, are huge time wasters and contribute little to either organizational or personal career goals. Discussing these behaviors with a trusted colleague may help identify those traits that can be easily modified. Others may require skilled counselling.

Planning, Personal Goal Setting

As Davidson (1978) points out, time that is consumed during the working day on items that do not serve organizational or personal professional career goals or priorities is primarily wasted time. Make a written list of *all* job activities that could be done now, as well as those that can be done in the near future. Break down any large projects into manageable parts. While considering the notions of importance and urgency discussed earlier, ask yourself, "What are the job responsibilities that absolutely have to get done today?" Cross them off your list and place them on your daily schedule. Then identify other items on the list that you would like to get accomplished today. Remember to choose items that are both important and urgent. Be realistic and do not overschedule.

Davidson (1978) labels the most important items the "aces" of the day; the other important items on your schedule for the day become your "kings." The two types of items left on the list of things to do are those responsibilities that you need to get done some time but will not get done because of the time available (the "jacks"); and, those items that are not really very important and do not contribute very much toward goals (the "deuces"). Each day a new schedule is made, and some items previously "kings" and "jacks" can become your "aces."

Although this system of daily scheduling is somewhat easier for the nurse leader in an educational setting, this basic concept of scheduling can be applied by the nurse leader in the clinical setting as well. For example, the nurse coordinator for several medical surgical units on which primary care nursing is implemented, may have certain routine responsibilities that must be accomplished daily, for example, clinical rounds. From the total list of responsibilities to be accomplished, the nurse coordinator selects as the "ace" the interviewing of a nurse applicant for a vacant position. In addition, one of the primary care nurses has assessed behavioral problems in a client for which a consultation from a psychiatric nurse expert is being sought. The coordinator plans to identify such a nurse expert and arrange for the consultation. This becomes a "king" for that day. In addition, she or he lists under the "kings" the responsibility of assisting the primary care nurses in utilizing nursing diagnoses as part of the nursing process. Among the items that remain as "jacks" on the list of things to do are: counselling a new nurse graduate who needs assistance in organizing work; providing input into the formulation of the nursing service department's budget for next year; and discussing with the unit manager ideas for reorganizing the storage of supplies for more convenience to primary care nurses.

As you survey your list of things to be done, have a good notion of the who, what, when, where, and how in relation to each responsibility. Delegate where possible. Attempt to work on the most important tasks during your high productivity periods of the day. Remember to refer to your schedule during the day and work on priority tasks so as to prevent getting immersed in detail and process without attention to goals. Obviously, there may be times, especially in the clinical setting, when clinical emergencies arise needing immediate and full attention. Decisions must thus be made regarding alternatives to accomplish the scheduled activities. In the example given, the interview with the nurse applicant could be conducted by the director of nursing service alone. A new appointment could be scheduled for the nurse applicant to meet with the nursing coordinator and the staff.

Recording, Reporting

Much time can be saved with reports and records that serve a purpose and are functional. Ask if this report is mandated and/or serving a useful purpose in the organization. If not, take steps to eliminate it, that is, eliminate all unnecessary reports. If needed, are there ways to simplify the report? For example, a standardized form requiring check marks can be developed to document the behavior of a patient treated by a behavior-modification program. In the same vein, work with the secretary to develop standardized letters and memos that can be used in recurring correspondence.

Likewise, the secretary, with assistance as needed, should set up an uncomplicated but organized filing system. Files should be organized into logical partitions but not too narrowly, otherwise knowing where to file materials will be difficult. Everyone having access to the file should be familiarized with the system. Enough storage space should be available for adequate record keeping, but, remember to purge the files periodically and dispose of items no longer needed or required legally to be kept. Finally, keep simplicity in mind when reporting, recording, and filing—it saves time.

Staffing, Staff Development

The nurse manager will most likely have input into selecting new nurse personnel. Selecting motivated staff, whose expertise closely matches the requirements of the position for which they are applying, will save much time in the long run. Staff development, *appropriate* delegation of responsibilities, and quality guidance and direction are necessary because they contribute to sound time management.

Utilizing Facilities, Nonhuman Resources, Budgeting

Time is conserved when adequate and functional supplies, equipment, and space (including storage areas) are available to nursing staff or faculty. With data from a comprehensive assessment, constructive change in the work environment can be initiated.

EVALUATION OF INTERVENTION STRATEGIES

After the selected strategies have been implemented for a reasonable period of time, evaluate the results. This can be done informally by discussing the impact with the work group. Formulate an overall evaluation of the results of the strategies used from everyone's observation of the degree to which time wasters have been reduced.

A more formal approach to evaluation can be taken by following a process similar to that during the original comprehensive assessment of time wasters. Limit the assessment tool, however, to the area of concern. Have work-group members keep time logs again. As before, analyze results, provide feedback, seek discussion, formulate diagnoses. Then select the most appropriate intervention strategies, if needed. Hopefully, findings will indicate, however, that the current intervention strategies are attaining the expected results.

SUMMARY

Time is a very valuable resource to the nurse leader, manager, and supervisor. Whether organizational or personal career goals are met depends in part on whether or not time is used wisely.

Time management means the effective and efficient use of time. It involves utilizing resources efficiently, engaging in activities selectively, and striving for the achievement of organizational goals in optimal time. Time wasters are those activities or tasks that require the use of time, but contribute little if anything to individual career or organizational goal achievement.

The process involved in time management involves: (1) systematic data collection about individual and organizational time wasters; (2) clarifying or formulating organizational goals; (3) analyzing the data collected; (4) providing feedback to work group members; (5) formulating diagnoses as to the major time wasters; (6) selecting appropriate intervention strategies; and finally, (8) evaluating the results.

Assessment tools and strategies are presented in this chapter. The content for both is organized under major components of the processes inherent in leadership, management, and supervision. These categories are: (1) communicating, (2) deciding, problem solving; (3) delegating; (4) directing, controlling, evaluating; (5) fostering constructive human interaction; (6) motivating; (7) managing the work environment; (8) organizing; (9) personal habits, traits; (10) goal setting planning; (11) recording, reporting; (12) staffing, staff development; and (13) utilizing facilities and nonhuman resources, budgeting.

Time wasters can be identified through systematic assessment in each of these categories. Likewise, intervention strategies can be selected and implemented that contribute to sound time management.

REFERENCES

Berlin, G. Time waits for no one. *Hospital Topics,* 1980, 58(1), 10–11.

Bliss, E. *Getting things done: The ABCs of time management.* New York: Scribner's, 1976.

Davidson, J. *Effective time management. A practical workbook.* New York: Human Sciences Press, 1978.

Fanning, T., & Fanning, R. *Get it all done and still be human: A personal time-management workshop.* Radnor, Penn: Chilton, 1979.

Ferner, J. *Successful time management.* New York: Wiley, 1980.

Kramer, M. *Reality shock: Why nurses leave nursing.* St. Louis: Mosby, 1974.

Lancaster, J. Making the most of meetings. *The Journal of Nursing Administration,* 1981, 11(10), 15–19.

LeBoeuf, M. Managing time means managing yourself. *Business Horizons,* 1980, 23, 41–46.

Love, S. *Mastery and management of time.* Englewood Cliffs, N.J.: Prentice-Hall, 1978.

Love, S. Increase your ability to accomplish more. *The Canadian Banker & ICB Review,* 1979, 86(5), 51–52.(b)

Mackenzie, R. *New time management methods.* Chicago: Dartnell, 1975.

Marriner, A. Time management. *Journal of Nursing Administration*, 1979, *9*(10), 16–18.

McCarthy, M. Managing your own time: The most important management task. *The Journal of Nursing Administration*, 1981, *11* (11–12), 61–65.

McDougle, L. Time management: Making every minute count. *Supervisory Management*, 1979, *24*, 35–40.

Rader, M. Suffering from information overload? *Management World*, 1979, *8*, 9–11.

Reynolds, H., & Tramel, M. *Executive time management.* Englewood Cliffs, N.J.: Prentice-Hall, 1979.

Schwartz, E., & Mackenzie, R. Time-management strategy for women. *Journal of Nursing Administration*, 1979, *9*(3), 22–26.

Smith, H., & Besnette, F. Effective time management: The forgotten administrative and nursing supervisor art. *Hospital Topics*, 1978, *56*(1), 32–37.

Volk-Tebbitt, B. Time: Who controls yours? *Supervisor Nurse*, 1978, *9*, 17–19; 21–22.

Yura, H., Ozimek, D., & Walsh, M. *Nursing leadership: Theory and process.* New York: Appleton-Century-Crofts, 1976.

Wiley, L. The ABCs of time management. *Nursing 78*, 1978, *8*(9), 105–112.

BIBLIOGRAPHY

Birckhead, L. Nursing and the technetronic age. *Journal of Nursing Administration*, 1978, *8*(2), 16–19.

Cercone, R. Measuring activity by "work sampling." *Dimensions in Health Service*, 1978, *55*, 34; 36.

Holliman, J. Analyzing faculty workload. *Nursing Outlook*, 1977, *25*(11), 721–723.

Isenberg, D. Some effects on time-pressure on vertical structure and decision-making accuracy in small groups. *Organizational Behavior and Human Performance*, 1981, *27*, 119–134.

Kliner, B. The productivity challenge—2. Managing yourself. *Management World*, 1980, *9*, 17–18; 36.

Love, S. How to be sure that priorities will serve your purposes. *The Canadian Banker & ICB Review*, 1979, *86*(6), 50–51.

Love, S. How to handle interruptions. *The Canadian Banker & ICB Review*, 1979, *86*(4), 44–45.(a)

Mahoney, T. The rearranged work week. *California Management Review*, 1978, *20*(4), 31–39.

McCullough, H. Utilize every moment: Plan ahead. *Hospital Financial Management*, 1980, *34*, 50–51.

McFarland, G., & Wasli, E. Psychiatric Nursing, Part 2. In L. Brunner & D. Suddarth, *The Lippincott manual of nursing practice.* Philadelphia: Lippincott, 1982.

McWilliams, C. Systems analysis can solve nursing management problems. *The Journal for Nursing Leadership and Management*, 1980, *11*, 17–26.

Moskowitz, R. *Assertiveness for career and personal success.* New York: AMACOM, 1977.

Nerone, B. Managing your time. *Imprint*, 1977, *24*, 32.

Roseman, E. How to manage time more effectively, *Medical Laboratory Observer*, 1978, *10*, 33–36.

Rotenbury, H. On time. *Management World*, 1979, *8*, 21.

Schilling, C. Time planning: How to divide up your day. *Supervision*, 1980, *42*, 12–15.

Sheppard, R. Nurses help conduct time study. *Hospital Topics*, 1975, *53*(3), 4–5.

Solomons, H., Jordison, N., & Powell, S. How faculty members spend their time. *Nursing Outlook*, 1980, *28*(3), 160–165.

Umiker, W. Six weeks to more effective time management. *Medical Laboratory Observer*, 1979, *11*, 60–66.

CHAPTER 20
STRESS MANAGEMENT

Stress researchers and theorists have offered varying definitions of stress, among them: (a) a situational condition, (b) a reaction, (c) a nonspecific response of the body to a demand on it, (d) a therapeutic force, (e) a debilitating force, (f) a general state type of phenomenon, and (g) a broad area of study (Blau, 1981; Greenwood & Greenwood, 1979; Selye, 1976).

It is acknowledged that "good stress," sometimes called "eustress," can be constructive and energizing and can increase productivity and efficiency.

> Stress is essential to life; any organic system without stress is dead and disintegrating. When, however, stress becomes excessive or uncontrolled, it can cause or contribute to mental or physical illness (Greenwood & Greenwood, 1979, p. 2) or other maladaptive behaviors.

There is no optimal level of stress. Each nurse manager must determine a stress level that is personally most appropriate and learn to utilize stress-management strategies to keep it at that level. At the same time, stress must be controlled in the manager's work group so that it is kept below the level beyond which individual and group performance and satisfaction will be adversely affected.

DEFINITIONS

Since nurses must frequently work in stress-producing work environments, the term "stress" in this chapter will be used to denote the negative aspects of stress. Stress is "a generic entity involving many variables working in concert" (Scott, Oberst, & Dropkin, 1980). *Stress* is thus defined as the neurocognitive, affective, physiologic, and behavioral response arising from environmental and/or internal demands which tax or exceed the person's perceived or actual available adaptive resources (Bailey, 1980; Scott et al., 1980). *Job stress* is defined as the response arising from job-related stressors which tax or exceed the worker's perceived or actual available coping/adaptive resources. The *stressor* is that internal or external stimulus or demand that helps bring about the stress.

A STRESS-ADAPTING MODEL

An open systems model of stress and adaptation is presented in Figure 20-1. The model depicts the person in continuous interaction with the environment. Stressors can arise from either external and/or internal sources. The person is alert to these stressors. The stressors are evaluated through neurocognitive activation and mental operations for

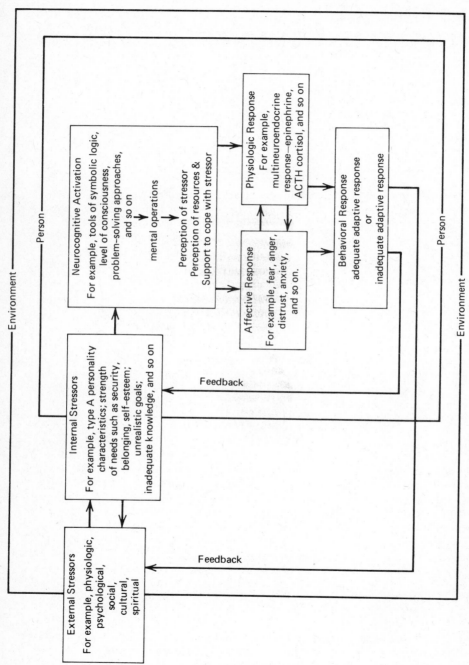

FIGURE 20-1. A STRESS-ADAPTING MODEL.

Adapted from Behling, O., & Holcombe, F. Dealing with employee stress, *MSU Business Topics*, 1981, 29, 54; McFarland, G., & Wasli, E. Psychiatric nursing. In L. Brunner & D. Suddarth, *The Lippincott manual of nursing practice*. Philadelphia: Lippincott, 1982, p. 910; Scott, D., Oberst, M., & Dropkin, M. A stress-coping model. *Advances in Nursing Science*, 1980, 3, p. 19; and Yates, J. *Managing stress*. New York: AMACOM, 1979, p. 19.

any threat to self-system survival. The *perception* of the stressor and the resources to cope with the stressor is the situation to which the person actually responds.

> It is the only view of the world a person possesses. It is an individualized, private view of the situation, and it may be very different from objective reality. (Behling & Holcombe, 1981, p. 56)

Cognitive functioning occurs after stressor impact and provides the initial direction for the entire stress response—"comprised of cognitive activity, emotions, and physiological response *in interaction*" (Scott et al., 1980, p.11), that is, the cognitive response to the stressor affects the emotional, physiologic, and outcome behavioral responses.

In the model, the outcome behavioral response includes all observable behaviors, such as expressive reactions and motor behaviors; self-reports of the person; and end-organ responses, such as cardiac changes, decreased peristalsis, and so forth (Scott et al., 1980). As these authors state,

> All neurocognitive, affective, and physiologic responses to the stress situation may be measured by direct observation of expressive and motor actions, self-report indices, or end-organ response levels. (Scott et al., 1980, p. 17)

The outcome behavioral response can be adaptive and serve to cope with the stressor in varying degrees. However, the behavioral response can be inadequate or maladaptive. In this latter response, the stressor continues to affect the person, and its impact may even be augmented.

In summary, the model depicts the human being as a dynamic open system in continuous interaction with the environment. The stress actually experienced, along with the resultant outcome behavioral responses, stem from multiple interacting variables. Adaptive behavioral responses result in (a) a constructive reappraisal of the significance of the stressor and the adequacy of related coping resources to deal with it, (b) the actual utilization of resources to cope with the stressor(s), (c) minimal impairment of functioning, (d) preservation of personal integrity through the control of emotional and physiologic responses, (e) learning and growth, (f) achievement of constructive goals, and/or (g) an augmented repertoire of coping strategies. Feedback—positive or negative—from either the adaptive or maladaptive behavioral response impacts on the actual and/or perceived stressor and the person reappraises the situation. The process of neurocognitive activation, affective response, physiologic response, outcome behavioral response, and feedback is again activated if the stressor continues to impact on the person.

External Stressors in the Nonwork Environment

Stressors can arise from the nurse leader's, manager's, or supervisor's nonwork environment. Although the focus here will be on the work environment, awareness of other environmental stressors is important for understanding the person's total stress response. It has been found, for example, that the accumulated exposure to stressors, within a given recent period of time, is associated with high levels of emotional and/or physical illness (Holmes & Rahe, 1967). There are 15 non-work-related stressors (with the potential for resulting in a maladaptive stress response, i.e., illness): death of spouse (100), divorce (73), marital separation (65), jail term (63), death of a close family member (63), personal injury or illness (53), marriage (50), marital reconciliation (45), retirement (45), change in health of family member (40), pregnancy (39), sex difficulties (39), gain of new family member (39), change in financial state (38), and death of a close friend (37). The numbers represent the scale values assigned to each of these potential stressors in the Social Readjustment Rating Scale developed by Holmes and Rahe (1967).

External Stressors in the Work Environment

Potential work-related stressors identified in the same Social Readjustment Rating Scale are fired at work (47), business readjustment (39), change to a different job (36), change in responsibilities at work (29), trouble with boss (23), and change in work hours or conditions (20).

Other research findings have identified sources of stress faced by managers in their work environment. In an American Management Association survey of top and mid-level managers (Kiev & Kohn, 1979), the major stressors were identified as (a) work and time pressures, (b) conflict between the personal goals of the manager and the expectations of the organization, (c) the "political" climate of the organization, (d) lack of feedback on job performance, (e) uncertainty about the organization's future, and (f) responsibility without authority. In relation to the political climate it was found that organizations "in which the prevailing atmosphere conveys the impression that 'it's not what you know but whom you know' are stressful places in which to work" (Kiev & Kohn, 1979, p. 3). It was also found that midlevel managers experience stress more frequently than top-level managers. In particular, midlevel managers found responsibility without authority to be a major source of stress. As Kiev and Kohn (1979) state:

> That senior managers appear to be under stress less frequently than middle managers is a common finding in management research and is generally attributed to their respective positions in the organizational hierarchy. Persons at or near the top have more power and control over the sources of stress than individuals at a lower echelon do; they are also more likely to have fulfilled their career aspirations. (p. 3)

Other research and literature identify additional potential stressors in the work environment of the manager—including nurse managers—that are included in the list below (Bailey, Steffen, & Grout, 1980; Beehr & Newman, 1978; Brief, 1980; Cohen & Orlinsky, 1977; Cooper & Melhuish, 1980; de Board, 1978; de Vries, 1979; Giammatteo & Giammatteo, 1980; Goodell, 1980; Greenberg & Valletutti, 1980; Greenwood & Greenwood, 1979; Hartl, 1979; Jacobson, 1978; Manuso, 1979; Parasuraman & Alutto, 1981; Preston, Ivancevich, & Matteson, 1981; Schmidt, 1978; Schwartz, 1980; Selverston, 1980; Yates, 1979). Any of these work-related factors have the potential of becoming stressors for the nurse leader, manager, or supervisor.

LIST OF POTENTIAL EXTERNAL STRESSORS IN THE WORK ENVIRONMENT OF NURSE MANAGERS

1. Organization/Institution's External Environment
   - Uncertainty about the organization's future
   - Rapidly changing technology and scientific developments
   - Inadequate available supply of adequately educated nursing staff or faculty
   - Pressures from consumers or from other social systems
   - Restrictive governmental laws or regulations

- Public complaints or lawsuits
- Fluctuating, uncertain, or decreasing student enrollment or patient admissions
- Competition from other social systems
- Fluctuating or decreasing sources of external funding
- Problems with suppliers of needed equipment, supplies, or services

2. Organizational Structure and Climate
- Bureaucratic pettiness, rumor, or harassment
- Lack of opportunity for participation in major decisions
- Lack of job security
- Pressures toward conformity
- Budget uncertainty or constraints
- Conflict between personal goals/values and organizational expectations
- Political climate, for example, cut-throat competition; reward for "whom you know and how you know them" rather than for what you know
- Inadequate information about career-advancement requirements
- Lack of adequate, or inconsistent, feedback on job performance
- Reorganization
- Inadequate staffing
- Inadequate training programs

3. Physical Work Environment
- Poor physical work conditions
- Lack of adequate resources
- Excessive, unpredictable noise
- Inadequate work space
- Open office space

4. Role/Job Demands and Expectations
- Role overload, that is, excessive time pressures, deadlines, and work responsibilities
- Role conflict, that is, simultaneous required conformance to a number of inconsistent and contradictory job expectations
- Role ambiguity, that is, unclear or vague job responsibilities and duties
- Other job characteristics, for example:
  - Decision making under time pressure
  - Changes in job responsibilities
  - Underutilization of expertise/skill
  - Lack of responsibility
  - Excessive job variability
  - Change in work hours or conditions
  - Responsibility without authority

5. Relationships at Work
- Poor relationship with own supervisor

- Poor relationships with colleagues including physicians
- Poor relationship with subordinates
- Inadequate support from own supervisor
- Inadequate job performance by own supervisor
- Inadequate job performance by subordinates
- Excessive interpersonal conflict
- Ongoing contact with "stress carriers"
- Responsibility for the job performance of inadequately prepared staff
- Unresponsive nurse leadership
- Communication problems/lack of information

6. Patient Care Demands
   - Death of patients
   - Critical/unstable or chronic patient conditions
   - Inadequate staffing
7. Other
   - Fired at work
   - Change to a different job, including promotion
   - Business/organization readjustment

Many of the stressors—similar to those identified in the work environment of the nurse manager—can also impact on nursing staff or faculty in the work group. For example, ambivalence, conflict, or overload in a nursing staff member's own role, or in a nursing faculty's own role, can be a stressor for that person. Since the nurse manager/supervisor must cope not only with his or her own stress, but should also assist in reducing stressors faced by subordinates, it is important that the potential stressors in various work environments of nurses be understood. For example, Friel and Tehan (1980) identify the following exogenous stressors in hospice home care:

> (1) All hospice patients are dying; (2) their disease process presents nurses with many distressful symptoms; (3) the work itself is physically and emotionally demanding; (4) many aspects of care cannot be controlled in the home due to inability of the family; (5) the process of integration of hospice into a health care system. (p. 287)

In another example, a study by Anderson and Basteyns (1981, p. 33) identified as most stressful for critical care nurses the following stressors: death of young patients, inadequate staffing, unavailable medical support in emergencies, medication errors, inadequate medical information provided to patients, inability to provide patient support due to other job pressures, demanding physicians, rotation to other hospital units, responsibility for the lives of patients, work overload, poor communications with physicians, dealing with death, and role conflict. Finally in a third example, Bailey et al. (1980) provide a detailed listing of the distribution of responses on sources of greatest stress faced by ICU nurses.

Internal Stressors

The stress-adapting model in Figure 20-1 also depicts internal stressors. A number of stress theorists and researchers identify these internal stressors. Yates (1979), for example, states:

> The various pressures or demands from your internal environment are called internal stressors. They include the pressures you put on yourself by being ambitious, materialistic, competitive, and aggressive. (p. 19)

Indeed, Friedman and Rosenman (1974) describe the Type A personality who becomes susceptible to coronary artery disease. This personality type is characterized by an excessive aggressive drive, a sense of time pressure and urgency, covert hostilities, impatience, the drive to accomplish more than one task simultaneously, extremely high goals, excessive competitive drives, and an extreme need for achievement. Although these personality characteristics are constructive in moderate degree, they can become internal stressors when excessive.

Davidson, Cooper, & Chamberlain (1980) found that females in senior managerial positions have a greater predisposition toward Type A personality characteristics and are more prone to higher stress levels, as well as stress-related illnesses, than the general population. What degree of the stress response results from self-imposed states versus work environments that enhance these characteristics, requires further investigation. Earlier research by Howard (1977) identified job conditions most responsible for eliciting the Type A characteristics as "(1) having supervisory responsibility for people; (2) feeling that you are working in competition with others; (3) excessive workloads; and (4) conflicting demands in the job" (p. 88). Howard states that "both personality and job conditions combine to produce behavior which, in its extreme, appears related to known risk factors in coronary heart disease" (1977, p. 88). In later research, Keenan and McBain (1979) found that persons with Type A personalities showed a stronger relationship between role ambiguity and tension at work than those with Type B personalities. Also, persons with an external locus of control showed a higher association between role ambiguity and experienced job tension than persons with an internal locus of control.

Other potential internal stressors have been identified (Bailey et al., 1980; Beehr & Newman, 1978; Goosen & Bush, 1979; Jacobson, 1978; Preston et al., 1981; Schmidt, 1978). Included are (a) inadequate knowledge and skill for the job; (b) lack of relevant experience; (c) strength of needs such as the need for self esteem, the need for belonging, and the degree of insecurity/fear of failure; (d) unrealistic goals/aspirations; (e) unconventional values; (f) need for clarity, that is, intolerance for ambiguity; (g) intrapersonal conflict; (h) typical anxiety level; and (i) high need for perfection.

Responses to Stressors and Stress: Neurocognitive Activation, Affective Response, Physiologic Response, and Outcome Behavioral Response

There are several components of neurocognitive activation that involve the cortical and subcortical areas of the brain. Components of thinking and reasoning include (a) the mental structure (e.g., long-term memory, short-term memory, abstraction, concept formation), and (b) mental operations (e.g., tools of symbolic logic such as induction or deduction, levels of consciousness/alertness, and problem solving) (Scott et al, 1980). These structures and operations evaluate the stressor–person impact to determine its degree of relevancy—irrelevant, relevant but benign, relevant and stressful—for that individual. As has been stated previously, the cognitive response resulting from this neurocognitive activation in turn affects the emotional, physiologic, and outcome behavior responses.

Although there is no consensus as to whether emotions are independent entities or secondary to cognition, there is an increasing awareness that the two are related (Izard, 1979; Scott et al., 1980) as is depicted in the proposed stress-adapting model in Figure 20-1. The affective response to stress can include a variety of emotions. Among them are anxiety, fear, anger, distrust, sadness, and numbness. Observable behavioral verbal and nonverbal reactions, along with related physiologic responses, are considered to be the observable behavioral manifestations of these emotions.

The physiologic response to stress involves multiple glandular secretory changes (e.g., from the hypothalamus, pituitary gland, pancreas, thyroid gland, or the adrenal cortex or medulla); sympathetic (autonomic) nervous system activation; and end-organ response. The "end-organ changes are considered to be behavioral outcomes of the process" (Scott et al., 1980, p. 16).

The final outcome of the stressor–person impact and the stress response is the behavioral response which can either be (a) an adaptive response or (b) an inadequate adaptive response. Included in the *outcome behavioral response*, as here defined, are (a) directly observable motor and expressive actions, (b) self-report indices, and (c) end-organ response levels that result from the interactive effects of the neurocognitive, affective, and physiologic responses. Outcome behavioral responses to stressors and stress in organizations have been identified by researchers, theorists, and experts on this phenomenon (Behling & Holcombe, 1981; Beehr & Newman, 1978; Buckalew & Gahan, 1979; Bullard, 1980; de Board, 1978; de Vries, 1979; Duemer et al., 1978; Greenberg & Valletutti, 1980; Greenwood & Greenwood, 1979; Humphrey, 1978; Kiev & Kohn, 1979; Mickel, 1981; Schuler, 1980; Tardy, 1977; Yates, 1979). A number of these outcome behavioral responses to stress appear in the accompanying list. Those listed are generally a component of a maladaptive, or at least a partially adaptive stress response.

Stress has been defined as the neurocognitive, affective, physiologic, and behavioral response arising from environmental and/or internal demands that tax or exceed the person's perceived or actual available adaptive resources. A stress-adapting model was presented in Figure 20-1. It must be kept in mind, however, that stress is a very complex phenomenon encompassing a large number of interacting and interrelated variables. Continuous system feedback and reappraisal occur until the stressor is neutralized or adaptation occurs. "The ultimate adaptation is unique for each individual and occurs within a range of effectiveness from maintenance of ideal integrity to death" (Scott et al., 1980).

OUTCOME BEHAVIORAL RESPONSES TO STRESSORS AND STRESS IN ORGANIZATIONS

	Yes	No
Absenteeism	☐	☐
Abrupt changes in grooming	☐	☐
Accident proneness	☐	☐

Apathy, resignation □ □
Apprehension, dread □ □
Asthma (long-term effect) □ □
Bizarre perceptions, reactions □ □
Boredom □ □
Callousness toward co-workers □ □
Change in smoking or drinking patterns □ □
Confusion about job role and duties □ □
Coronary thrombosis (long-term effect) □ □
Declining job performance □ □
Decreased appetite or compulsive eating □ □
Depression □ □
Diarrhea or other gastrointestinal disturbances □ □
Difficulty concentrating □ □
Disorganization □ □
Disorientation □ □
Emotional instability □ □
Emotional tension, alertness, being "keyed up" □ □
Excessive daydreaming □ □
Excessive defensiveness □ □
Feelings of persecution □ □
Feelings of unreality □ □
Floating anxiety, irrational fears □ □
Forgetfulness □ □
Frequent urination □ □
Frigidity, impotence □ □
General adaptation syndrome—(a) alarm reaction; (b) □ □
  countershock phase; (c) resistance state; (d) stage of
  exhaustion (If stressors persist and defenses prove in-
  adequate, adaptation energy is depleted. Death may
  eventually occur.)
Hay fever, other allergies (long-term effect) □ □
Hopelessness in coping with life □ □
Hyperactivity □ □
Hypersensitivity □ □
Hypertension (long-term effect) □ □
Immature behavior □ □
Impulsiveness □ □
Increased use of tranquilizers or other drugs □ □
Insomnia □ □
Intense itching □ □

Intolerance for ambiguity	☐	☐
Irritability	☐	☐
Job turnover (voluntary)	☐	☐
Lack of concern for co-workers	☐	☐
Lack of concern for employing organization	☐	☐
Loss of contact with reality	☐	☐
Lower back pain, neck pain, chest pain	☐	☐
Migraine headache	☐	☐
Mistrustfulness	☐	☐
Negativism, critical, argumentative	☐	☐
Nervous, high-pitched laughter	☐	☐
Neurosis	☐	☐
Overdependency	☐	☐
Physiologic responses as increased heart rate, blood pressure, respiration, sweating	☐	☐
Preoccupation with busywork	☐	☐
Psychosis	☐	☐
Rheumatoid arthritis (long-term effect)	☐	☐
Rigidity of thought	☐	☐
Ritualistic behavior	☐	☐
Sense of powerlessness	☐	☐
Sleeping too much	☐	☐
Suicidal thoughts	☐	☐
Trembling, nervous tics	☐	☐
Tunnel vision	☐	☐
Ulcer (long-term effect)	☐	☐
Vacillation in decision making	☐	☐
Weakness, excessive fatigue	☐	☐
Weight gain or loss (sudden)	☐	☐

ASSESSMENT

There are a number of tools available to assess one's stress level or "behavioral response" to stress. One of the most familiar is the Social Readjustment Rating Scale developed by Holmes and Rahe (1967) which was previously described. Other tools can be found in major texts on stress and stress management. Bullard (1980), for example, includes two assessment tools—Health Problems Often Related to Stress (pp. 124–126) and Behavior Change Checklist (pp. 132–134). Yates (1979) includes a tool titled "Symptoms of Type A Behavior" (p. 67) that can be used to determine to what degree one possesses Type A personality characteristics. Also presented are two checklists—The Physical and Mental Signs of Stress (p. 89)—that can be used as a cursory assessment of signs of stress. Warning signs of stress that can be used to review one's own level are listed by Greenberg and Valletutti (1980, pp. 70–72). An assessment of job-related stressors can be done by using the listing of factors appearing in Exhibits 9 and 10 in *Executive Stress* (Kiev & Kohn, 1979, pp. 21–22). Goldberg (1978) advocates keeping a daily log for two weeks to identify stressors. A scale for assigning scores to activities is provided (pp. 23–24). In addition, a stress symptom checklist is noted (pp. 37–38). Additional guidelines are provided for self-evaluation of (a) signs of fight-or-flight (p. 39), (b) psychological warnings (pp. 41–42), (c) cardiovascular warnings (pp. 44–45), (d) diabetic warnings (p. 53), the Glazer Stress-Control Life-Style Questionnaire (pp. 98–100), and a tool for detecting the Type A behavior pattern (p. 105). Johnson and Sarason (1979) have reproduced a life experiences survey. This tool measures life changes and their impact on a person. Finally, the outcome behavioral responses checklist can be used to give some indications of whether one is experiencing partially adaptive or maladaptive outcome behavioral responses to stressors and stress in organizations. Review the responses. Check whether or not they are being experienced personally. "Yes" responses may indicate inadequate personal coping with external or internal stressors. The same tool can be used formally or informally to assess outcome behavioral responses to stressors and stress in organizations experienced by members of the work team.

STRESS ADAPTING/COPING STRATEGIES

A number of strategies can be employed to reduce the stressor–person impact and to increase one's adaptive responses in coping with the stressor and stress response (Barash, 1980; Bullard 1980; Cooper & Crump, 1978; Douglass, 1977; Greenberg & Valletutti, 1980; Greenwood & Greenwood, 1979; Kiev & Kohn, 1979; Tardy, 1977; Willis, 1979; Yates, 1979). Strategies can be utilized to (a) eliminate stressors, (b) increase one's resistance to their impact, (c) improve problem-solving skills or alter perceptions, (d) preserve self-integrity by regulating affective responses, (e) preserve self-integrity by regulating physiologic responses, and/or (f) improve adaptive motor or expressive behaviors designed to neutralize the stressor. The stress coping/adapting strategies will be organized under the headings where they appear to belong most logically. It must be stressed, however, that any given coping/adapting strategy can have impact on any combination of the six purposes just outlined. As was noted earlier, the components of the stress-adapting model are interrelated.

Eliminate Stressors

The work and nonwork environments should be examined to identify and eliminate as many stressors as possible. Some sources of external stress can be eliminated. For example, role clarification through clear and specific job descriptions and delineation of responsibilities can eliminate the stressor of role ambiguity. Other sources of external stress can be reduced. For example, through appropriate delegation and use of time management strategies the stressor—role overload—can be reduced. Other external stressors cannot be eliminated or reduced, consequently, other coping strategies must be used. For example, the stressor—open space—can perhaps not be eliminated, so other adaptive strategies will need to be used to cope with this source of stress. In summary, "analyze stress-producing situations and decide what is worth worrying about and what isn't" (Kiev & Kohn, 1979, p. 40).

Increase Resistance to Stressor Impact

As has been described, the impact of stressors can affect numerous body subsystems. A healthy lifestyle, in general, aids in a person's ability to cope with stressors. Greenberg and Valletutti (1980) state that (a) "physical exercise has been recognized as an effective tool in reducing and coping with stress" (p. 77), (b) that physicians and researchers agree that there is a relationship between diet and stress, and (c) that "sound mental health practices are as important to coping with and reducing stress as are good physical health practices" (p. 87). The following are some suggestions:

1. Eat a well-balanced nutritious diet
2. Reduce caffeine consumption
3. Reduce/eliminate smoking
4. Use alcohol in moderation
5. Engage in a constructive exercise program
6. Develop regular eating and sleeping habits
7. Take vacations when needed
8. Allocate some time for rest and relaxation each day
9. Avoid being a perfectionist
10. Appreciate some of the simple things in life
11. Obtain regular physical check-ups
12. Avoid using drugs to deal with stress unless prescribed by a doctor
13. Make good use of leisure time. Engage in enjoyable hobbies

Increase Problem-Solving Skills and Alter Perceptions

Talking with a trusted colleague or friend is recognized by many as a strategy for looking at and altering one's perception of the stressor and/or one's available coping strategies, as well as a way to regulate one's affective response to stress. As Cooper and Crump (1978) state, personal control of the objective conditions can be regained—if lost through a lack of control over a stressor—"in subjective terms by incorporating a potentially threatening event into a cognitive plan, thereby reducing anxiety" (p. 422). This tends to lessen the stress response. Nurse managers must learn to recognize their need for such personal support when the need arises. Discussing sources of stress in the work environment with another nurse manager in whom one can confide aids in developing a realistic appraisal of the situation and may lead to the discovery of new coping strategies.

Cognitive options to alter perception of stressors and reduce stress reactions can be engaged in individually:

1. Distance yourself emotionally and/or physically from "stress carriers"
2. Separate your professional life from your personal life
3. Memorize and repeat affirmative sentences and positive thoughts
4. Attempt to reduce/eradicate self-defeating thoughts, substituting positive thoughts in their place

5. Without denying reality, focus and accentuate the positive elements of a job
6. Have a clear set of values and overall life goals with which to place stressors into their proper perspective

Sometimes, however, professional help is advisable. Greenwood and Greenwood (1979) identify four psychotherapeutic approaches "easily relatable to executive stress research" and which are claimed "to aid in reducing stress on the individual executive" (p. 196). These are transactional analysis, rational-emotive therapy (RET), reality therapy and assertive theapy. RET, especially, uncovers irrational ideas and can give insight into a manager's internal stressors.

Finally, the strategies of problem solving, decision making, idea generation, and logical analysis are useful in analyzing stressors, available coping skills, and stress reactions. These skills can be used by the nurse manager to define problems, to identify alternative coping strategies, to select the most appropriate strategy, and to evaluate the results after implementation.

Regulate Affective and Physiologic Responses

In addition to the strategies already mentioned, there are a number of additional strategies to regulate the affective and/or physiologic responses in order to reduce them to a level that preserves self-integrity.

Biofeedback is one example.

Basically, biofeedback is simply a process of monitoring one or more physiological functions of the human body with some type of instrumentation and translating the recorded activity into audio or visual signals (negative feedback) which are transmitted directly to the individual whose functions are being monitored. The theory is that the individual may, by observing these signals, learn to exercise some degree of control over the particular function being monitored. (Greenwood & Greenwood, 1979, p. 175)

Another stress-management strategy that is increasing in popularity is meditation, one example being transcendental meditation (TM). In TM, techniques are used to temporarily escape from logical mental processes. The person selects a quiet environment and separates self from thoughts by focusing on a secret word which is repeated. The eyes are closed and breathing is done in a slow, relaxed manner. In addition, to TM, there are the techniques of progressive relaxation, self-directed relaxation, and controlled breathing. Each of these strategies can be learned in order to cope with stressors and regulate their impact.

Engage in Other Adaptive Behaviors to Cope with Stressors

Any number of other strategies can be employed to cope with stressors. One may choose to:

1. Strengthen personal and professional skills and qualifications
2. Practice sound leadership, management, and supervision
3. Develop a network of professional colleagues, as well as a confidante
4. Take constructive action to eliminate the stressor
5. Enroll in courses on stress management

6. Utilize constructive outlets for emotions such as physical exercise, talking it out, and so forth
7. Take appropriate breaks at work
8. Utilize such strategies as conflict management, time management, constructive use of power-oriented behavior, planned change, and communication skills

BURNOUT

Continuous exposure to work environment stressors and other external or internal stressors, along with inadequate coping/adapting skills can lead to burnout (Patrick, 1979; Pines & Maslach, 1978). Burnout is manifested by emotional and physical exhaustion, increasing negative and critical attitudes towards the job, and an increasing sense of personal devaluation and low self-esteem. Burnout can be prevented by employing appropriate stress-management strategies. Burnout intervention and management approaches, in fact, utilize many of the same strategies. Patrick (1979) summarizes these approaches to deal with burnout:

1. Improve problem-solving and decision-making skills
2. Clarify values and set realistic personal goals
3. Develop coping strategies to deal with emotions
4. Employ assertive communication skills
5. Practice good health habits
6. Engage in regular exercise and recreational activities
7. Acquire relaxation skills
8. Practice meditation
9. Decrease stressors in the work environment

EVALUATION

The effectiveness of stress-management strategies is measured in terms of their impact on adaptive behavioral responses and a decrease in the negative outcome behavioral responses to stressors and stress in organizations. Tools to assess the stressor–person impact can again be administered. For example, have the number of personal indicators of stressors and stress in organizations been reduced after completing the outcome behavioral response checklist?

SUMMARY

Stress was defined in this chapter as the neurocognitive, affective, physiologic, and behavioral response arising from environmental and/or internal demands that tax or exceed the person's perceived or actual available adaptive resources. An open systems model of stress and adaptation was presented. Stressors that stem from a variety of internal and external sources were identified. Sample assessment tools were identified and one tool was included. Finally, a variety of stress adapting/coping strategies were described.

REFERENCES

Anderson, C., & Basteyns, M. Stress and the critical care nurse reaffirmed. *The Journal of Nursing Administration*, 1981, *11*(1), 31–34.

Bailey, J. Stress and stress management: An overview. *Journal of Nursing Education*, 1980, *19*(6), 5–7.

Bailey, J., Steffen, S., & Grout, J. The stress audit: Identifying the stressors of ICU nursing. *Journal of Nursing Education*, 1980, *19*(6), 15–25.

Barash, D. Organizational stress in nursing. *Kansas Nurse*, March 1980, *55*, 6–8.

Beehr, T., & Newman, J. Job stress, employee health, and organizational effectiveness: A facet analysis, model, and literature review. *Personnel Psychology*, 1978, *31* 665–699.

Behling, O., & Holcombe, F. Dealing with employee stress. *MSU Business Topics*, 1981, *29*, 53–61.

Blau, G. An empirical investigation of job stress, social support, service length, and job strain. *Organizational Behavior and Human Performance*, 1981, *27*, 279–302.

Brief, A. How to manage managerial stress. *Personnel*, 1980, *57*, 25–30.

Buckalew, M., & Gahan, N. *Learning to control stress*. New York: Richards Rosen, 1979.

Bullard, P. *Coping with stress: A psychological survival manual*. Portland, Oregon: Pro Seminar, 1980.

Cohen, H., & Orlinsky, N. Work stress on critical care units. *Emergency Medical Services*, 1977, *6*, 27–28, 30–31.

Cooper, C., & Crump, J. Prevention and coping with occupational stress. *Journal of Occupational Medicine*, 1978, *20*(6), 420–426.

Cooper, C., & Melhuish, A. Occupational stress and managers. *Journal of Occupational Medicine*, 1980, *22*(9), 588–592.

Davidson, M., Cooper, C., & Chamberlain, D. Type A coronary-prone behavior and stress in senior female managers and administrators. *Journal of Occupational Medicine*, 1980, *22*(12), 801–805.

de Board, R. The anxious organization. *Management Today*, 1978, 58–61; 114.

de Vries, M. Organizational stress: A call for management action. *Sloan Management Review*, 1979, *21*, 3–14.

Douglass, M. Stress and personal performance. *The Personnel Administrator*, 1977, *22*, 60–63.

Duemer, W., Walker, N., & Quick, J. Improving work life through effective performance planning. *The Personnel Administrator*, 1978, *23*, 23–26.

Friedman, M., & Rosenman, R. *Type A behavior and your heart*. Greenwich, Conn.: Fawcett, 1974.

Friel, M., & Tehan, C. Counteracting burn-out for the hospice care-giver. *Cancer Nursing*, 1980, *3*(4), 285–293.

Giammatteo, M., & Giammatteo, H. *Executive well-being: Stress and administrators*. Reston, Va.: National Association of Secondary School Principals, 1980.

Goldberg, P. *Executive health: How to recognize health danger signals and manage stress successfully*. New York: McGraw-Hill, 1978.

Goodell, A. Responses of nurses to the stresses of caring for pediatric oncology patients. *Issues in Comprehensive Pediatric Nursing*, 1980, *4*, 1–6.

Goosen, G., & Bush, H. Adaptation: A feedback process. *Advances in Nursing Science*, 1979, *1*(4), 51–65.

Greenberg, S., & Valletutti, P. *Stress and the helping professions*. Baltimore: Paul H. Brooks, 1980.

Greenwood, J., & Greenwood, J. *Managing executive stress: A systems approach*. New York: Wiley, 1979.

Hartl, D. Stress management and the nurse. *Advances in Nursing Science*, 1979, *1*(4), 91–100.

Holmes, T., & Rahe, R. The social readjustment rating scale. *Journal of Psychosomatic Research*, 1967, *2*, 213–218.

Howard, J. The Type A manager. *Management Today*, 1977, 87–88; 134.

Humphrey, R. Are you a stress carrier? *Training and Development Journal*, 1978, *32*, 38–41.

Izard, C. Emotions in personality and psychopathology: An introduction. In C. Izard (Ed.), *Emotions in personality and psychopathology*. New York: Plenum, 1979.

Jacobson, S. Stressful situations for neonatal intensive care nurses. *American Journal of Maternal Child Nursing*, 1978, *3*, 144–150.

Johnson, J., & Sarason, I. In V. Hamilton & D. Warburton (Eds.), *Human stress and cognition*. New York: Wiley, 1979.

Keenan, A., & McBain, G. Effects of Type A behaviour, intolerance of ambiguity, and locus of control on the relationship between role stress and work-related outcomes. *Journal of Occupational Psychology*, 1979, *52*, 277–285.

Kiev, A., & Kohn, V. *Executive stress*. New York: AMACOM, 1979.

Manuso, J. Executive stress management. *The Personnel Administrator*, 1979, *24*, 23–26.

McFarland, G., & Wasli, E. Psychiatric nursing. In L. Brunner & D. Suddarth. *The Lippincott manual of nursing practice*. Philadelphia: Lippincott, 1982.

Mickel, F. Stress: Race to the bottom line. *Management Accounting*, 1981, *62*, 15–20.

Parasuraman, S., & Alutto, J. An examination of the organizational antecedents of stressors at work. *Academy of Management Journal*, 1981, *24*(1), 48–67.

Patrick, P. Burnout: Job hazards for health workers. *Hospitals*, 1979, *53*(22), 87–90.

Pines, A., & Maslach, C. Characteristics of staff burnout in mental health settings. *Hospital and Community Psychiatry*, 1978, *29*(4), 233–237.

Preston, C., Ivancevich, J., & Matteson, M. Stress and the OR nurse. *AORN Journal*, 1981, *33*(4), 662–671.

Schmidt, W. Basic concepts of organizational stress—Causes and problems. In *Proceedings of occupational stress conference, Los Angeles, November 3, 1977*. Washington, D.C.: U.S. Government Printing Office, 1978.

Schuler, R. Definition and conceptualization of stress in organizations. *Organizational Behavior and Human Performance*, 1980, *25*, 184–215.

Schwartz, G. Stress management in occupational settings. *Public Health Reports*, 1980, *95*(2), 99–108.

Scott, D., Oberst, M., & Dropkin, M. A stress-coping model. *Advances in Nursing Science*, 1980, *3*, 9–23.

Selverston, H. Stress. *Critical Care Update*, 1980, *7*, 28–29.

Selye, H. *Stress in health and disease*. Boston: Butterworth, 1976.

Tardy, W. Ways to cope with stress in your working environment. *Black Enterprise*, 1977, *8*, 39–42; 44.

Willis, R. Options in managing stress. *Pediatric Nursing*, 1979, *5*, 24–27.

Yates, J. *Managing stress*. New York: AMACOM, 1979.

BIBLIOGRAPHY

Adams, J. *Understanding and managing stress: A book of readings*. San Diego: University Associates, 1980.

Alexander, C. Counteracting burnout. *AORN Journal*, 1980, *32*(4), 597–604.

Allen, R., & Kraft, C. From burn-out to turn-out. *Hospital Forum*, 1981, *24*, 18–20; 23–24; 27–28.

Anderson, C., Hellriegel, D., & Slocum, J. Managerial response to environmentally induced stress. *Academy of Management Journal*, 1977, *20*(2), 260–272.

Antonovsky, A. *Health, stress, and coping*. San Francisco: Jossey-Bass, 1979.

Asken, M. Psychological stress in ICU affects both patients, staff. *Pennsylvania Medicine*, 1979, *82*, 40–42.

Bailey, J., Walker, D., & Madsen, N. The design of a stress management program for Stanford intensive care nurses. *Journal of Nursing Education*, 1980, *19*(6), 26–29.

Baldwin, A., & Bailey, J. Work-site interventions for stress reduction. *Journal of Nursing Education*, 1980, *19*(6), 48–53.

Barstow, J. Stress variance in hospital nursing. *Nursing Outlook*, 1980, *28*(12), 751–754.

Benson, H., & Allen, R. How much stress is too much? *Harvard Business Review*, 1980, *58*, 86–92.

Berg, M. Tune in, turn on, drop out? A look at burnout. *Imprint*, 1980, *27*, 11–12; 24–25.

Blake, R., & Mouton, J. *Grid approaches to managing stress*. Springfield: Charles C Thomas, 1980.

Borland, J. Burnout among workers and administrators. *Health and Social Work*, 1981, *6*, 73–78.

Bright, D. *Creative relaxation: Turning your stress into positive energy*. New York: Harcourt Brace Jovanovich, 1979.

Brosnan, J., & Johnston, M. Stressed but satisfied: Organizational change in ambulatory care. *Journal of Nursing Administration*, 1980, *10*(11), 43–48.

Brown, B. *Stress and the art of biofeedback*. New York: Harper & Row, 1977.

Burnout: Beyond executive stress. *Management Review*, 1981, *70*, 4–5.

Calhoun, G. Hospitals are high-stress employers. *Hospitals*, 1980, *54*(12), 171–176.

Clark, C. Burnout: Assessment and intervention. *Journal of Nursing Administration*, 1980, *10*(9), 39–43.

Cook, R. Helping critical care nurses with work-related stress. *Critical Care Update*, 1980, *7*, 32–35.

Donnelly, G. "Relax? That's easy for you to say!" *RN*, 1980, *43*(6), 34; 75–78.

Donnelly, G. "Stop driving yourself crazy!" *RN*, 1981, *44*(2), 55; 100–104.

Donnelly, G. Why you "just can't take it anymore!" *RN*, 1980, *43*(5), 34; 36–37.

Donovan, M. Study of the impact of relaxation with guided imagery on stress among cancer nurses. *Cancer Nursing*, 1981, *4*, 121–126.

Dornstein, M. Organizational conflict and role stress among chief executives in state business enterprises. *Journal of Occupational Psychology*, 1977, *50*, 253–263.

Fly, R. Why rotating shifts sharply reduce productivity. *Supervisory Management*, 1980, *25*, 16–21.

Forbes, R. *Corporate stress*. Garden City, N.Y.: Doubleday, 1979.

Francis, B. A nursing network to battle burnout. *The Journal of Practical Nursing*, 1980, *30*(11), 25–27.

Garbin, M. Conceptualizations of stress and adaptation. *Advances in Nursing Science*, 1979, *1*(4), 101–104.

Gmelch, W. Stress: Management's twentieth-century dilemma. *Supervisory Management*, 1978, *23*, 30–36.

Greenberg, H. *Coping with job stress*. Englewood Cliffs, N.J.: Prentice-Hall, 1980.

Grout, J. Occupational stress of intensive care nurses and air traffic controllers: Review of related studies. *Journal of Nursing Education*, 1980, *19*(6), 8+.

Hamilton, V., & Warburton, D. *Human stress and cognition: An information processing approach*. New York: Wiley, 1979.

Hefferin, E. Life-cycle stressors: An overview of research. *Family Community Health*, 1980, *2*, 71–101.

Hover, W. Emotional stress and how to respond. *Occupational Health Nursing*, 1979, *27*, 14–16.

How companies cope with executive stress. *Business Week*, August 21, 1978, 107–108.

Huckabay, L., & Jagla, B. Nurses' stress factors in the Intensive Care Unit. *Journal of Nursing Administration*, 1979, *9*(2), 21–26.

Jacobson, E. *You must relax*. London: Souvenir, 1977.

Johnson, J. More about stress and some management techniques. *Journal of School Health*, 1981, *51*, 36–42.

Johnston, R. The holistic experience of stress: Opportunity for growth or illness. *Occupational Health Nursing*, 1980, *28*, 15–18.

Keelan, J. Nine tips for beating stress. *AORN Journal*, 1979, *30*(1), 138–148.

Kjervik, D., & Martinson, I. *Women in stress: A nursing perspective*. New York: Appleton-Century-Crofts, 1979.

Kövecses, J. Burnout doesn't have to happen. *Nursing '80*, 1980, *10*, 105+.

Kutash, I., & Schlesinger, L. *Handbook on stress and anxiety*. San Francisco: Jossey-Bass, 1980.

La Grand, L. Reducing burnout in the hospice and the death education movement. *Death Education*, 1980, *4*, 61–75.

Latack, J. Person/role conflict: Holland's model extended to role-stress research, stress management, and career development. *Academy of Management Review*, 1981, *6*(1), 89–103.

Lecker, S. *The natural way to stress control*. New York: Grosset & Dunlap, 1978.

Lenhart, R. Faculty burnout—And some reasons why. *Nursing Outlook*, 1980, *28*(7), 424–425.

Levinson, H. When executives burnout. *Harvard Business Review*, 1981, *59*, 73–81.

Little, J. Stress during the human life-cycle. *Health Visitor*, 1980, *53*, 373; 376.

Madders, J. *Stress and relaxation*. New York: Arco, 1979.

Marshall, R., & Kasman, C. Burnout in the neonatal intensive care unit. *Pediatrics*, 1980, *65*(6), 1161–1165.

McConnell, E. How close are you to burnout? *RN*, 1981, *44*(5), 29–33.

McGaffey, T. New horizons in organizational stress prevention approaches. *The Personnel Administrator*, 1978, *23*, 26–32.

McLean, A. *Work stress*. Reading, Mass.: Addison-Wesley, 1979.

Melhuish, A., & Cooper, C. The stresses that make managers ill. *International Management*, 1980, *35*, 51; 55.

Morano, R. How to manage change to reduce stress. *Management Review*, 1977, *66*, 21–25.

Nelson, J. Burnout—Business's most costly expense. *Personnel Administrator*, 1980, *25*, 81–87.

Newman, J., & Beehr, T. Personal and organizational strategies for handling job stress: A review of research and opinion. *Personnel Psychology*, 1979, *32*, 1–43.

Odiorne, G. Executives under siege: Strategies for survival. *Management Review*, 1978, *67*, 7–13.

Page, J. Burnout: The most probable causes and the most likely solutions. *EMT Journal*, 1980, *4*, 52–54.

Pendleton, B. Coping with managerial stress. *Management World*, 1981, *10*, 25–27.

Potter, E., & Fiedler, F. The utilization of staff member intelligence and experience under high and low stress. *Academy of Management Journal*, 1981, *24*(2), 361–376.

Pritchard, M., & Proudfoot, M. An introduction to stress management: Theory and practice. *Washington State Journal of Nursing*, 1980, *52*, 14–18.

Rader, M. Dealing with information overload. *Personnel Journal*, 1981, *60*, 373–375.

Ross, A. Managing executive stress and other related subjects. *Journal of Ambulatory Care Management*, 1980, *3*(4), 1–10.

Rummel, R. Coping with executive stress. *Personnel Journal*, 1978, *57*, 305–307; 332–334; 336.

Sanders, M. Stressed? Or burnt out? *The Canadian Nurse*, 1980, *76*(9), 30–33.

Schwettman, J., Shepard, J., & Sampson, K. Hassle management workshop. *EMT Journal*, 1980, *4*, 49–50.

Scully, R. Stress in the nurse. *American Journal of Nursing*, 1980, *80*(5), 912–918.

Selye, H. *The stress of life*. New York: McGraw-Hill, 1976.

Sethi, A. Using meditation in stress situations. *Dimensions in Health Service*, 1980, *57*, 24–26.

Shubin, S. Burnout: The professional hazard you face in nursing. *Nursing '78*, 1978, *8*, 22–27.

Skinner, K. Support group for ICU nurses. *Nursing Outlook*, 1980, *28*(5), 296–299.

Smith, M., & Selye, H. Reducing the negative effects of stress. *American Journal of Nursing*, 1979, *79*(10), 1953–1964.

Speich, P. Taking a psychosocial stress "pulse." *Journal of Emergency Nursing*, 1979, *5*, 43–47.

Stillman, S., & Strasser, B. Helping critical care nurses with work-related stress. *The Journal of Nursing Administration*, 1980, *10*(1), 28–31.

Storlie, F. Burnout: The elaboration of a concept. *American Journal of Nursing*, 1979, *79*(1), 2108–2111.

Swagger, G. Toward understanding stress: A map of the territory. *Journal of School Health*, 1981, *51*, 29–35.

Tillman, K., & Feinman, J. Stress reduction through movement. *Point of View*, 1981, *18*, 4–7.

Troxler, R., & Cook, R. Synergy: A technique for managing stress. *Critical Care Update*, 1980, *7*, 34–37.

Warrick, D. Managing the stress of organizational development. *Training and Development Journal*, 1981, *35*, 37–41.

Zindler-Wernet, P. Coping with stress through an "on-site" running program for Stanford ICU nurses. *Journal of Nursing Education*, 1980, *19*(6), 34–37.

Zindler-Wernet, P., Bailey, J., Walker, D., & Holzemer, W. Personalogical measures to assess program effects: A case study. *Journal of Nursing Education*, 1980, *19*(6), 38–42.

CHAPTER 21
CONFLICT AND
CONFLICT MANAGEMENT

Nurse leaders and nurse managers find themselves functioning in a rapidly changing, and at times turbulent, health care and academic environment. Economic pressures and scarcity of resources pit individuals and groups against each other in their quest for adequate resources. External regulatory agencies and other groups apply their own unique pressures. The legal profession, with its increasing interest in health care litigation, is an example. As a result, far-reaching changes have already occurred in the health care arena.

The knowledge explosion along with rapidly changing technology has led to ever-increasing specialization. This in turn has led to the introduction of more professionals and paraprofessionals, each with their own set of values, goals, and expertise. The result is increasing interprofessional interfacing and intersection, along with potential conflict.

Within the nursing profession itself, clear differentiation among the various levels of nursing personnel, especially in the work environment, does not yet exist. In addition, the number of nursing specialties is increasing. The result is intraprofessional inter-facing and intersection, role ambiguity, role confusion, and potential conflict.

Nurses themselves are changing in their new expression of assertiveness. They are becoming more actively involved in bringing about change for themselves and their patients. In addition, other forces are producing change for the nursing profession (see chapter 22—The Future: Forces, Issues, and Trends). Such a changing and turbulent environment is a conflict producing environment.

CONFLICT: A CHANGING CONCEPT

There are three categories of conflict: intrapersonal, interpersonal, and intergroup (Lewis, 1976). *Intrapersonal conflict* refers to discord occurring within a person. It is a struggle among incompatible or differing values, beliefs, allegiances, or choices. *Interpersonal conflict* arises between two or more people, while *intergroup conflict* refers to discord between two or more groups of people, departments, or organizations. Inter-personal or intergroup conflict is the "expressed struggle between at least two inter-dependent parties, who perceive incompatible goals, scarce rewards, and interference from the other party in achieving their goals. They are in a position of opposition in conjunction with cooperation" (Frost & Wilmot, 1978, p. 9). In interpersonal conflict, "parties" refers to two or more people. In intergroup conflict, "parties" refers to two or more *groups* of people, departments, or organizations.

Intrapersonal Conflict

Values, beliefs, sentiments, motives, assumptions, and perceptions certainly do affect a person's behavior including one's interpersonal interactions, such as how one deals with interpersonal or intergroup conflict. Intrapersonal conflict, however, "relates to discord within an individual" (Lewis, 1976, p. 19). It is conflict originating from within the person and remains an internal struggle. Reality shock, a conflict between school-bred professional values and work-world bureaucratic values, is an intrapersonal conflict frequently occurring in new graduates (Kramer, 1974; Schmalenberg & Kramer, 1979). The new nurse graduate possesses and prizes such beliefs and values as comprehensive, individualized patient care; the whole-task system of work; functioning autonomously; utilizing professional judgment and decision-making skills; and basing nursing interventions on scientific knowledge. The work setting, on the other hand, often approaches patient care through functional assignments or a part task system of work organization. Such bureaucratic values as efficiency, organization, cost-effectiveness, cooperation, and responsibility are stressed.

These two different value sets can lead to intrapersonal conflict in the new nurse graduate. This source of intrapersonal conflict may decrease, however, for future nurse graduates as (a) nursing schools increase their efforts to help nurse graduates cope with this potential conflict; and (b) health care settings move toward a whole-task system of care, for example, primary care nursing in hospitals.

Intrapersonal conflict occurs in ethical, as well as in other dilemmas, faced by many nurse leaders and managers today. Smith and Davis (1980) identify *five* types of intrapersonal conflict faced by nurses in ethical dilemmas. Other kinds of intrapersonal conflict can be categorized using this five-category scheme.

The *first type* is an intrapersonal conflict which involves a conflict between two ethical principles in which the nurse leader believes. For example, the head nurse on a psychiatric unit must provide leadership for the provision of quality care to psychiatric patients, many of whom have a history of criminal behavior. The head nurse experiences intrapersonal conflict, because crime is perceived as unethical behavior. At the same time, this head nurse holds the ethical professional conviction of providing quality care to all patients, regardless of their choice of lifestyle, through leadership and management skills.

In a second example, a nurse faculty coordinator's role is affected by the ethical dilemmas experienced by nursing students. An increased religious consciousness in a nursing student can create an intrapersonal conflict between the student's values and the humanist values inherent in psychiatric mental health treatment approaches (Slimmer, 1980). In this example, the faculty coordinator's assistance and expertise is sought by a newly employed nurse faculty member who must assist such a student to deal with this intrapersonal conflict while at the same time facilitating the student's ability to empathize effectively.

Similar intrapersonal conflicts between two sets of beliefs occur in dilemmas other than ethical ones. A nursing coordinator, for instance, believes very strongly in the inherent potential of the nursing staff. Much time and effort has been spent by this coordinator in assisting a particular staff nurse cope with the nursing role. The assistant director of nursing, the coordinator's supervisor, has now suggested that the employment of this staff nurse be terminated. Over time, the nurse coordinator has come to value and trust the assistant director's judgment and expertise. The nurse coordinator is now experiencing intrapersonal conflict stemming from a personal belief in human potential, while at the same time valuing the supervisor's expertise and viewpoints.

The *second type* of intrapersonal conflict involved in ethical dilemmas is the conflict that stems from the need to make a decision and take action based on inconclusive data both *for* and *against* taking that action. This type of intrapersonal conflict also occurs in other than ethical dilemmas. For example, a head nurse in agency A has been offered the position of department clinical manager in Agency B. The head nurse finds that data are favorable, but not conclusive, for accepting the position. On the other hand, the head nurse is satisfied with agency A and there is evidence, although not conclusive, that a promotion opportunity may exist in agency A. Because of the inconclusive reasons for either accepting, or not accepting, the job offer, the head nurse begins to experience intrapersonal conflict.

The *third type* of intrapersonal conflict stems from the need to take immediate action and the need to reflect before taking that action, because the nurse has had insufficient preparation for the situation. Mr. Johnson, a nurse, has just accepted his first nursing supervisory position in a large nursing home in which he has never worked before. During his first week in this position, two nursing assistants report to him that Mr. Jones, also a nursing assistant, has been drinking whiskey and request that Mr. Johnson, their supervisor, talk to Mr. Jones immediately. Mr. Johnson is not yet familiar with the informal structure in the new agency, however, he has observed behavior among the nursing assistants that appears indicative of scapegoating Mr. Jones. Mr. Johnson is not certain, though, because he does not have enough data.

Mr. Johnson has never encountered a similar request from nursing staff before. He experiences intrapersonal conflict, as there is the desire and need to explore the employees' request. Yet, on the other hand, not knowing enough about the actual interpersonal group dynamics among the nursing assistants, the request by the two nursing assistants may be a ploy to undermine Mr. Jones. Immediate action is difficult, given the conflicting nature of the situation.

The *fourth type* of intrapersonal conflict is one between two alternative causes of action that are equally unsatisfactory. A clinical coordinator has implemented primary care nursing some time ago on the clinical units. A number of the primary care nurses has moved out of the geographical area with their families. As a result, a severe shortage of qualified registered nurses exists on the units. There is a general shortage of registered nurses in this geographical area making recruitment very difficult. The shortage of qualified registered nurses is jeopardizing the continuation of primary care nursing, while a sufficient supply of nursing assistants and licensed practical nurses would support a return to a functional assignment of clinical care responsibilities. The clinical coordinator does not want to continue primary care nursing under the present conditions, but, neither does the coordinator want to return to a functional assignment pattern on the clinical unit. As a result, the coordinator experiences intrapersonal conflict.

The *fifth type* of intrapersonal conflict is one existing between the nurse's own ethical beliefs and the requirements of the position. A similar type of intrapersonal conflict, which has been described previously, occurs in a nurse, who adhering to professional values about nursing care, is in conflict because of the bureaucratic demands of the nursing position. This type of intrapersonal conflict can also occur in the nurse manager who believes in a democratic approach to leadership while being confronted by demands for an authoritarian approach by a very rigid and highly controlled nursing service organization.

Intervening in Intrapersonal Conflicts

The process of structuring an ethical dilemma involves the exploration of three elements—data base or situational facts, decision making, and underlying ethical theories (Aroskar, 1980). In seeking clarification of the situational facts, the nurse manager/supervisor should raise questions about the proposed and alternative actions, purpose, and consequences of these actions, the context of the situation, and the actors involved. Under the decision-making element, she or he should ask about who ought to decide, what the bases for selecting a given course of action are, and what ethical values are enhanced or diminished by the decision. In the third element—underlying ethical theories—she or he should determine which ethical position is being utilized.

The nurse manager can utilize the process of structuring ethical dilemmas that are being *personally* experienced to resolve the related intrapersonal conflict. This three-step structuring process can also be utilized by the nurse manager in assisting a staff nurse who faces an ethical dilemma and experiences related intrapersonal conflict. The expected result of this exploration of situational facts, decision questions, and ethical theories, is the clarification of the ethical dilemma, the management of the intrapersonal conflict, and the selection of a sound decision and course of action.

An adaptation of this three-step process of analysis appears to be applicable to the management of intrapersonal conflicts. In step 1, determine the actor or actors involved and their past involvement in the situation. Clarify the action, alternatives, and consequences. In the example above, Mr. Johnson, the new nursing supervisor in the nursing home, utilizes this part of the process when he seeks to clarify his own experienced intrapersonal conflict. Who are the actors in the situation? What does he know about the past involvement of the two nursing assistants with Mr. Jones? What is the ward "culture" really like among the nursing staff? What is the motivation of the nursing assistants making the proposed request? What are the consequences for Mr. Johnson, himself, for the nursing assistants, and, for Mr. Jones, if the decision is made to confront Mr. Jones immediately? What other alternative actions are possible?

In step 2, ask decision-making questions. Mr. Johnson queries himself as to who should really decide on the immediacy and type of action needed. What management principles or other facts should he use to make the decision? What principles of management would be supported or negated with a given course of action?

In step 3, articulate the underlying values, beliefs, and goals inherent in the situation. What are Mr. Johnson's goals, beliefs, and values relevant to the situation described? Is it important for him to be well liked by his employees? Is his ultimate goal quality nursing care delivered by a motivated, well-functioning work team?

Mr. Johnson reasons through these steps, albeit somewhat quickly, given the nature of the situation and request. Being aware of the possibility of scapegoating as a motive, Mr. Johnson makes the decision to tell the nursing assistants that he is deeply concerned with the optimal performance of every member on his work team, including that of Mr. Jones. He tells them that he will observe the situation and determine what is happening to Mr. Jones or to any other staff member appearing to experience difficulties. Mr. Johnson then proceeds to observe Mr. Jones, as well as other nursing staff members, in their delivery of patient care services, as part of his ordinary supervisory responsibilities. In this manner he can determine the facts in the situation and can make certain that safe patient care is delivered. Thus, the action taken was that of not meeting the direct requests of the nursing assistants to confront Mr. Jones, but rather to delay such an action until more concrete factual data are available.

While many intrapersonal conflicts may be resolved by traditional rational means, such as suggested by Aroskar (1980), other intrapersonal conflicts have strong emotional aspects that defy traditional rational analysis. The task of intrapersonal conflict resolution would be far easier if we only had a left cerebral hemisphere.

Interpersonal and Intergroup Conflict

Interpersonal or intergroup conflict is the

> expressed struggle between at least two interdependent parties, who perceive incompatible goals, scarce rewards, and interference from the other party in achieving their goals. They are in a position of opposition in conjunction with cooperation. (Frost & Wilmot, 1978, p. 9)

The parties may also perceive an incompatibility in methods of goal achievement. In interpersonal conflict, "parties" refers to two or more *people*. In intergroup conflict, "parties" refers to two or more *groups* of people, departments, or organizations.

Intrapersonal conflict, or an internal struggle within the person, has been described. Intrapersonal conflict may occur at the same time that an *interpersonal* or *intergroup* conflict is taking place. A major differentiation is that interpersonal or intergroup conflict is an *expressed* struggle between at least *two* parties. Interpersonal or intergroup conflict is

> communicative behavior; it is impossible to have conflict without either verbal or nonverbal behavior, or both. The "expression" may be very subtle, but it must be present for the activity to be interpersonal conflict. (Frost & Wilmot, 1978, p. 10)

Interdependence, in various degrees, exists in all interpersonal or intergroup conflict. The conflict occurs precisely *because* there is a degree of interdependence, that is, the decisions made by one party impact on the decisions made by the other party or parties. Conflict cannot occur between or among parties who do not interact in any way, who do not have any common interests or related goals, or who do not share access to, or have an interest in, common resources. For example, staff nurses and nurse supervisor/managers interact frequently, have similar goals (e.g., to provide quality patient care), and share an interest in common resources (e.g., the budget available for staff development). Conflicts between the two groups—employees and management—can readily occur. On the other hand, staff nurses working in a hospital, and staff engineers working on aircraft design in an aerospace company, generally do not interact professionally, nor do they share common goals, or access to similar resources.

The nature of interdependence and the degree of interdependence between parties in a conflict varies. Sometimes the interdependence is because of the party's own choice. Sometimes the interdependence is forced. The *degree* of interdependence varies in conflicts depending on how the parties perceive it. However, the parties involved in interpersonal or intergroup conflict are all interdependent to some degree.

> Their perceptions of the interdependence affects the choices they make. They will decide whether they are acting as (1) *relatively independent agents* or (2) relatively interdependent agents. . . . In all conflicts . . . interdependence carries elements of cooperation and elements of competition. (Frost & Wilmot, 1978, p.13)

Some goals between parties involved in a conflict are truly incompatible, even if higher-order goals are considered. Oftentimes however, the incompatibiliy of goals among conflicting parties is a *perceived* conflict. Although subgoals may appear to be incompatible, overall goals or higher-order goals held by the parties involved in the conflict may be actually, or at least partially, compatible.

The parties in an interpersonal or intergroup conflict may perceive or actually experience a scarcity of rewards or of resources. These rewards or resources can be economic (e.g., money), physical (e.g., space), or social (e.g., power). In "interpersonal conflicts, regardless of the content issue involved, the parties usually perceive a shortage of power and/or self esteem rewards. And, the key is the perception of the scarcity" (Frost & Wilmot, 178, p. 12).

Source of Interpersonal and Intergroup Conflict

Sources of interpersonal or intergroup conflict for nurse managers or leaders in service or academic settings can be categorized into four broad areas: (a) perceived or actual incompatibility of goals; (b) perceived or actual interference from the other party in achieving the goals; (c) perceived or actual incompatibility of methods of goal achievement; and (d) perceived or actual scarcity of resources or rewards.

Certain conditions existing within a social system are conducive to the development of interpersonal or intergroup conflict. Goldsmith (1977) documents a number of these: (a) when nurses in an organization violate confidentiality, lowering trust among work group members, and setting members against one another; (b) when nurse managers and supervisors do not use consistent and rational policies for selection, termination, evaluation, and promotion of their nursing staff or faculty; (c) when necessary information, useful in the achievement of system or subsystem goals, is withheld or deliberately distorted; (d) when change is unplanned or improperly conducted, especially when the "costs" of the change is unequally distributed among individuals or among groups; (e) when there are no approved methods in an organization for nursing staff or faculty to influence their work environment or to have input into the decision-making process; (f) when the nurse manager, leader, or supervisor feels no responsibility in serving as a "role model" for expected group member behaviors, for example, managing conflict, making decisions, or collaborating with each other; and (g) when the "lid" is kept on the expression of feelings, such as anger, and employees are prevented from resolving their differences.

Additional conditions in social systems that are conducive to conflict development occur when system or subsystem goals are not clearly delineated, when individuals or groups interfere with each other's efforts at goal attainment, when one party's methods of goal attainment encroaches upon the territory of another party, or when resources to achieve goals or consequential rewards for goal attainment are very scarce. Eldridge (1979) states that when perceived or actual relative deprivation (a discrepancy between what a particular group feels that they deserve and what they actually obtain in rewards and resources) exists between groups, intergroup conflict can occur. There is also some evidence to suggest that work-group solidarity and cohesiveness can be a source of intergroup conflict. On the other hand, work-group cohesiveness can be potentiated through experienced intergroup conflict (Eldridge, 1979).

Other sources of interpersonal or intergroup conflict for nurse managers and leaders in academic or service settings have been identified. Specialization has grown rapidly in the health service delivery arena. Specialization accentuates differences between groups of people in preparation, expertise, areas of interest, and territorial claims (Sexton, 1980). Yet, since specialists are interdependent with other groups of specialists, and with generalists, there is the potential for interpersonal and intergroup conflict.

Kalisch and Kalisch (1977) provide an excellent analysis of the sources of conflict between physicians and nurses. Conflict can occur because physicians believe that they have a right to intervene in, or control, the independent aspects of professional nursing. Nurses also resent the often nonsupportive attitude from physicians regarding advanced education for nurses. Indeed, the different levels of nurse preparation is confusing to physicians. Unfortunately, nurses prepared at the doctoral level, as well as those with the most experience, are generally not found collaborating with physicians in the provision of *direct* patient care. Nurses and physicians bring different educational backgrounds, perspectives, and values, to the health care arena. Frequently, the two groups have difficulty in comprehending the other group's viewpoints. Physician dominance and devaluation of nursing also leads to conflict. Many physicians still view the nurse in a handmaiden role and place minimal value on the nurses' contribution to health care through their independent role components.

Indeed Hite (1977) predicts an irrepressible conflict between nurses and physicians. While the autonomy and dominance of the physician are beginning to shrink somewhat, nurses are seeking expanded roles. Nurses are requesting more responsibility and authority, desiring and seeking more education, desiring to formulate nursing diagnoses, and wanting a larger voice in the decision-making process. Hite views the inevitability of conflict as stemming "from the tendency of humans to assume that because roles are intertwined there is an automatic sequence: if one gains, it will be at the expense of the other" (1977, p. 15).

Another major source of conflict is dysfunctional communication. When two or more individuals or groups do not transmit and receive verbal and nonverbal messages clearly, without distortion, then the potential for conflict exists. Perceptual differences and distortions can likewise generate conflict.

Organizational size and structure can generate conflict. An increase in size increases the *number* of interactions between groups and individuals that become necessary, thus making conflict possible. Increase in size also places physical distance between groups or departments that must work closely together, thus increasing the chance for misunderstandings.

Additionally, conflict can arise from an organizational structure in which the director of nursing and the nursing staff receive directives from both the hospital administrator and the physician or department of medicine. Other sources of conflict stemming from organizational structure are inadequate and rigid channels of communication, inconsistent reward systems, and adherence to rigid and outmoded policies and procedures.

Personality differences between individuals can be a source of conflict. Differences in the desire for control, affection, and inclusion, as well as the mode of expression of these needs, can be a potential source of conflict (Schutz, 1967). Conflict can also readily occur between a team and nurse manager during the counterdependent stage of maturation of the team.

Conflicts between nursing faculty members often result from differences in philosophy and conceptual frameworks, differences in values, personality clashes, and problems in communication (O'Connor, 1978). The diversity of the nursing student population with the need for individualization of instruction, the evaluation process, the tendency of nursing students to challenge the instructor, and the teaching–learning process can all lead to interpersonal conflicts between students and nursing faculty. Finally, many sources of conflict exist between nurse faculty and administration (nurse faculty coordinators, assistant deans, deans). Among these sources are scarce and/or inequitable distribution of resources, misuse of power, as well as differences in perception of performance evaluations, goals, means to achieve goals, assignment of responsibilities, and desired rewards including salary.

Indeed, O'Connor (1978) maintains that "faculty members in schools of nursing are continually involved in conflict situations" (p. 35). Rakich, Longest, and O'Donovan (1977) contend that the management of organizational conflict is one of the primary problems confronting hospitals. Myrtle and Glogow (1978) state that, "conflict is one of the most prevalent issues facing nursing administrators today" (p. 103). Furthermore, Fenn (1977) makes this observation:

> The conflicts for nursing administration are weighty. They arise from increasing government regulations, proliferating external organizations, changing values, internal realignments, power-base struggles, changes in institutional philosophy, instability in physician-agency relationships, and racism and sexism. (p. 17).

Leininger (1975) believes that effective conflict management is dependent on the expertise and skills of nursing managers. Finally, Kleiner (1978) refers to a study in which middle managers were found to spend 25% of their time and effort managing conflict, while it is speculated that first-line supervisors spend 30% of their time in the management of conflict. Such research indicates that conflict management skills are important to the nurse leader, manager, and supervisor.

Evolving Views of Conflict

The earliest view of conflict was the traditionalist philosophy which continued into the mid-1940s. The behavioral philosophy dominated the latter 1940s and the early 1950s. The period from the late 1950s to the present time is marked by the interactionist philosophy (Lewis, 1976; Robbins, 1978). The hallmark of the traditionalists was that conflict was viewed as destructive and abnormal, while harmony was seen as normal. Therefore, it was thought that conflict should be eliminated. The nurse manager's role in this era would have been to rid the individual, group, or larger social system of any conflict, perhaps through avoiding it, by keeping the lid on any conflict-related behaviors, or at best, by resolving it.

The traditionalists gave way to the behavioralists. The behavioralists softened the stance toward conflict, by recognizing and rationalizing its existence. Social systems were viewed as experiencing built-in conflict, so acceptance of conflict was heavily emphasized by these scholars. Emphasis remained on resolution, however. Therefore, conflict-resolution techniques were developed to achieve the *resolution* of conflict which was the desired outcome. Nursing managers, operating under this perspective, identified and recognized conflict among their nursing staff. Their approach to conflict was the use of intervention strategies to resolve it.

The current philosophy of conflict is the interactionist philosophy. The interactionist approach

> recognizes the absolute necessity of conflict, explicitly encourages opposition, defines conflict management to include stimulation as well as resolution, and considers the management of conflict as a major responsibility of all administrators. (Robbins, 1974, pp. 13–14.)

According to the interactionists, the input, throughput, output, and feedback process within a social system becomes most functional when there is an optimal amount of conflict, that is, the level of conflict within a work group or organization may be too high. In this case, excess conflict hinders organizational effectiveness and becomes dysfunctional. It then becomes necessary to intervene with conflict-resolution strategies.

organization. The danger to the manager is "group think" and the unquestioned satisfaction with the status quo. As has been discussed in previous sections of this volume, a social system, in order to survive, must adapt to its environment. Its input, throughput, output, and feedback processes must be effective and efficient so that organizational goals are met. The organization must likewise maintain goals that keep abreast of environmental change and demands. Literature and research both suggest that an appropriate level of conflict is conducive to organizational survival and adaptation, because functional levels of conflict lead to a higher level of productivity and more innovation (Robbins, 1978). Thus, the interactionists are of the opinion that in some work groups or organizations conflict levels are too low. Conflict will have to be stimulated in order to reach the desired optimal level. Conflict is generally cyclical in nature (Frost & Wilmot, 1978). However, neither too much or too little conflict over time is functional.

Nurse leaders, managers, and supervisors using the interactionist philosophy recognize the functional aspects of an appropriate level of organizational conflict. Interestingly, in a research study by Myrtle and Glogow (1978), nursing administrators made more positive (51%) than negative (49%) comments about conflict.

> This finding perhaps signifies that these nursing administrators are in concert with current organization theory which suggests that conflict is necessary for organizational growth and not automatically symptomatic of organizational pathology. (p. 105)

Positive aspects of conflict that were reported by these nursing administrators in descending rank order were: enhances personal self-awareness and understanding; develops and builds teams; clarifies staff member's own view; increases interaction and participation in groups; fosters personal growth; offers challenges; produces new leaders; stimulates communication; stimulates and motivates individuals; generates healthy anxiety; fosters competition; reduces intrapersonal tension; augments trust; and can be pleasant for the individual.

Drawing from a variety of resources, King (1981) identified a number of positive group outcomes of functional conflicts. Conflict can foster the development and maintenance of group identity, strength, and cohesion. Conflict can bring about change by bringing issues to the surface, mobilizing energy in a system, and generating creativity. It can improve performance and can develop skills useful in future conflict situations. In addition, conflict can improve communication and eventually resolve unproductive relationships and result in constructive coalitions.

Therefore, if the assessment of the nursing service organization's level of conflict indicates that it is too low, the nurse manager may want to seek strategies for stimulating conflict to a more functional level. An appropriate level of conflict contributes to the achievement of organizational goals.

The skilled nurse manager, adhering to the interactionist philosophy of conflict, must assess the organization and determine when conflict becomes excessive and dysfunctional. Conflict is identified as dysfunctional when it fails to contribute to the achievement of organizational growth. Excessive conflict can result in lowered morale among nursing personnel, absenteeism, job dissatisfaction, job turnover, and lowered productivity. The input, throughput, output, and feedback process is affected and the achievement of organizational goals is hindered. The nurse leader must select the most appropriate conflict resolution strategy in order to reduce conflict.

In summary, some level of conflict appears desirable. Albeit, the optimal level of conflict for a given work group during any given time is difficult to determine. An adequate assessment of the level of conflict becomes a necessity.

ASSESSMENT OF INTERPERSONAL AND INTERGROUP CONFLICT

Conflict assessment can be catergorized into four component parts—assessment of potential conflict; assessment of actual conflict; assessment of functional conflict versus dysfunctional conflict; and assessment of conflict levels that are too low or too high. The assessment guides which appear in the following were formulated from a variety of sources (Bacon, 1980; Calhoun & Perrin, 1979; Collins, 1978; Derr, 1978; Frost & Wilmot, 1978; Goldsmith, 1977; Hein, 1981; Meux, 1980; Robbins, 1978; Tappen, 1978; Wehr, 1979).

Assessment of Potential Conflict

A number of sources of interpersonal and intergroup conflict were identified and discussed previously in this chapter. The presence of any one or a combination of these sources can result in conflict. Whether the conflict results in functional or dysfunctional conflict depends on such factors as the type of issue at stake, as well as its clarity; the distribution of power; the communication skills employed; skills available or outside resources sought in conflict management; and the matching of the most appropriate conflict-management strategy with the nature of the conflict occurring.

Assessment of Actual Conflict

Nurse leaders, managers, and supervisors will be confronted with interpersonal and intergroup conflict arising from a variety of sources. A comprehensive analysis of interpersonal or intergroup conflict that is taking place is a critical step in the process of conflict management.

Conflict assessment can help formulate a conflict diagnosis in the organization and/or subsystem. That is, does a potential for conflict exist? What is the nature of the conflict occurring? Is the conflict functional, or dysfunctional? Is the conflict level too high, or too low?

The assessment can be used individually prior to intervening with conflict management strategies, or, depending on the circumstances, the parties involved in the conflict, or the entire work group, can be involved in completing the assessment. (See the accompanying assessment guide for actual conflict).

ASSESSMENT GUIDE FOR ACTUAL CONFLICT

1. Who?
   - Who are the primary individuals or groups involved? Characteristics (values; feelings; needs; perceptions; goals; hostility; strengths, as past history of constructive conflict management; self-awareness)?
   - Who, if anyone, are the individuals or groups that have an indirect investment in the result of the conflict?
   - Who, if anyone, is assisting the parties to manage the conflict constructively?
   - What is the history of the individuals' or groups' involvement in the conflict?

- What is the past and present interpersonal relationship between the parties involved in the conflict?
- How is power distributed among the parties?
- What are the major sources of power used?
- Does the potential for coalition exist among the parties?
- What is the nature of the current leadership affecting the conflicting parties?

2. What?
   - What is/are the issue/issues in the conflict?
   - Are the issues based on facts? Based on values? Based on interests in resources?
   - Are the issues realistic?
   - What is the dominant issue in the conflict?
   - What are the goals of each conflicting party?
   - Is the current conflict functional? Dysfunctional?
   - What conflict management strategies, if any, have been used to manage the conflict to date?
   - What alternatives in managing the conflict exist?

3. How?
   - What is the origin of the conflict? Sources? Precipitating events?
   - What are the major events in the evolution of the conflict?
   - How have the issues emerged? Been transformed? Proliferated?
   - What polarizations and coalitions have occurred?
   - How have parties tried to damage each other? What stereotyping exists?

4. When/Where?
   - When did the conflict originate?
   - Where is the conflict taking place?
   - What are the characteristics of the setting within which the conflict is occurring?
   - What are the geographic boundaries? Political structures? Decision-making patterns? Communication networks? Subsystem boundaries?
   - What environmental factors exist that influence the development of functional versus dysfunctional conflict?
   - What resource persons are available to assist in constructive conflict management?

Assessment of Functional Versus Dysfunctional Conflict

The differentiation between functional and dysfunctional conflict is difficult. Robbins (1978) states:

> The demarcation between functional and dysfunctional is neither clear nor precise. No level of conflict can be adopted at face value as acceptable or unacceptable. The level that creates healthy and positive involvement toward one group's goals may, in another group or in the same group at another time, be highly dysfunctional, requiring immediate conciliatory attention by the manager. (p. 70)

However, major characteristics exist that set functional conflict apart from dysfunctional conflict. The assessment guide (see accompanying chart) can be used to determine whether a given conflict is functional or dysfunctional.

ASSESSMENT OF FUNCTIONAL VERSUS DYSFUNCTIONAL CONFLICT

	Yes	No
Does the conflict support the goals of the organization?	☐	☐
Does the conflict contribute to the overall goals of the organization?	☐	☐
Does the conflict stimulate improved job performance?	☐	☐
Does the conflict increase productivity among work group members?	☐	☐
Does the conflict stimulate creativity and innovation?	☐	☐
Does the conflict bring about constructive change?	☐	☐
Does the conflict contribute toward the survival of the organization?	☐	☐
Does the conflict improve initiative?	☐	☐
Does job satisfaction remain high?	☐	☐
Does the conflict improve the morale of the work group	☐	☐

A yes response to the majority of the question indicates that the conflict is probably functional. If the majority of responses are no, then the conflict is most likely a dysfunctional conflict.

Assessment of Too-Low Conflict Level

At times, the level of conflict in a system may be too low. It may then become necessary for the nurse manager to stimulate conflict. But, how does one assess a "too-low conflict level"? An affirmative response to the questions in the accompanying assessment guide, can be indicative of such a state. However, as with the task of differentiating functional and dysfunctional conflict, determining whether the conflict level in a work group is too low is difficult.

ASSESSMENT OF WHETHER THE CONFLICT LEVEL IN A WORK GROUP IS TOO LOW

	Yes	No
Is the work group consistently satisfied with the status quo?	☐	☐
Are no or few opposing views expressed by work-group members?	☐	☐
Is little concern expressed about doing things better?	☐	☐
Is little or no concern expressed about improving inadequacies?	☐	☐
Are the decisions made by the work group generally of low quality?	☐	☐
Are no or few innovative solutions or ideas expressed?	☐	☐
Are many work-group members "yes men"?	☐	☐
Are work-group members reluctant to express ignorance or uncertainties?	☐	☐
Does the nurse manager seek to maintain peace and group cooperation regardless of whether this is the correct intervention?	☐	☐
Do the work-group members demonstrate an extremely high level of resitance to change?	☐	☐
Does the nurse manager base the distribution of rewards on "popularity" as opposed to competence and high job performance?	☐	☐
Is the nurse manager excessively concerned about not hurting the feelings of the nursing staff?	☐	☐
Is the nurse manager excessively concerned with obtaining a consensus of opinion and reaching a compromise when decisions must be made?	☐	☐

A yes response to the majority of these questions can be indicative of a too-low conflict level in a work group.

Assessment of Too-High Conflict Level

At other times, the level of conflict in a system can be too high. It then becomes necessary for the nurse manager to employ conflict resolution strategies. But, how does one assess a "too-high conflict level"? An affirmative response to the questions in the assessment guide (see accompanying chart), can be indicative of such a state. But, again the task of determining whether the level of conflict is too high in a group is not easy.

ASSESSMENT OF WHETHER THE CONFLICT LEVEL
IN A WORK GROUP IS TOO HIGH

	Yes	No
Is there an upward and onward spiralling escalation of the conflict?	☐	☐
Are conflicting parties stimulating the escalation of conflict without considering the consequences?	☐	☐
Is there a shift away from conciliation, minimizing differences, and enhancing goodwill?	☐	☐
Are the issues involved in the conflict being increasingly elaborated and expanded?	☐	☐
Are false issues being generated?	☐	☐
Are the issues vague or unclear?	☐	☐
Is job dissatisfaction increasing among the work-group members?	☐	☐
Is work-group productivity being adversely affected?	☐	☐
Is energy being directed to activities that do not contribute to the achievement of organizational goals (e.g., destroying opposing party)?	☐	☐
Is the morale of the nursing staff being adversely affected?	☐	☐
Are extra parties getting dragged into the conflict?	☐	☐
Is a great deal of reliance on overt power manipulation noted (threats, coercion, deception)?	☐	☐
Is there a great deal of imbalance in power noted among the parties	☐	☐
Are the individuals or groups involved in the conflict expressing dissatisfaction about the course of the conflict and feel that they are losing something?	☐	☐
Is absenteeism increasing among staff?	☐	☐
Is there a high rate of turnover among personnel?	☐	☐
Is communication dysfunctional, not open, mistrustful, and/or restrictive?	☐	☐
Is focus being placed on nonconflict relevant sensitive areas of the other party?	☐	☐

A yes response to the majority of these questions can be indicative of a conflict level in a work group that is too high.

FORMULATING A CONFLICT DIAGNOSIS

Analyze the data collected by using the assessment guide and formulate a conflict diagnosis. The data is analyzed to determine the nature of the conflict, whether the conflict is functional or dysfunctional, and whether the conflict is too high or too low. The conflict diagnosis can be stated to include the type of conflict and the related source, for example, dysfunctional interpersonal conflict related to differences in values, functional intergroup conflict related to differing subgoals, or too-high interpersonal conflict related to unequal access to essential resources. Such conflict diagnostic statements, along with an in-depth understanding of the nature of the conflict, can give direction to the selection of conflict-management strategies that are appropriate to the situation.

In many conflict situations, it is proper to provide conflict-management assistance to individuals experiencing interpersonal conflict. Sometimes, especially in intergroup conflict, it may be helpful to obtain the assistance of an outside expert. The psychiatric nurse specialist, psychologist, or organizational consultant can be a valuable resource in diagnosing and intervening in conflict situations.

INTERPERSONAL AND INTERGROUP CONFLICT-MANAGEMENT STRATEGIES

The interactionist philosophy of conflict proposes that the optimal level of conflict for any work group or organization be maintained. In order to achieve this goal, it is no longer possible to rely solely on conflict-resolution strategies. Certainly, many conflict situations exist in which conflict resolution strategies are the most appropriate intervention techniques, but, in social systems where the conflict level is too low, conflict may need to be stimulated. Hence, the term conflict management is most appropriate.

Interpersonal or Intergroup Conflict Stimulation Strategies

Once the diagnosis has been made that the level of conflict in a work group is too low, the decision must be made whether to stimulate conflict in the subsystem. There are several strategies available to the nurse manager to stimulate conflict (Lewis, 1976; Robbins, 1974, 1978).

The structure of the social system or subsystem can be altered in a number of ways to generate conflict. The nursing manager can redefine job responsibilities or alter tasks assigned to the nursing staff. This can be done either through a formal change in the nursing position descriptions, or, it can be done informally by changing responsibilities and tasks among the nursing staff while staying within the boundaries and scope of the current position descriptions. As an example of the latter, a nursing coordinator decides to stimulate conflict by reassigning the responsibility of developing a diabetic patient teaching program from the head nurse to the clinical specialist.

Job responsibilities can be specifically altered to introduce role ambiguity, incongruence, and role conflict. Assigning overlapping and ambiguous responsibilities to nursing staff or faculty can definitely serve as a strategy to stimulate conflict. For example, the nursing coordinator plans to have a diabetic patient teaching program initiated, developed, and implemented. To stimulate conflict, overlapping and unclear responsibilities for this program are assigned to both the head nurse and clinical specialist.

Other structural changes can be used as techniques to stimulate conflict. Conflict can be stimulated by the directive to alter the goals, activities, and structure of a clinical unit or that of a faculty teaching team. The size of the unit or team can be increased, thereby increasing required interaction and coordination along with enhancing the possibility of conflict. Increasing the physical distance between interdependent work groups through an actual physical move makes smooth communication more difficult thereby enhancing the possibility of conflict. Rewards and resources can be unequally or inconsistently allocated among work teams thus stimulating intergroup conflict. New work-group members can be added or old members removed and transferred. In particular, adding a "devil's advocate" or a known "change agent" can arouse a work group from its satisfaction with the status quo. Requirements of increasing standardization of job performance and peer review can likewise stimulate conflict.

The flow of communication in a subsystem and system can be specifically altered to stimulate conflict. Among the strategies available to the nurse manager are to (1) deviate from the traditional channels of communication; (2) foster communication overload; (3) transmit threatening information; (4) transmit ambiguous information; (5) skip the chain of command in transmitting information; (6) withhold needed and desired information; and (7) transmit incomplete information.

An example of each strategy follows. Introduce information through the informal social structure or "grapevine" in your nursing organization (strategy 1). Transmit excessive information about any given issue (strategy 2). Inform staff nurses that their roles are going to be redefined (strategy 3). As a faculty coordinator, communicate several different ambiguous versions of teaching assignments (strategy 4). As a nursing coordinator, discuss with staff nurses plans to revise a unit policy, thus skipping the head nurse in the communication chain (strategy 5). As the nurse manager, withhold all information about an impending reorganization of the teaching faculty (strategy 6). As a faculty coordinator, inform faculty about a critical meeting which will affect everyone and is to be held in two weeks, while withholding any further details (strategy 7).

Combining nursing staff or faculty with certain leadership or personality traits can be used to stimulate conflict.

> Leadership roles in an organization can be utilized to stimulate discord. This can be accomplished by altering an individual's leadership style or by interchanging individual leaders among units. (Lewis, 1976, p. 22)

The preferable method is for the nurse leader to change leadership style as opposed to exchanging nurse leaders among the various subsystems of an organization.

In summary, a word of caution is in order. Conflict stimulation must be monitored and managed very closely to prevent a level of conflict that is too high or becomes dysfunctional. The selection of conflict stimulation strategies must be carefully considered. Some strategies allow for quick escape valves. For example, conflict stimulated through withholding information can be reduced rather quickly by providing that information. Whereas conflict aroused by such strategies as formally changing job descriptions, or geographical moves, will not so readily be reduced since such strategies are more permanent in nature.

Interpersonal or Intergroup Conflict-Resolution Strategies

When the diagnosis has been made that the level of conflict in the work group is too high, the most appropriate conflict-resolution strategy and process of intervention must be selected. Decisions will need to be made related to whether or not to personally intervene, what process of intervention to utilize, and what conflict resolution strategies to employ.

The nature of the conflict must be thoroughly assessed. The assessment guide for actual conflict, discussed previously, can be used for this purpose. At the same time, the manager should be equally aware of personal modes of handling conflict. Answers to the following questions can help formulate the course of action: Are you skilled and comfortable in using a broad range of conflict-resolution skills while in the role of intervenor? Is the conflict worth the risk of your involvement? What are the possible consequences for your work group if you function in the role of interventionist? Are the parties involved in the conflict likely to resolve the conflict constructively themselves without any outside intervention? What is the best timing for intervention? Should a third party be called in to assist in resolving the conflict? Once the decision to intervene has been made, select the conflict resolution strategy most appropriate for the nature and type of conflict. Some of the conflict-resolution strategies described in the following lend themselves well, when engaging in the conflict interventionist role. All can be appropriately adapted to deal with interpersonal or intergroup conflict in which one is personally involved.

Avoidance

Avoidance is a temporary, short-term, conflict "resolution" strategy in which the nurse manager engages in a nonassertive behavior pattern and refrains from openly expressing issues, feelings, and differences. Concern for both people and production tends to be low.

There are several tactics for achieving avoidance (Frost & Wilmot, 1978). The conflict can be avoided by *leaving the conflict situation*, as, for example, by adjourning a meeting and walking out of the room. This tactic is useful when not wishing to become involved in or participate in a given conflict situation, as when physically threatened, or when greatly outnumbered.

Conflict can be avoided through *postponement*. After acknowledging the emotional aspect of the conflict, request that the issues central to the conflict be put off for discussion until a later time. A reasonable and realistic time interval must be selected. Postponement allows tempers to "cool down," or buys time so that issues can be studied in more depth, but it can have negative results if the nursing staff feels they are being put off or when staff energy and time are available to work through the conflict when it occurs.

Fogging, or *sidestepping*, is another avoidance tactic. Agreement is voiced about one part of a conflicting issue while at the same time ignoring a major portion of the issue. The tactic can be useful if one is in a low-power position or does not want to get involved in a conflict.

Conflict can be avoided through *denial*, by refusing to recognize it, by ignoring it, or by being indifferent to it. These tactics can be used as power ploys when the desire is to remain in control of a given situation. They can have a very negative effect on employees. Nonrecognition of the conflict by the nurse leader can be disconfirming and painful for nurse staff or faculty members.

Resorting to formal rules or *arbitrary break tactics* avoids immediate conflict but does not work out underlying power issues. Calling for a vote, the use of formal rule structures as Roberts' Rules of Order, calling for coffee or lunch breaks, or tabling a motion, are examples.

Withdrawal from conflicts too frequently reflects poor leadership. Avoidance does not resolve conflicts permanently. This strategy offers no effective resolution in the long run since conflicts that are avoided may later erupt into more major discord.

On the other hand, avoidance is a natural, easy reaction and can be useful in certain situations. As Tappen (1978) puts it,

> You should "pick your fights" rather than dissipating your energy on many minor conflicts which distress no one. These minor conflicts can sometimes be handled best by ignoring them. (p. 49)

Chief executives reported the use of avoidance to be positive in situations when (a) time is needed for people to "cool" tempers, (b) the need for more data is critical, (c) issues are nonimportant or tangential, (d) potential disruption outweighs the constructive consequences of resolution, (e) there is minimal chance of attaining any part of personal goals, or (f) when others can resolve the conflict better (Thomas, 1977).

Smoothing

Smoothing is a conflict-resolution strategy in which differences are played down, common interests are emphasized. Concern for people is high while concern for production is low. This is a temporary intervention strategy. Since in smoothing, differences are not confronted and dealt with openly, the real issues in a conflict are not addressed and resolved permanently. The conflict frequently resurfaces later.

Smoothing does recognize the commonality in conflict situations and reinforces cooperation. By identifying areas of agreement, areas of disagreement may gain a clearer focus. Smoothing is particularly important when the preservation of a relationship is more important than dealing with the conflicting issue. It is also useful when (a) stability, harmony, and maintaining cooperation are important; (b) the conflict issues are more important to others; (c) social credits are being built for later use; or (d) when one is losing or outmatched in a conflict.

Forcing

Forcing is a conflict-resolution strategy in which one party uses its superior power to impose its conflict solution on the other party, thus attaining a win–lose outcome. The concern for production is high while concern for people is low.

The source of power can be that vested in a nurse manager or supervisor, who, for example, holds formal positional authority. In such a case the nurse manager uses her formal positional power to force subordinates to accept a decision. Power may also come from persuasive parties in the conflict who form coalitions, thus getting others to join their cause, gain more power, and attain their goals. Conversely, for a nurse manager trying to maintain a power position it may become necessary to prevent coalitions from forming (Frost & Wilmot, 1978). This can be achieved, for example, by making certain everyone in a meeting is included in the decision-making process. Finally, the source of power in forcing may also take the form of majority rule, as in voting. In any case, the outcome includes winners and losers.

Forcing does not bring about agreement, because the losers frequently do not support the final decision. It is a temporary measure which eliminates discord momentarily, but does not necessarily resolve the conflict. Future interactions of the parties may be marred because of the presence of the unresolved conflict, remaining resentment, and withdrawal of cooperation with, and commitment to the solution by the loser, along with efforts to retaliate.

Forcing is useful in conflicts where other strategies are inappropriate. This can include conflict situations when (a) a quick decision is critical, as in emergencies; (b) unpopular courses of action such as disciplining, enforcing unpopular rules, or budget slashing measures need to be implemented by management; (c) a need for protection exists against a party that takes advantage of nonforcing conflict strategies; and (d) when controversial issues that are critical to the organization's welfare need to be implemented (Thomas, 1977).

Compromising, Negotiating, Bargaining

Compromise is a conflict-resolution strategy in which a middle-ground solution that falls somewhere between opposing positions is sought. Each party in the conflict is required to give up something of value, yet gains something through the final outcome. Compromise falls between cooperativeness and assertiveness as an approach. Concern for both production and people is moderate. In the process of compromise, issues are addressed more directly than in avoiding or forcing, but are not explored in as much depth as in collaboration.

Bargaining and *negotiations* are involved in order to search for a solution that offers some degree of satisfaction to all parties involved in a conflict and for partial fulfillment of the needs of each party . The bargaining or negotiations involved in compromise may be undertaken by the parties themselves or can take place with the assistance of an interventionist or third party.

Compromise is a strategy in which there is no clear winner. Parties engaging in compromise may assume an initially inflated position as a buffer against loss since they know that they will have to give up something. The outcome of the bargaining itself depends to an extent on the balance of power between parties. The compromise solution may yield less than optimum results and may be so weakened that it will not be very effective.

> The problem with the compromise style is that persons sometimes give in too easily and fail to seek a solution that gives significant gains to either party. The "giving in" can become so habitual that it becomes a goal in itself. (Frost & Wilmot, 1978, p. 31)

But, compromise can be useful in settling an immediate issue. With its use, there are no real losers, and it is consistent with our democratic values. Compromise is useful when (a) resources are limited; (b) it is necessary to forestall a win-lose outcome; (c) temporary resolution of complex conflict issues is essential; (d) other conflict resolution strategies are not successful; (e) solutions are needed under time limitations; (f) goals are not important enough to risk the disruption caused by such strategies as forcing; and (g) parties support mutually exclusive goals and possess an equal amount of power (Thomas, 1977).

Collaboration, Confrontation, Consensus

Collaboration is a conflict-resolution strategy in which parties seek conflict resolution through confrontation, problem solving, and consensus. Concern for both production and people is high. Solutions that satisfy goals and are acceptable to the parties involved in the conflict are sought. In fact, conflict is viewed as natural and helpful and the conflicting parties work to find new and creative solutions in which the goals of all parties involved in the conflict are maximized. Through direct open confrontation and problem solving the alternative solution that is worked out often synthesizes the original positions and is superior to them.

Collaboration involves rational problem solving. Feelings and facts are shared in a climate of openness. Mutual understanding and definition of the conflict issues are sought. After mutual problem definition, alternative solutions are proposed and analyzed. The best and mutually acceptable alternative is selected.

Collaboration through concensus decision making can be very time-consuming. It also requires considerable interpersonal skills. It has been found to be of limited usefulness in values conflicts.

Although collaboration is perhaps the most difficult method of resolving conflict, it is judged to be one of the most successful conflict-resolution strategies. Labovitz (1980) states that this method of conflict resolution seems "to be the hallmark of both effective organizations and effective supervisors" (p. 35). Several studies exist in which collaboration was reported to give the best results in conflict resolution. Indeed the outcome of collaboration is a win–win position. Parties tend to share a commitment to the solution developed and establish a basis for working together constructively in future conflicts.

In particular, collaboration as a conflict-resolution strategy is useful when (a) conflicts are based on misunderstandings; (b) intergroup conflict is present; (c) both sets of issues and goals are too important for compromise; (d) feelings that interfere with conflict resolution need to be resolved; (e) commitment to the solution is important; and (f) the merging of different perspectives is important.

Other Interpersonal and Intergroup Conflict Resolution Strategies

Some authors (Lewis, 1976; Robbins, 1978) identify additional conflict-resolution strategies. Included are superordinate goals, expansion of resources, altering the human variable, and altering the structural variables. Superordinate goals are global goals that are highly valued and commonly sought by both parties in a conflict. In expansion of resources, more resources are made available so that both parties in a conflict can win. In altering human variables, attitudes and behaviors of the conflicting parties are changed through such means as sensitivity training. Altering structural variables includes such tactics as expanding or contracting boundaries, adding or removing work-group members, and creating new roles. Each one of these four techniques, however, can be part of the outcome of the major conflict-resolution strategies already described, especially as part of the outcome of collaboration.

In summary, conflict-resolution strategies should be selected that are the most appropriate for a given conflict situation at a given point in time. It becomes important to develop a repertoire of conflict-resolution skills that can be readily applied when the situation calls for them.

The Interventionist Role

As a nurse leader, manager, or supervisor, it will at times becomes necessary to intervene in interpersonal or intergroup conflict involving nursing staff or faculty. The first prerequisite is to have a thorough understanding of the nature of the conflict (see the assessment guideline for actual conflict).

The actual decision to intervene, and when, should be based on the following criteria (Wehr, 1979; Frost & Wilmot, 1978):

1. Do you have enough credibility to gain entry?
2. Is successful intervention a possibility?

3. Can the conflict be fragmented into smaller segments that become more manageable?
4. Is the timing correct? Or is it too early or too late?
5. Is nonintervention riskier than intervention in relation to a constructive outcome?
6. Do you have sufficient analytical abilities and communication skills to intervene constructively in the conflict?
7. What choices are available to you in negotiating your role as a third party?

As an interventionist, it is important to understand the nature of the conflict so that neutrality can be maintained and one does not become enmeshed in the conflict itself. Analysis of the conflict should assist in formulating a conflict diagnosis and in selecting appropriate conflict-management strategies. Finally, it is critical to be aware of both the relational and the content issues involved in the conflict.

EVALUATION OF CONFLICT MANAGEMENT

Evaluation must follow assessment and diagnosis of conflict and selection and implementation of conflict-management strategies. Evaluation data collection centers about two critical questions:

Are organizational/unit goals being met?
Are the relationships among work-group members constructive and conducive to high-level performance?

Data supporting affirmative responses to these questions lends support to the assumption that the conflict management strategies implemented resulted in the desired outcomes.

SUMMARY

In today's rapidly changing health care arena and larger social structure, sources of intrapersonal, interpersonal, and intergroup conflict are in abundance. Conflict is no longer viewed as negative by contemporary theorists. Rather, the interactionists conceptualize conflict as having constructive potential for social systems.

Within this perspective, the notion of conflict management has evolved. Inherent in this notion is the importance of conflict resolution as well as conflict stimulation. The contemporary nurse leader, manager, or supervisor must be skilled in a variety of conflict-stimulation and conflict-resolution strategies. It must be kept in mind that interpersonal and intergroup conflict do not occur in isolation but rather within the context of a larger social system. The manner in which conflict within or among subsystems is managed has system-wide ramifications. It is thus realized that successful conflict management contributes to a functional input, throughput, output, and feedback process, the attainment of social system goals, and most importantly to the organization's survival under changing conditions.

REFERENCES

Aroskar, M. Anatomy of an ethical dilemma: The theory. *American Journal of Nursing*, 1980, *80*(4), 658–660.

Bacon, C. Conflict management in the systems environment. *Journal of Systems Management*, 1980, *31*(2), 32–37.

Calhoun, G., & Perrin, M. Management, motivation and conflict. *Topics in Clinical Nursing*, 1979, *1*, 71–80.

Collins, P. Strategies for dealing with conflict. Crisis intervention. *Journal of Nursing Education*, 1978, *17*(5), 39–46.

Derr, C. Managing organizational conflict: Collaboration, bargaining, and power approaches. *California Management Review*, 1978, *21*, 76–83.

Eldridge, A. *Images of conflict*. New York: St. Martin's, 1979.

Fenn, M. "Male-female" and other games we play. In National League for Nursing, *Conflict management-flight, fight, negotiate?* (Pub. No. 52-1677). New York: National League for Nursing, 1977.

Frost, J., & Wilmot, W. *Interpersonal conflict*. Dubuque, Iowa: Wm. C. Brown, 1978.

Goldsmith, D. Interpersonal conflict in organizations. In National League for Nursing, *Conflict management—flight, fight, negotiate?* (Pub. No. 52-1677). New York: National League for Nursing, 1977.

Hein, E. Conflict. *Critical Care Update*, February 1981, *8*, 22–24; 26–27.

Hite, R. New radicalism in nursing: Prelude to an irrepressible conflict. *Supervisor Nurse*, 1977, *8*(3), 14–16.

Kalisch, B., & Kalisch, P. An analysis of the sources of physician–nurse conflict. *Journal of Nursing Administration*, 1977, *7*(1), 51–57.

King, D. Three cheers for conflict! *Personnel*, 1981, *58*, 13–22.

Kleiner, B. How to make conflict work for you. *Supervisory Management*, 1978, *23*, 3–6.

Kramer, M. *Reality shock: Why nurses leave nursing*. St. Louis: Mosby, 1974.

Labovitz, G. Managing conflict. *Business Horizons*, 1980, *23*, 30–37.

Leininger, M. Taft-Hartley amended: Implications for nursing—Conflict and conflict resolution. *American Journal of Nursing*, 1975, *75*(2), 292–296.

Lewis, J. Conflict management. *Journal of Nursing Administration*, 1976, *6*(10), 18–22.

Meux, M. Resolving interpersonal value conflicts. *Advances in Nursing Science*, 1980, *2*, 41–69.

Myrtle, R., & Glogow, E. How nursing administrators view conflict. *Nursing Research*, 1978, *27*(2), 103–106.

O'Connor, A. Sources of conflict for faculty members. *Journal of Nursing Education*, 1978, *17*(5), 35–38.

Rakich, J., Longest, B., & O'Donovan, T. *Managing health care organizations*. Philadelphia: Saunders, 1977.

Robbins, S. *Managing organizational conflict: A nontraditional approach*. Englewood Cliffs, N.J.: Prentice-Hall, 1974.

Robbins, S. "Conflict management" and "conflict resolution" are not synonymous terms. *California Management Review,* 1978, *21*, 67–75.

Schmalenberg, C., Kramer, M. Bicultural training: A cost-effective program. *Journal of Nursing Administration*, 1979, *9*(12), 10–16.

Schutz, W. *Fundamental interpersonal relation orientation behavior*. Palo Alto, Calif.: Psychologists Press, 1967.

Sexton, D. Organizational conflict: A creative or destructive force. *Nursing Leadership*, 1980, 3(3), 16–21.

Slimmer, L. Helping students to resolve conflicts between their religious beliefs and psychiatric-mental health treatment approaches. *JPN and Mental Health Services*, 1980, 18(7), 37–39.

Smith, S., & Davis, A. Ethical dilemmas: Conflicts among rights, duties, and obligations. *American Journal of Nursing*, 1980, 80(8), 1463–1466.

Tappen, R. Strategies for dealing with conflict. Using confrontation. *Journal of Nursing Education*, 1978, 17(5), 47–52.

Thomas, K. Toward multi-dimensional values in teaching: The example of conflict behaviors. *Academy of Management Review*, 1977, 2, 484–490.

Wehr, P. *Conflict regulation*. Boulder, Colo.: Westview, 1979.

BIBLIOGRAPHY

Cochran, D., & White, D. Intraorganizational conflict in the hospital purchasing decision making process. *Academy of Management Journal*, 1981, 24(2), 324–332.

Crisham, P. Measuring moral judgment in nursing dilemmas. *Nursing Research*, 1981, 30(2), 104–110.

Devine, B. Nurse–physician interaction: Status and social structure within two hospital wards. *Journal of Advanced Nursing*, 1978, 3, 287–295.

Glenn, E., & Pood, E. Groups can make the best decisions, if you lead the way. *Supervisory Management*, 1978, 23, 2–6.

Hart, L. *Learning from conflict: A handbook for trainers and group leaders*. Reading, Mass.: Addison-Wesley, 1981.

Haw, M. Conflict resolution and the communication myth. *Nursing Outlook*, 1980, 28(9), 566–570.

Heineken, J. The team scapegoat. *Supervisor Nurse*, 1980, 11, 36–37.

Hoh, A. Consensus-building: A creative approach to resolving conflicts. *Management Review*, 1981, 70, 52–54.

Hughes, E. Helping staff to manage conflict well. *Hospital Progress*, 1979, 60(7), 68–71; 83.

Kilmann, R., & Thomas, K. Four perspectives on conflict management: An attributional framework for organizing descriptive and normative theory. *Academy of Mangement Review*, 1978, 3, 59–68.

Kramer, M., & Schmalenberg, C. Conflict: The cutting edge of growth. *Nursing Digest*, 1978, 5(4), 59–65.

Mariano, C. The dynamics of conflict. *Journal of Nursing Education*, 1978, 17(5), 7–11.

Marriner, A. Conflict resolution. *Supervisor Nurse*, 1979, 10(5), 46; 49; 52–54.

Nichols, B. Dealing with conflict. *The Journal of Continuing Education in Nursing*, 1979, 10(6), 24–27.

Perspectives: Resolving an ethical dilemma. *Nursing 80*, 1980, 10(5), 39–43.

Phillips, E., & Cheston, R. Conflict resolution: What works? *California Management Review*, 1979, 21,(4), 76–83.

Preston, P. Creative conflict management. *Supervisory Management*, 1979, 24, 7–11.

Roseman, E. How to overcome intergroup conflict. *Medical Laboratory Observer*, 1980, 12, 41–44.

Seidl, A. Gaming: A strategy to teach conflict resolution. *Journal of Nursing Education*, 1978, 17(5), 21–28.

Sheane, D. When and how to intervene in conflict. *Personnel Journal*, 1980, 59(6), 515–518.

Sheard, T. The structure of conflict in nurse–physician relations. *Supervisor Nurse*, 1980, *11*, 14–15; 17–18.

Stafford, L. Scapegoating: How and why scapegoating occurs. *American Journal of Nursing*, 1977, *77*(3), 406–409.

Thamhain, H., & Wilemon, D. Leadership, conflict, and program management effectiveness. *Sloan Management Review*, 1977, *19*, 69–89.

This, L. *A guide to effective management: Practical applications from behavioral sciences.* Reading, Mass.: Addison-Wesley, 1974.

Thurkettle, M., & Jones, S. Conflict as a systems process: Theory and management. *Journal of Nursing Administration*, 1978, *8*(1), 39–43.

Veninga, R. The management of conflict. *Nursing Digest*, 1977, *5*(3), 72–74.

CHAPTER 22
THE FUTURE: FORCES, ISSUES, AND TRENDS

Forces, issues, and trends can be identified that will probably have an impact on nursing during the remainder of this century. In this chapter, we will attempt to identify *some* of the forces that may affect nurse leaders, managers, and supervisors as we move into the twenty-first century. Obviously, attempting to make inclusive, accurate predictions about the next 20 years is difficult for even the most experienced futurologist. But, being informed about major forces, issues, or trends that have been identified will arm nurse leaders with the data base essential for contributing to the shaping of the nursing profession as we prepare ourselves to meet the challenges of the 21st century.

SELECTED SOCIAL FORCES

A few of the major social forces that are predicted to affect the future of nursing have been selected for comment. The selection is not intended to be all inclusive nor does it speculate about the relative strength or impact of each of these driving societal forces for change.

Women in the Work Force

The number of women in the work force continues to increase. By 1990, it is predicted that two-thirds of the married women in America below the age of 55 will be employed outside the home (Fraser, 1980/1981). A strong motivator for these women to work is economic, particularly in times of general societal economic constraints. Other equally important motivators include professional fulfillment, a desire for involvement in the occupational community, as well as broadened horizons, a need to achieve a personal identity outside the home, and a need to contribute to society through a profession or occupation.

Many more professions are now opening up to women than the traditional fields of teaching, social work, and nursing. Professionals are seeking appropriate rewards. Other more lucrative disciplines are attracting women (Ellis, 1980). Some of our brightest young womem are electing to enter such fields as law, medicine, and corporate management. The predictions are that the position of women in the work place will continue to evolve and progress over the next several decades (Fraser, 1980/1981). Through such strategies as political action and collective bargaining nurses are bringing about change in conditions of employment and in the delivery of nursing care. Can the profession of nursing continue to attract some of our most able young men and women in the future?

Consumerism

Contemporary citizens are more knowledgable about health care and demand accessible quality care at reasonable costs. Patients are seeking an active role and a new partnership in health care (Sovie, 1978). Questions are being raised about ways to maintain good health and about the nature of any illness encountered. Requests to participate in treatment decisions are being voiced.

This momentum of consumerism is likely to continue into the twenty-first century and may become very militant. The consumer movement is identified as a major driving societal force shaping nursing's future (Sovie, 1978).

The Economy and Cost Containment

The evolution of nursing will to some extent depend on the growth of the economy as a whole. The growth of the economy will be in part affected by how the United States manages its present shift from what Naisbitt (1982) identifies as our self-sufficient national economy to becoming part of an interdependent global economy. As Ginzberg (1981) notes, the success of a professional group depends to a large degree on the health of the economy and of the industry to which it is most closely aligned. The issue of cost containment began to become prevalent as the growth of the economy began to slow down in the 1970s. It is expected that there will be relatively slow *real* economic growth in the future, that inflationary pressures will continue, that taxpayers will resist enlarged government expenditures, and that there may be a continued shift in federal outlay from human resources to defense.

From this scenario, Ginzberg (1981) predicts that little or no new money will be available in the future to expand or improve the health care system. Pressures will be brought to bear on health care providers to economize and to control and reduce the outlays of hospitals and nursing homes. Ginzberg (1981) also projects that the economic realities may not be conducive to gains in salaries, fringe benefits, or employment opportunities for nurses in institutional settings in the future.

It would seem reasonable to speculate, at any rate, that cost containment in the health care industry will remain a viable issue well into the twenty-first century.

Knowledge and Technology Explosion

More knowledge and technology are available to us than ever before in history. Naisbitt (1982) describes America's shift to an information society. It is predicted that knowledge and technology will continue to expand at an explosive rate (Sovie, 1978). With this expansion of technology "must be in a counterbalancing human response—that is, high touch" (Naisbitt, 1982, p. 39). The challenges to nurses then become: knowing how to cope with the vast sources of available information; coping with more rapid obsolescence of existing knowledge and skills; learning how to learn; maintaining competence through continuing education; and resolving the ethical dilemmas stemming from the increased use of technology (Barnard, 1980; Christman, 1978, 1979). Finally, the challenge remains to continue to utilize knowledge from the psychosocial sciences and to seek ways to creatively introduce more "high touch" into our health care delivery system.

Health Care Policy

Shifting federal emphasis on the health care industry and nursing in terms of legislation, authorizations, and appropriations impacts on the nursing profession. New legislation can change the focus in personnel preparation and the delivery of health care services. It is critically important that nurse leaders study legislative proposals that impact on nursing, health care delivery, and health care work force preparation. It is even more important that nurses voice their opinions to legislators and become politically active in other ways. Finally, it is important for nurse leaders to remain cognizant of new legislation and authorization levels and analyze the potential impact on the nursing profession.

Organizational Structures

In a classic article, Bennis (1978) predicted the decline of bureaucracies over the next 25 years, along with a reconsideration of new organizational structures. Four forces are identified as bringing about this change in organizations: psychological forces; rapid, unexpected change; growth in size; and increasing complexity of modern technology. A change in the philosophy of management behavior views people more positively, emphasizes collaboration, and values humanistic–democratic ideals. Organizations are becoming larger, more complex, and international in focus. Traditional activities of the organization may not be enough to sustain its growth. Because of the complexity of modern technology, persons with diverse and highly specialized skills are needed.

These changing forces have created issues—integration, social influence, collaboration, adaptation, revitalization—for which bureaucratic solutions have been found to be nonexistent or inadequate (Bennis, 1978). Organizations of the future must find ways to integrate the employee's own career and personal needs with the goals of the organization. Coercive power and formal authority can no longer be explicitly relied upon to influence employees in an organization. The constructive resolution of conflict through collaboration will become increasingly important.

The next 25–50 years will continue to confront organizations with turbulent, less predictable, and changing external environments. Organizations of the future will need to learn to adapt. Likewise, organizational revision and revitalization will become imperative as rapid changes are faced in the social norms and values, tasks, human and nonhuman resources, and needs of society. As Naisbitt (1982) points out, "Just as we seek a greater voice in political decisions, through initiatives and referenda, we are reformulating corporate structures to permit workers, shareholders, consumers, and community leaders a larger say in determining how corporations will be run" (p. 175).

What will organizations be like at the turn of the century? Bennis (1978) makes several predictions. Organizations will become more interdependent with each other and partnerships with government will be common. Organizations will continue to grow in size and complexity and become multinational in scope. Organizational survival will depend on the effective utilization of brain power. Managers will need to accommodate employees who will be more committed to their professional careers and require more involvement, autonomy, and participation.

Organizational tasks will increase in complexity requiring the collaboration of specialists in a project or team form of organization or in a matrix structure that combines both the traditional hierarchy and project teams. Organizational goals will become more complex, encompassing adaptation, revitalization, and creativity. Metagoals may be needed to provide a framework for the goal structure. Indeed, Naisbitt (1982) points to the shift away from short-term managerial planning to *long-term* planning. The social structure of organizations of the future may be temporary.

> There will be adaptive, rapidly changing *temporary systems*. These will be "task forces" organized around problems-to-be-solved by groups of relative strangers who represent a diverse set of professional skills. The groups will be arranged on an organic rather than mechanical model; they will evolve in response to a problem rather than to programmed role expectations. The "executive" thus becomes a coordinator or "linking pin" between various task forces. (Bennis, 1978, p. 287)

Naisbitt (1982) continues in this vein: "In policymaking, we are giving up the grand, top-down strategies imposed from above and substituting bottom-up approaches, that is, limited, individual solutions that grow naturally out of a particular set of circumstances" (p. 102). With the shift occurring from centralization to decentralization, networking and informal linkages are becoming more important.

Predictions for future organizational structures can also be drawn from variables that appear to be contributing to the success of current organizations. A major recent study of the "most excellent" companies (those that are highly successful in providing products and services that are well received by society) in the United States was conducted by Peters and Waterman (1982). The results of this study are reported in their book *In Search of Excellence*. There were several attributes that were found to characterize these highly successful companies:

1. *A bias for action.* Environments are set up where new ideas can be tried. Ad hoc committees and other small temporary work groups are utilized, instead of standing committees, for specific purposes or goals. These committees and groups are composed of people empowered to make relevant decisions. Managers get out of their offices and talk to their employees and clients, keeping in touch with the input → throughput → output process of the organization. The organizational structures are fluid and managers may have face-to-face contacts across levels in the hierarchy. Somewhat fluid budgets are developed, permitting subsystems in the organization to "squirrel away" resources to work on small pilot projects. Lengthy and formal procedures are avoided. Brief written communication is encouraged or demanded. Rich, frequent, and effective informal communication within the organization and among team members is strongly encouraged. Coffee breaks, large tables in cafeterias, small conferences rooms with chalkboards, as well as other provisions, are made to encourage the exchange and development of ideas.

2. *Close to the client/customer.* The excellent organizations have an "obsession" with serving the client or customer. Service excellence goes well beyond what could reasonably be justified on a profit basis. The long-term benefits of the value of a reputation for being the best in the field is highly valued. The client or customer is the focus in designing services or products in order to meet the client's or customer's needs. In fact, customer/clients are involved in designing the service or product.

3. *Autonomy and entrepreneurship.* Employees who are innovators and creative are encouraged and protected. Newly designed services or products are supported and protected in all phases of their development. Autonomy and control is placed very far down in the organization, creating more divisions with potential duplication of effort than was conventionally considered wise.

4. *Productivity through people.* The excellent organizations believe very deeply in having respect for the individual employee and this attitude pervades the organization.

Employees are treated as adults. Labels or titles are used to upgrade the status of the employee. Efforts are made to create an atmosphere of "meaning and a sense of family." Job security is considered important and protected in times of economic decline. Employees at all levels are made to feel a part of a "winning team." Organizational information is made available to the employees to give them a sense of involvement.

5. *Hands-on, value driven*. The excellent organization has a few clearly delineated values that were made known to everyone and were restated over and over again. Generally, these values were developed and put into action by an earlier leader. The values then became ingrained and supported throughout the organization. The values generally related to the quality of the service or product output of the organization. These organizations went to great lengths to socialize new employees to these values.

6. *Stick to the knitting*. The organizations did not expand into large conglomerates. The hands-on involvement by top managers was critical to success and this was per-ceived as being lost when large acquisitions occurred.

7. *Single form, lean staff*. There were few layers in the organizational hierarchy. A great deal of autonomy and a number of support functions were placed down into the individual divisions.

8. *Simultaneous loose–tight properties*. The organizations appear to have simultaneous contradictory attributes. The day-to-day executive decisions are decentralized, but tight control is maintained around core values. Employees are provided with a great deal of responsibility and trust, but will be quick to confront those who abuse trust. Provision of quality services or products is an obsession yet cost control and efficient management practices are supported.

CHANGING HEALTH CARE NEEDS AND HEALTH CARE DELIVERY SERVICES

The health care needs of society are becoming increasingly complex. Many changes are occurring.

Health Problems

An international study of industrialized countries was conducted to predict how health care would be organized by 1990 (Selby, 1974). The study reported that societies have been less successful in combating illnesses resulting from the impact of the environment and living habits. The major health problems confronting people until about the turn of the century will be cardiovascular diseases, mental disorders, and malignant diseases. Other prevalent health problems will include: chronic health problems associated with old age, genetically determined diseases, viral diseases, and venereal disease.

Leininger (1978) points to an increase in chemical, electrical, nuclear, and technologi-cal accidents. She predicts a widespread increase in organ transplants, as well as limb and tissue transplants related to increased car and chemical accidents and shootings, bombings, and other acts of violence. Leininger concurs with Selby in that a marked increase in cardiovascular and emotional disease is projected for the United States, stemming from fast-paced lifestyles. In addition, chronic ailments will become an increasingly greater concern to health professionals as medical advances continue to prolong life (Barnard, 1980; Christman, 1979; Maxmen, 1976).

Health Care Delivery and Nursing Services

A shift in health care from a medical to a health care model and to an increased focus on health care maintenance and disease prevention are predicted for the future (Leininger, 1978; Selby, 1974). Greater emphasis will be placed on health education in schools and to the public via mass media, and on occupational health, immunizations, and mass screening for the early detection of disease. Automated and computerized methods will be used for disease detection and diagnoses (Selby, 1974).

Maxmen (1976) goes so far as to predict the medic-computer model of health care delivery in the United States for the twenty-first century. That is, computers will be used to make diagnoses and treatment decisions that are presently made by physicians. Medics would assume responsibility for supportive and technical tasks, eventually replacing physicians. Whether or not his predictions materialize, it would appear a realistic prediction that the use of technology, such as computers, monitoring and maintenance equipment, and audiomedia technology, will continue to increase as we move toward the twenty-first century.

Maxmen (1976) also predicts that prior to reaching this medic-computer health care delivery model, the United States will enter into the health team model. In the health team model, the physician coordinates, supervises, and consults with a variety of health team members and carries out the most complex and specialized procedures. The more routine diagnostic and treatment tasks will be performed by nurses and allied health care workers.

It seems reasonable to predict that interdisciplinary teamwork and collaboration will become increasingly important and necessary in the next two decades. Role complementation will be stressed in future work arrangements. That is, multidisciplinary functions will complement and facilitate the actions of team members and stress interdisciplinary interdependence, responsibility, equality, and colleagueship (Christman, 1978; Leininger, 1978). Nurses will become true partners with other health care professionals and will eventually receive direct financial reimbursement for their services (Leininger, 1978).

Types of services and modes of delivery are predicted to change in other ways. Ambulatory care, outpatient care, self-care consumer clinics, home care, and care in other noninstitutional settings will increase. Primary health care will become increasingly available to all citizens by the year 2000. Hospital inpatient care will focus increasingly on acute and specialized care, with university health science centers organizing rural satellite centers for primary care and health maintenance services. Rehabilitation will take on an expanded focus, becoming accepted as an essential treatment component. Mechanisms to insure an acceptable quality of nursing care will be increasingly utilized as a result of pressures from consumers, legal liability, governmental regulations, and voluntary regulatory agencies (Christman, 1978).

What will occur in nursing and health care by 1992? In a research study by Hill (1982), a nursing education administrator sample was surveyed to investigate these questions. Included in the findings (a median of probability of over 50% was established to indicate probability of occurrence) were the following:

1. An increasing focus on health maintenance in the health care delivery system.
2. Clients will be offered incentives to choose a given health care agency for its service.
3. Counselors will be increasingly utilized to assist persons to maintain healthier lifestyles.

4. Technical and professional nurses will be utilized according to uniform position descriptions designed for each level.
5. Computers will be used by the majority of staff nurses in making autonomous patient care decisions.
6. Technical nurses will provide the majority of inpatient nursing care.

Other specific predictions are made for nursing practice in the next several decades (Christman, 1979; Leininger, 1978). More independent and expanded nursing roles will exist, with more emphasis on patient teaching and guidance. Cost-effectiveness, productivity, accountability, and audits will become increasingly important in nursing practice.

Major recommendations for the nursing profession are made by the National Commission for the Study of Nursing and Nursing Education (Lysaught, 1974). Nurse managers are encouraged to reduce nurse turnover and increase retention of nurses in clinical practice. Identified strategies to achieve this were: improving salaries, rewarding clinical practice through advancement in clinical career ladders, clarifying clinical nursing roles, establishing opportunities for nurses to provide optimal nursing care through organizational and staffing practices, and providing for planned inservice education, flexible employment schedules, and assistance with continuing education. In essence, strategies must be implemented to permit nursing to practice at its very highest capacity.

The National Commission on Nursing (1983) was charged with the task of developing and implementing action plans for nursing for the future. Primary attention focused on hospital nursing. Major issues and concerns that are identified include: increasing interdependence and collegial relationships among health professionals, movement to multi-institutional arrangements for health care, effective management of nursing resources to increase job satisfaction (staffing, salaries, schedules, career development, support services, modes of care delivery), improving nurse–physician relationships, enhancing the image and status of nurses, enabling the nurse to participate in organizational decision making related to patient care, and fostering career mobility.

The National Commission on Nursing (1983) was charged with the task of analyzing contemporary nursing issues and problems in the United States. Primary attention focused on hospital nursing. The following are selected recommendations made by the National Commission on Nursing (1983):

1. A suitable practice environment for nurses must be established, including the involvement of nursing in decision making and policy development in a health care organization.
2. Authority over the management process, including responsibility for identifying and managing resources needed to assure high quality nursing care, is needed by nursing.
3. "Nurse executives and nurse managers of patient care units should be qualified by education and experience to promote, develop, and maintain an organizational climate conducive to quality nursing practice and effective management of the nursing resource" (p. 9).
4. "Effective nursing practice is found where conditions of nurse employment foster professional growth and development. Approaches such as flexible scheduling, appropriate staffing patterns, career advancement programs like a career ladder, and recognition for achievement should be explored and developed" (p. 9).
5. "Current trends in nursing toward pursuit of the baccalaureate degree as an achiev-

able goal for nursing practice and toward advanced degrees for clinical specialization, administration, teaching, and research should be facilitated. . . . Educational mobility and reentry opportunities should be promoted within the educational system" (p. 15).

6. "To provide adequate clinical education for nursing students, strong affiliations between academic institutions and practice settings should be developed" (p. 16).

A study of 41 hospitals in the United States considered to be good places to practice nursing and to work was conducted by the American Academy of Nursing (1983). This study is certain to become a classic and to impact on nursing management. Among the variables identified in these hospitals that produced a satisfying professional environment for registered nurses were

1. Competitive salaries, benefits, opportunities for promotion, and flexible scheduling patterns
2. Opportunities for professional development (e.g., financial assistance for education, availability of in-service and continuing education programs, management and clinical ladders, nursing research opportunities)
3. Sufficient numbers of well-qualified registered nurses to provide quality nursing care
4. Decentralized department structures, permitting budgeting and staff scheduling at the department level
5. A positive image of the nursing service within the institution and in the community
6. Organizational placement of the nursing director at the executive level of the hospital, demonstrating support by hospital administration
7. Opportunities to maximize professional nursing practice by such means as autonomy, availability of consultation, availability of resource personnel, and primary care

PREDICTIONS FOR HIGHER EDUCATION AND NURSING EDUCATION

Changes that are occurring, or are projected to occur, will affect higher education and nursing education in the next two decades.

Projections for Higher Education

The Carnegie Council on Policy Studies in Higher Education (1980) makes some enlightening observations and predictions for the next 20 years in higher education. A number of contemporary trends are identified by this Council. Students are concentrating in increasing numbers in public institutions (with public community colleges being the greatest gainers) and in large institutions. Higher education is being subjected to more and more regulation by governmental agencies. Changes in sources of financial support are noted with more dependence on public sources of financial support for higher education. An increasingly older faculty remains on staff as the rate of new hires decreases. Although public confidence in higher education is again at a comparatively high level, it could be threatened by the declining reputation for integrity of student conduct. Fluctuating rates of enrollment growth, along with changing faculty acquisition rates and declining federal research dollars in selected areas are creating uncertainties in higher education.

Students with generally lower levels of developed aptitudes that in the past are enrolled. Some of the other student trends include: more concentration on professional and vocational subjects, less political activity, less interest in academic reforms, more interest in trade-union efforts (for example, better counselling services, no tuition increase), less respect for regulations and rules of conduct, and more confidence about their own futures. In the next two decades, student (consumer) sovereignty will most likely prevail in institutions of higher learning.

The Carnegie Council (1980) predicts a decline in undergraduate enrollment over the next 20 years, since there will be a substantial decrease in the number of young persons. A number of factors will impact on actual enrollments however: the new phenomenon of drop-outs/drop-ins, decreased student dependence on parents for financial support, increasing enrollment of adults, increase in part-time students, increase in students with commitment of attendance linked to shifting personal circumstances, changing financial inducements to attend college, changing perceived value of actual worth of college education, changing military recruitment policies, and increase in nontraditional institutions catering to specialized student markets. A slight increase, however, is predicted in the next two decades for graduate enrollment in relation to undergraduate enrollment.

Internally, the Council notes that institutions are changing to a defensive stance or an emphasis on survival. This includes the utilization of such strategies as (a) lowered admission requirements, (b) recruitment of nontraditional students, (c) increased emphasis on student retention, (d) raising level of grades to attract and retain students in courses, (e) introduction of vocational and professional subjects based on student demand, (f) introduction of courses that are popular with students, (g) increasing faculty interest in collective bargaining to protect tenure and income, and (h) recruitment of administrators and managers for survival with skills in cost accounting, recruitment of students, and fund raising.

The impact of this defensive stance is that it is more difficult to start anything new. Persons in top leadership are being more cautious and less visible. The search for consensus within the institution becomes more important, with internal tensions, nevertheless, exacerbated. Departments compete to survive and coalitions form around decisions related to cuts and elimination of programs. The avoidance of alienation of important external constituencies is becoming critically important. "The ambiance was once one of overall excitement; now it is more one of tenacity, of holding on within each little academic fortress" (Carnegie Council on Policy Studies in Higher Education, 1980, p. 27).

Institutions of higher learning will need to take action to lessen the secondary impact of this changing student enrollment pattern on faculty employment and retention, as well as on their other financial expenditures (Carnegie Council on Policy Studies in Higher Education, 1980). Threats of reduction in personnel and a decline in real income will stimulate collective bargaining, which in turn will have a potential impact on traditional forms of academic governance. In any case, adaptations within the system will be made to absorb most of the impact. The most vulnerable institutions will be the less selective, general liberal arts colleges and private two-year colleges.

Projections for Nursing Education

Major recommendations relevant to nursing education are made by the National Commission for the Study of Nursing and Nursing Education (Lysaught, 1974). Among these are (a) the need to investigate problems encountered in nursing education in order to utilize the resulting data to develop the most functional, effective, and economic approaches in educating nurses in the future; (b) the need for more qualified nursing faculty; (c) the need to use new educational technology and media to increase learning efficiency and effectiveness, as well as extend the impact of the individual faculty member; (d) the need for state and regional areas to share resources; (e) the need to recruit more disadvantaged persons and minorities into nursing; and (f) the need to increase counselling services and recruitment efforts for mature females seeking initial entry into nursing programs.

The National Commission on Nursing (1981), in its task of developing and implementing action plans for nursing for the future, includes some recommendations for nursing education:

1. The promotion of educational mobility in nursing for undergraduate and registered nurses in the higher-education system (baccalaureate) by means of articulation among components of the system
2. The achievement of baccalaureate education for professional nursing practice
3. The allocation of nursing educational resources to prepare adequate numbers of nurses in basic and graduate programs
4. The development of collaborative relationships between schools of nursing and health care agencies to develop continuing education offerings for nurses
5. The development of strong affiliations between academic and practice settings in order to provide adequate clinical education for nursing students
6. The appropriate utilization of nurses related to competencies obtained in educational programs

The Institute of Medicine conducted a two-year study of nursing and nursing education in order to determine "the need for continued federal support of nursing education programs, to make recommendations for improving the distribution of nurses in medically underserved areas, and to suggest actions to encourage nurses to remain active in their profession" (Institute of Medicine, 1983, p. xv). The following are among the IOM report's recommendations:

1. Financial aid should be provided to postsecondary students so that prospective nursing students will have the ability to enroll in generalist nursing education programs.
2. Student financial and institutional support should be maintained by a variety of sources to "assure that generalist nursing education programs have capacity and enrollments sufficient to graduate the numbers and kinds of nurses commensurate with state and local goals for the nurse supply" (p. 5).
3. "To assure a sufficient continuing supply of new applicants, nurse educators and national nursing organizations should adopt recruitment strategies that attract not only recent high school graduates but also nontraditional prospective students, such as those seeking late entry into a profession or seeking to change careers, and minorities" (p. 6).
4. State education agencies, employers of nurses, and nursing education programs should share responsibility for developing programs to enable licensed nurses to upgrade their education, enhancing their career opportunities.
5. "Closer collaboration between nurse educators and nurses who provide patient

services is essential to give students an appropriate balance of academic and clinical practice perspectives and skills during their educational preparation" (p. 8).

6. Federal financial funding should be provided to graduate programs in nursing to increase the number of nurses with master's and doctoral degrees in nursing.

7. "The proportion of nurses who choose to work in their profession is high, but examination of conventional management, organization, and salary structures indicates that employers could improve both supply and job tenure by the following: providing opportunities for career advancement in clinical nursing as well as in administration; ensuring that merit and experience in direct patient care are rewarded by salary increases; assessing the need to raise nurse salaries if vacancies remain unfilled; encouraging greater involvement of nurses in decisions about patient care, management, and governance of the institution; identifying the major deterrents to nurse labor force participation in their own localities and responding by adapting conditions of work, child care, and compensation packages to encourage part-time nurses to increase their labor force participation and to attract inactive nurses back to work" (p. 17).

What will occur in nursing education by 1992? Hill's (1982) research also surveyed nursing education administrators to investigate this question. Among the findings were the following:

1. The increase of faculty to student ratio in clinical education to 1:15
2. The utilization of computers in the development and analysis of nursing education programs
3. The innovative utilization of faculty

What other predictions and recommendations are being made for nursing education for the next two decades?

1. The changes anticipated in the health care delivery system will require well-prepared nurses who can act independently, cope with responsibility, and possess excellent clinical and research skills (Scott, 1979).
2. Nursing educators and nurses in practice settings need to participate in joint planning and seek ways to unify nursing practice and education (MacPhail, 1979; Werner, 1980).
3. University health science centers will develop new models for multidisciplinary education (Leininger, 1978).
4. Many more areas of generalized and specialized education than the four traditional areas of nursing are projected (Leininger, 1978).
5. Satellite communications will be utilized to enable leading nurse educators to teach nursing students (Abdellah, 1980).
6. Nursing faculties will need to address the following issues/concerns: the practice readiness of graduates, first-job adjustment problems, professional socialization, clinical expertise of faculty, dialogue with nursing service personnel, research on what students actually learn from teachers, and preparing nurses to work on the emerging systematic problems of nursing (Felton, 1980).
7. Increasing enrollment of students with earned liberal arts degrees in collegiate nursing programs will occur (Christman, 1978; MacPhail, 1979).

8. In an era of cost containment and retrenchment, the number of nursing programs in each state will need to be examined and the concept of master planning operationalized (MacPhail, 1979).

9. Centers of "excellence in nursing" may come into existence characterized by excellence in practice and the cultivation of an outstanding learning milieu for students (Christman, 1978).

10. Nursing school enrollments may continue to decline with a continued and sustained reduction in the number of new graduates. (An increase in older students has lessened this decrease in enrollments.) (Aiken, Blendon, & Rogers, 1981; Schlotfeldt, 1981).

IMPLICATIONS FOR NURSING LEADERS MANAGERS, AND SUPERVISORS

What then are the implications of these forces and trends for nurse leaders, managers, and supervisors during the next two decades? What skills and abilities will be needed?

We predict a changing, somewhat turbulent, external environment and a scarcity of resources confronting nurse managers during the next several decades. The exercise of political astuteness, economics, trend analysis (Hill, 1982), planned change, problem solving, decision making, understanding of complex systems, planning, forecasting, and goal setting will all be important for coping with the system's input processes.

Increasing organizational complexity, changing organizational structure, increasing availability of information, increased use of technology, interdisciplinary teamwork or collaboration, competition for scarce resources, internal conflict and power struggles, and problems needing creative solutions are predicted to characterize organizational systems in which nurse leaders or managers will find themselves in the future. Managing a system's throughput process in such a milieu will demand abilities in computer usage, program analysis via computer usage, information systems knowledge, coping with organizational complexity, cost-effective budgeting (Hill, 1982), team building, problem solving, idea generation, decision making, communication skills, conflict management, use of power-oriented behavior, stress management, time management, system diagnosis with more precision, as well as such traditional management skills as organizing, directing, staffing, and developing adaptive organizational structures.

SUMMARY

Multiple forces—social and professional—have the potential to change the nursing profession and to affect the functional roles of nurse managers. A selected number of these forces have been discussed—women in the work force, consumerism, cost containment, knowledge/technology explosion, health care policy, organizational structures, health problems, trends in health care delivery and nursing services, trends in higher education, and trends in nursing education.

It is important to realize, however, that the future is not purely a random happening. It is largely a matter of choice, a result of planned change. Sovie (1978) so nicely summarizes this:

> As planners of the future, nurses must help promote the coalescence of these multiple forces and use the resulting dynamic energies to attain carefully determined goals and objectives. In

its efforts to shape the future and realize planned change, nursing must remain flexible and prepared to respond to the unexpected. . . . Nursing's structure must be such that it fosters intellectual creativity and facilitates a readiness to respond to the unanticipated problems that will certainly emerge as society moves into the next century. (p. 366)

REFERENCES

Abdellah, F. *Future directions of nursing from a national perspective*. Paper presented at DHHS Region VII Conference on Nursing Education and Nursing Service, Kansas City, Missouri, August 15, 1980.

Aiken, L., Blendon, R., & Rogers, D. The shortage of hospital nurses: A new perspective. *American Journal of Nursing*, 1981, *81*(9), 1612–1618.

American Academy of Nursing. *Magnet hospitals: Attraction and retention of professional nurses*. Kansas City: American Nurses' Association, 1983.

Barnard, K. Knowledge for practice: Directions for the future. *Nursing Research*, 1980, *29*(4), 208–212.

Bennis, W. Organizations of the future. In W. Natemeyer (Ed.), *Classics of organizational behavior*. Oak Park, Ill.: Moore, 1978.

Carnegie Council on Policy Studies in Higher Education. *Three thousand futures: The next twenty years for higher education*. San Francisco: Jossey-Bass, 1980.

Christman, L. Alternatives in the role expression of nurses that may affect the future of the nursing profession. In N. Chaska (Ed.), *The nursing profession: Views through the mist*. New York: McGraw-Hill, 1978.

Christman, L. The future of nursing practice: The next century. *Imprint*, 1979, *26*, 30–31; 63.

Ellis, B. Winds of change sweep nursing profession. *Hospitals*, 1980, *54*(1), 95–98.

Felton, G. Is academic nursing preparing practitioners to meet present and future societal needs? (Publication Series 81, No. 1). Washington, D.C.: American Association of Colleges of Nursing, 1980.

Fraser, E. Working women in America: The changing outlook. *The Collegiate Career Woman*, Winter 1980/81, 22–25; 46.

Ginzberg, E. The economics of health care and the future of nursing. *The Journal of Nursing Administration*, 1981, *11*(3), 28–32.

Hill, B. Probable future managerial response by nursing education administrators to trends in health care: A Delphi application (Doctoral dissertation, Ball State University, 1982). (University Microfilms No. 82–23, 575)

Institute of Medicine. *Nursing and nursing education: Public policies and private actions*. Washington, D.C.: National Academy Press, 1983.

Leininger, M. Futurology of nursing: Goals and challenges for tomorrow. In N. Chaska (Ed.), *The nursing profession: Views through the mist*. New York: McGraw-Hill, 1978.

Lysaught, J. (Ed.). *Action in nursing: Progress in professional purpose*. New York: McGraw-Hill, 1974.

MacPhail, J. The future of nursing education. *Imprint*, 1979, *26*, 32–33; 73.

Maxmen, J. *The post-physician era*. New York: Wiley, 1976.

Naisbitt, J. *Megatrends: Ten new directions transforming our lives*. New York: Warner, 1982.

National Commission on Nursing. *Summary report and recommendations*. Chicago: The Hospital Research and Educational Trust, 1983.

Peters, T., & Waterman, R. *In search of excellence. Lessons from America's best-run companies*. New York: Harper & Row, 1982.

Schlotfeldt, R. Nursing in the future. *Nursing Outlook*, 1981, *29*(5), 295–301.

Scott, J. Nursing at the national level. In National League for Nursing, *The emergence of nursing as a political force* (Pub. No. 41–1760). New York: National League for Nursing, 1979.

Selby, P. *Health in 1980–1990: A predictive study based on an international inquiry*. Basel: S. Karger, 1974.

Sovie, M. Nursing: A future to shape. In N. Chaska (Ed.), *The nursing profession: Views through the mist*. New York: McGraw-Hill, 1978.

Werner, J. Joint endeavors: The way to bring service and education together. *Nursing Outlook*, 1980, *28*(9), 546–550.

BIBLIOGRAPHY

Aydelotte, M. The future health delivery system and the utilization of nurses prepared in formal educational programs. In N. Chaska (Ed.), *The nursing profession: Views through the mist*. New York: McGraw-Hill, 1978.

Barnard, C. The environment of decision. *The Journal of Nursing Administration*, 1982, *12*(3), 25–29.

Erickson, E. The nursing service director, 1880–1980. *The Journal of Nursing Administration*, 1980, *10*(4), 6–13.

Hill, M., Gortner, S., & Scott, J. Educational research in nursing—An overview. *International Nursing Review*, 1980, *27*(1), 10–17.

Humphrey, C. Introduction: Mandate for nurses: Involvement in health policy. In National League for Nursing, *The emergence of nursing as a political force* (Pub. No. 41–1760). New York: National League for Nursing, 1979.

Kramer, M. Philosophical foundations of baccalaureate nursing education. *Nursing Outlook*, 1981, *29*(4), 224–228.

Leininger, M. Political nursing: Essential for health service and educational systems of tomorrow. *Nursing Administration Quarterly*, 1978, *2*, 1–16.

Lippitt, G. Power begins with you. In National League for Nursing, *Assuring a goal-directed future for nursing* (Pub. No. 52–1814). New York: National League for Nursing, 1980.

McNally, J. Toward anticipating possible needs for nursing services that might emerge from anticipated social and technological developments: A demonstration of a use of the Delphi method (Doctoral dissertation, Columbia University, 1974). (University Microfilm No. 75–6473)

Mechanic, D. *Future issues in health care*. New York: Free Press, 1979.

National Commission on Nursing. *Summary of the public hearings*. Chicago: The Hospital Research and Educational Trust, 1981.

Parrish, D., & Cleland, V. Characteristics of a professional nursing practice climate: A survey. *The Journal of Nursing Administration*, 1981, *11*(4), 40–45.

Roberts, M. Economic forecast for health care. In National League for Nursing, *The emergence of nursing as a political force* (Pub. No. 41–1760). New York: National League for Nursing, 1979.

Schlotfeldt, R. The nursing profession: Vision of the future. In N. Chaska (Ed.), *The nursing profession: Views through the mist*. New York: McGraw-Hill, 1978.

Smith, G. Nursing beyond the crossroads. *Nursing Outlook*, 1980, *28*(9), 540–545.

Spekke, A. (Ed.). *The next 25 years: Crisis and opportunity*. Washington, D.C.: World Future Society, 1975.

This, L. Critical issues confronting managers in the '80s. *Training and Development Journal*, 1980, *34*, 14–17.

INDEX